THE POLITICAL ECONOMY OF HEALTH CARE

A clinical perspective

Julian Tudor Hart

First published in Great Britain in April 2006 by

The Policy Press
University of Bristol
Fourth Floor
Beacon House
Queen's Road
Bristol BS8 1QU
UK

Tel +44 (0)117 331 4054
Fax +44 (0)117 331 4093
e-mail tpp-info@bristol.ac.uk
www.policypress.org.uk

British Library Cataloguing in Publication Data
A catalogue record for this book is available from the British Library.

Library of Congress Cataloging-in-Publication Data
A catalog record for this book has been requested.

ISBN-10 1 86134 808 8 paperback
ISBN-13 978 1 86134 808 1
ISBN-10 1 86134 809 6 hardcover
ISBN-13 978 1 86134 809 8 hardcover

Cover design by Qube Design Associates, Bristol.
Front cover: photograph supplied by kind permission of Hugh Turvey/Science Photo Library.
Printed and bound in Great Britain by MPG Books, Bodmin.

To Mary, for everything

I think it is a sad reflection that this great Act, to which every Party has made its contribution, in which every section of the community is vitally interested, should have so stormy a birth. I should have thought, and we all hoped, that [the doctors] would have realized that we are setting their feet on a new path entirely; that we ought to take pride in the fact that, despite our financial and economic anxieties, we are still able to do the most civilized thing in the world – put the welfare of the sick in front of every other consideration.

Aneurin Bevan, Minister of Health, speaking in the House of Commons debate on the National Health Service, February 1948 (quoted from Foot, 1973, p 191)

A massive transfer of NHS services into private sector management is planned throughout England under the Government's £2.5bn independent sector procurement programme. Confidential documents sent to potential bidders … show that rather than supplementing NHS provision, many of the five-year contracts will … involve 'significant volumes of transferred activity' and movement of staff out of the NHS. While 'wave one' contracts have focused mainly on routine elective surgery, second wave contracts will include renal dialysis and cardiology services…. Doctors in many specialties will therefore be forced to work for the private sector, or face redundancy.

Melanie Newman, *Hospital Doctor*, 22 September 2005

Over more than half a century, health professionals followed Bevan's new path, away from private trade into public service. Politicians still claiming to be his heirs are now driving all NHS staff into a new marketplace, not as self-employed entrepreneurs, but as employees of giant multinational corporations. You, readers of this book, will help to decide where they go next.

Contents

Preface

I wrote this book mainly to provide students of health and caring sciences with a big picture of their work: how the National Health Service (NHS) now functions in the society we have, and how it might help to create a more civilised society in the future. Every student needs such a big picture within which to work, and all of them have such a picture – either the one passively accepted from conventional assumptions, or one they build for themselves. Both the conventional picture and apparent alternatives are now losing their landmarks.[1,2] News of the reality of a health service driven ever faster and at over 100% capacity toward constantly shifting management targets, by forces apparently outside anyone's control, is now reaching even those just starting their professional careers. Twenty years ago, virtually all students of health sciences expected to work their whole lives in the NHS, in one or other specialist or generalist capacity determined partly by their own interests, but mainly by patterns of state investment directed toward perceived population needs. Today, needs are increasingly assumed to be sufficiently represented by wants – anything for which there is consumer demand, or for which such demand may by media promotion be created. The health workers' employer may now be either some NHS body fighting for economic survival, or any corporate provider competing in the new public health care market.

My aim is to provide a big picture useful for people who want to make health sciences available for the whole of society. Not just for customers who can make their demands heard, but a framework that can sustain critical thought where most staff and patients actually live, work and try somehow to survive, not only in approved centres of excellence with exceptional resources, but in the real world of often almost impossible tasks. Though this may entail swimming against the tide of fashion, I still believe it follows the prevailing winds and currents of history. This is not a consensus book, because today we have no consensus, except perhaps among people without personal responsibility for giving health care, or substantial personal experience of receiving it. Applied health sciences are going through hard times.

I write from personal experience. In 1948, when Nye Bevan made the speech quoted at the opening of this book,[3] I was a second-year medical student at Cambridge. Inside medical schools as well as the real world outside (of which most medical students then knew little) a battle was raging between Bevan as Minister of Health in Britain's postwar Labour government, and the British Medical Association (BMA). The BMA mainly represented established general practitioners who feared losing ownership of health care as self-employed small businessmen. The government had been elected by landslide majority to make health care a national public service, rather than a rag-bag assortment of private enterprise, underfunded local government, and hand-to-mouth charity. Like the war that preceded it, to contemporary participants the outcome of this struggle was uncertain. Unlike most of his cabinet colleagues and established media opinion, Bevan was confident that a large majority of patients[4] would rise to the occasion, and use the free service as responsible citizens. More surprisingly, he was also confident that doctors – a notoriously conservative profession – when freed from chasing fees in the medical marketplace and allowed to treat people according to their needs, would discover possibilities for their work they had never previously imagined. With an optimism as amazing then as it still seems today, he regarded doctors, and health workers generally, as a politically ignorant but educable class. All that was needed was time, and experience of the social relations of health production that would emerge when care was removed from the marketplace.

Bevan's roots lay in the inclusive solidarity of South Wales mining communities. He tried to extend the lessons he had learned there to all communities everywhere. He knew that people didn't have to be rich to be generous – quite the contrary. Then a country almost on its knees could take brave decisions, of which we, with our present wealth, are presumed to be incapable.

He was right: the sceptics (then, as now, in confident majority wherever respectable opinion is formed) were wrong. The NHS soon established itself as Britain's most successful and overwhelmingly popular nationalised undertaking, an institution so close to the nation's heart that not even Margaret Thatcher ever dared openly to hand it over to corporate business.[5] Her successors, first in Conservative, now in New Labour government, have continued her costly privatisation of public services.[6] They have had to do so by stealth, proclaiming each successive capitulation to commerce as support for otherwise declining NHS standards, still within a dwindling concept of gift economy.[7] No open electoral battle has ever been fought, but the slide back to the market continues, driven by its own idiot logic of the bottom line, where profit stands proxy for every other outcome.

Bevan had indeed set the feet of doctors, patients and everyone else involved one way or another in the NHS, on a new path entirely. The social forces he set in motion could still prove irreversible.[8] Over the half century following 1948, the NHS became an independent subset economy, threatening to legitimise an entirely new set of economic rules, creating new dimensions for public expectations. How this occurred, and how it created opportunities for us to get back on the road toward a more civilised, generous and sustainable society, this book tries to explain.

Why economics?

My explanation is organised around an economic analysis. I assume that the hard work of NHS professionals, together with the often even harder work of their patients, should have a useful product. If this product is real, it must somehow be measurable. The leading edge of medicine got past wishful thinking around 1935, and the leading edge of nursing passed it several centuries earlier (the trailing edges of both have yet to consider the matter at all). Many people are so accustomed to all economic arguments being used only against humane ideas rather than to support them, that they reject economic terms altogether. They assume that human progress depends on defiance of economic laws, rather than on questioning the laws we have, and developing new ones better fitted to the real world they claim to explain. Economic laws are not laws of nature, but descriptions of human behaviour. As individuals we have no real choice as to our economic behaviour, but as collective groups we can organise change – as we did in my lifetime during the Second World War, when both Britain and the United States partially reorganised their economies around a consensus social objective. Germany, despite all the coercive power of a dictatorship, failed to do so. For a few years, we dared to rewrite economic laws, and got away with it. All who care about the future of the NHS as a humane service for all of the people, rather than a profitable business for some of the people, need to understand and present their argument in economic terms, but they also must find the courage and imagination to see economic possibilities invisible to most current experts, confident that what they may lack in formal knowledge will be more than compensated for by their familiarity with actual points of production. Without some understanding of the economics of health care derived not from classical theory but from experience of the real health care economy, with clinical decisions as its principal units, those trying to oppose continued commercialisation and industrialisation of the NHS can only wring their hands and agonise, leaving all real decisions to the industrialisers and commercialisers.

This argument is presented in outline in Chapter 1. Like any skeleton, this is a bit dry. The next four chapters add flesh, so far as possible drawing their real examples from work I have either done myself, or been associated with closely enough to know its limitations as evidence. I hope this will make this combination of clinical, political and economic argument more lively and interesting for readers, who can then decide for themselves how far its conclusions are justified (it's much easier to see what's wrong than what's right). Finally, the last chapter considers how these conclusions might begin to be developed in practice, starting from where we actually are, with the people we actually have, against the immense resistance we shall certainly face in the future, no less than in the past.

Economics concerns wealth and power, and who holds them. President George W. Bush has inadvertently taught the world a lesson that each generation must always learn for itself from its own experience: that the rich and powerful never willingly release their hold on what they have, and never cease to demand more. Our only asset is that we are many, they are few. Unity and solidarity are the keys, but they depend on understanding, and confidence that we know where we're going, and really can make a better world by thoughtful human decision than by the tidal waves of avarice released by market forces. Our present defencelessness in the face of arrogant riches derives from the collapse of the understanding and confidence we had in 1948, when Bevan set our feet on his new path. Much of the understanding of those days proved illusory. Though loss of illusion is painful, it is a necessary advance. No truth is ever final, whether in science, or in social thought. For people who want a world planned and shared rather than plotted and grabbed, a fundamental revision of thought was necessary and inevitable. During that interruption in progress, existing wealth and power have enjoyed themselves and bullied their opponents into submission, but they can have no lasting victory. We need a new big picture of where we have come from, where we want to go, and how we can get there. I hope this book can help to provide at least an outline sketch from which to begin.[9]

Some apologies

This work has serious limitations. It has altogether the wrong tone for an academic work, but admits too many uncertainties for a polemic missile. Anger is a necessary ingredient of education in times like these, but without intelligent direction and discipline it becomes mere cursing, letting off steam. Health professionals need a book that helps them to work and make sense of their experience, and avoid that demoralising sense of hardworking futility that has always threatened those in public service, and is now reaching crisis levels.[10] I hope this book will also be useful to patients interested in making the NHS work better, both for themselves and for other patients whose problems they share. That eventually includes virtually everybody.

Any book that looks at the world must start from somewhere, why not from where we actually are? I have written unashamedly from my own point of view as a doctor (not some other sort of health worker), as a community-based general practitioner (GP), not a hospital-based specialist, who worked in a South Wales coal-mining community, with substantial research interests and commitments, not at all typical of my contemporary colleagues. Useful experience must be specific, because to be verifiable (or falsifiable) truth must be concrete. To generalise beyond specific experience always entails some error, but it is less dangerous (in our present increasingly dangerous circumstances) than doing nothing, providing it is done cautiously and carefully. I think the world needs books along essentially similar lines to this one, for other health care systems and other cultures, but others must write them. As the industrial revolution (of which our care system is a late product) began in Britain, and reached its zenith on the eve of the First World War in the South Wales mining valleys (which also created embryonic models for the NHS) this standpoint may have some advantages, even for a global view. I am aware that this omits the hungry half of the world, which contains most of the world's ill health and least of its health care services. I am aware also that it omits other developed industrial economies, some of them having packed into four decades what took Britain four centuries to develop. There is quite a lot about the US, simply because it is the relatively new US corporate model that is now being imposed throughout the world by marketisation of health care, but I do not pretend to have written a book that can be of much use to students in that country, if they do not have good background knowledge or experience of the NHS. For both health care and education, national traditions are of huge significance. Each country must find its own path, knowing that the nature of its national health care is a centrally important part of its identity. The patriotism of the rich, rolled out at every opportunity to intimidate dissent, is entirely false, as their shifting investments to wherever life and labour are cheapest shows every day in the stock market. True patriotism does exist, nowhere more clearly than in public health care, and remains an extremely powerful potential force. For health workers it is most effectively expressed through service to the people they know best.

Finally, the fact that I have chosen the NHS as the main vehicle for my argument does not imply that other fields might not have served almost as well. Most obvious of these is education, but I think similar arguments could probably be applied to virtually any field of creative work dealing with people more than with things. However, at least in Britain, I believe the NHS provides the most readily available and most effective initial spearhead for fundamental political change, because it is the most socially inclusive, has the widest and most resilient popular base and deepest cultural roots, and because transformation of life itself into a commodity can most easily be recognised by the broadest majority of people as a basic threat to civilisation.

No single author can have all the skills or experience needed to provide more than a first outline of so large a subject, which is itself only at an early stage of development. Though a better book could surely have been written as a collective enterprise, to wait for that might have meant it was not written at all. As a compromise, I have had immense help from critical colleagues who struggled through many earlier drafts stretching over the past eight years. My more recent advisers are listed in my acknowledgements. I hope it will provide enough material to encourage a new generation with contemporary experience and less encumbered with obsolete ideological luggage, to complete the picture and embark on the new tasks it implies.

Julian Tudor Hart MB DSc DCH FRCGP FRCP
30 September 2005

julian@tudorhart.freeserve.co.uk, www.juliantudorhart.org

Notes

[1] Doyal and Pennell, 1979.

[2] Navarro, 1976.

[3] My original title for this book was 'A new path entirely', from the passage in Bevan's speech quoted earlier, because it provides a connecting thread throughout my argument. My editors thought this would be incomprehensible to most of the people otherwise likely to be interested in reading it, so I bowed to their view. The new title is probably better.

[4] The word 'patient' remains useful, despite its many obvious disadvantages. For reasons explained later, I cannot accept 'consumer' or 'customer' as appropriate substitutes, except in the special circumstances of commercial provider–consumer transactions, which any NHS worthy of the name would exclude. 'Client' is little better. If doctors and nurses must take their terms from another field, teachers are surely more appropriate than lawyers, but nobody has suggested 'pupils' or 'students'. Apart from the fact, verified by opinion polls, that patients generally prefer 'patient' to any alternatives, and that this is an established term everyone understands, patience remains a virtue that almost all of them must either possess or acquire, simply to function effectively in an always imperfect service. I wish all health care professionals (including myself) could learn to be as patient as most of our patients.

[5] Though Margaret Thatcher provides the obvious marker for the shift in Britain from welfare capitalism to more aggressive deregulated markets, this has happened everywhere, with little resistance from socialist or social democrat parties where they were in power, and often the shift has been led by them. New Zealand, the birthplace of state welfare, was an outstanding example of this.

[6] NHS care bought in from or contracted out to the private health care sector has increased ten-fold since the last Conservative government in 1997, despite average procurement costs 15% higher from the private sector than from within the NHS itself (Lister, 2005).

[7] Titmuss (1997) provided a comparative analysis of the economics of blood for transfusion in Britain, where blood was available only as a free gift from volunteer donors, and the US, where almost all blood

for transfusion came from paid donors through commercial enterprises. The UK National Blood Transfusion Service (NBTS) was a government service created during the Second World War, organising and recruiting on a mass scale in peacetime as a natural development parallel to the NHS. Using data from the 1960s, Titmuss found good evidence of greatly reduced costs and very much higher quality in the UK programme, with much lower risks of the then known contaminants, mainly hepatitis viruses (this was long before the AIDS pandemic). In Britain at least, few then challenged his conclusions (Darnborough, 1974). By the 1980s, commercial providers were hammering on the door everywhere, and illicit insider trading in high-value blood products (not blood for transfusion, but plasma derivatives) was becoming a serious problem within state services. In New Zealand, when government was about to impose market competition on its hitherto gift economy in blood for transfusion, 345 consecutive donors were questioned, with a 98% response rate. Over half were opposed to profits being made from blood, 71% were concerned about blood quality in a commercialised service, 41% would no longer give blood if profits were made from selling blood products, and 10% were reconsidering giving blood in future (Howden-Chapman et al, 1996). Since then blood products derived from blood for transfusion have become an extremely profitable byproduct for the NBTS, creating fears that the UK system will soon be indistinguishable from that in the US (Oakley, 1996). Even human body organs are now being seriously proposed by some health economists as an effective or even morally superior legal market (Cherry, 2005; J.S. Taylor, 2005).

[8] First hopeful signs of renewed organised resistance appeared during the last few weeks before my final draft was completed. The NHS Support Federation, the NHS Consultants Association, and a huge, growing and unprecedentedly wide-ranging number of senior health professionals and NHS trade unions are gathering around a movement to Keep Our NHS Public, to be officially launched in October 2005. Most NHS staff are only now beginning to understand what is being done to them.

[9] Some critical understanding of economics is central to understanding health care as a social function. Many economists – notably Galbraith, Polanyi, Shonfield and Hutton – have grappled with the problem that classical economics, which starts from the market, is unable to include hugely important economic activities that produce value, but not in commodity form; not only public health care, but bringing up children

and all sorts of other work within families. On the other hand, perversely, classical economics does include production not of goods but of bads – commodities that are profitable but damaging to society, and byproducts of commodity production such as pollution and environmental degradation. These are addressed by measures of net economic welfare, and many other attempts to tackle the areas ignored by the economic orthodoxy embraced by neoconservatives in the US, and abjectly accepted by New Labour.

Acknowledgements

My wife Mary gave up a large part of her life to this book, and to its many preceding component parts developed over our 43 years together, of which eight went into its production through a long and often uncomfortable gestation. I cannot thank her enough. Tony Beddow, John Bunker, Iain Chalmers, Anna Donald, John Ivor Lewis, Colin Leys and Graham Watt all took immense trouble, and time they could hardly spare, to give extremely helpful advice on earlier drafts, and critical support without which I would certainly have abandoned this project as over-ambitious and unworkable. I also thank the following colleagues who contributed critical comments, and did their best to make me develop the argument clearly and keep to the point: Hixinio Beiras, Ros Bryar, June Clark, Franco Delzotti, Jane Elliott, Ron Frankenberg, Trisha Greenhalgh, Ajey Hardeekar, John Horder, Ben Hart, Adrian Hastings, Andrew Herxeimer, Mauri Johanssen, Pat Lewis, Irvine Loudon, Theo Macdonald, John Meisel, Ian Millington, Ann Oakley, Gianluigi Passerini, Malcolm Rigler, John Robson, Ron Singer, Tomi Spenser, Steve Tomlinson and Morton Warner. None is responsible for anything in this final version. Finally, I thank librarians in many places for their unfailing patience and courtesy, and Philip de Bary at The Policy Press for leaving my final draft virtually unchanged.

Abbreviations and acronyms

ADHD	attention-deficit hyperactivity disorder
BBC	British Broadcasting Corporation
BMA	British Medical Association
BMJ	*British Medical Journal*
BUPA	British United Provident Association
CE	chief executive
EBM	evidence-based medicine
EU	European Union
FDA	Federal Drugs Administration
GATS	General Agreement on Trade in Services
GATT	General Agreement on Tariffs and Trade
GNP	gross national product
GP	general practitioner
HMO	health management organisation
ICC	International Cochrane Collaboration
ILP	Independent Labour Party
IMF	International Monetary Fund
IT	information technology
ITC	Independent Treatment Centre
JAMA	*Journal of the American Medical Association*
MRC	Medical Research Council
NICE	National Institute for Clinical Excellence
NHS	National Health Service
NPfIT	National Programme for Information Technology
OECD	Organisation for Economic Cooperation and Development
PFI	private finance initiative
PPP	public–private partnership
RCGP	Royal College of General Practitioners
RCN	Royal College of Nursing
SHA	Socialist Health Association
SMA	Socialist Medical Association
SMSA	State Medical Service Association
UN	United Nations
WB	World Bank
WHO	World Health Organisation
WTO	World Trade Organisation

ONE

The National Health Service as a creative system

One of the few advantages of being 78 years old is that I now have enough experience of alleged crises to understand that all but a few are illusory. There has never been a time when, according to conventional wisdom, the country was not going to the dogs, institutions and professions were not losing public respect, and patients were not looking back to good old days when doctors knew not just their patients' names, but those of their children, their grandchildren, their dogs, cats and budgerigars, and even visited them in their own homes when they were sick, without making a big song and dance.

For most of my 40 years of patient care, almost everything about it got steadily better: more effective, more humane and less authoritarian. Until about 20 years ago, resistance to this advance was weakening on almost all fronts. Progress was real, visible to everyone, and this sustained the morale of both health care professionals and patients, because all of them worked within a big picture shared by a general consensus, toward consensus objectives. Obviously much of this improvement depended on expanding knowledge, which will continue to increase exponentially as a progressive social force; but both health professionals and patients were also undergoing a sea change in their social behaviour that depended not on knowledge, but on learning – learning from their practical experience of work in the gift economy Bevan had created, aiming to identify needs and meet them, rather than make money. For both these reasons, health professionals of all kinds have become more knowledgeable, more humane, more imaginative, less arrogant, less opinionated, and more willing to acknowledge and learn from their own errors, from the scientific literature (itself based mainly on successive recognitions of error), and from their patients' opinions and experience. For the same reasons, patients generally became less ignorant, less credulous, less fearful of truth and less prone to denial, and more understanding of their own real needs, the needs of others, and even – though to a far more limited extent

– of the nature of medicine as an inexact science rather than either magic or human engineering.

For its first three decades, both professional and patient experience of the NHS was overwhelmingly positive – not because it was free from all the ancient greeds, cruelties, crass errors, despotisms and desperate material shortages besetting every public medical care system grudgingly funded by government from taxes, but because all these faults (except the last) were so obviously in decline. Despite all its shortages, in popular experience the pre-'reform' NHS worked more efficiently than either the dog's dinner of public, private and charity provision before 1948, or what UK citizens found if they, or their friends or relatives fell sick in the US (its opposite in political and economic terms) or elsewhere in the European Union (EU) (with more bureaucratic insurance-based systems).[1] And so, despite over two decades of vigorously promoted market competition, consumerism, contempt for public service, and resurrection of superstition and antiscience, a majority of voters of all persuasions still believes that we need a single national service available to all of the people, all of the time, according to their need and scientific evidence of effectiveness, therefore somehow defying all the laws of the market. Of course, there are still many greedy doctors and selfish patients, but in my experience at least, both were always a minority, and even today are less numerous than they seemed in 1952, when I qualified. Undeniably they now have a louder voice than before 1979 (when they had sunk to a barely audible whisper) because Margaret Thatcher restored greed and selfishness to their pre-war dominance as drivers for a wealth-creating economy: but we still have no evidence, either from elections or opinion polls, that this is what most people ever wanted, or that this was a rising social trend in the pre-'reform' days of consensus.[2]

The crisis is real

However, the crisis today is real, getting worse, and of a fundamental nature. The natural and still-continuing progress of health professionals and patients that I have already described has since the early 1980s been forced by government to flow through channels modelled not from experience of meeting public needs through public service, but from experience (mainly US experience) of commodity distribution in markets led by consumer demand. As exponentially rising possibilities and expectations funnel into narrowing NHS pipelines, the overflow spills to a rapidly growing private sector that few people want and even fewer voted for, but government is determined to create. The result is confusion, turbulence and a general feeling that health professionals are just corks in the ocean, and that patients are becoming mutually competitive consumers, looking each to their own interest. A growing proportion of staff has given up trying to work rationally in a service that no longer makes intuitive sense. Staff seem to face ever-increasing fragmentation and bureaucratisation of their work, dwindling job security, rising cost competition, time-pressures, personal threats of litigation and collective threats of unit bankruptcy, from patients encouraged by government to act as acquisitive consumers rather than responsible citizens. Though an immense majority of NHS patients still report positive personal experience of care, the NHS they see on television, hear about on radio or read about in newspapers seems for the past two or three decades to have been in terminal decline, with resort to the private market as the only way out. With no political party close to power offering any positive alternative to continued relentless subordination of the NHS to industrialisation on business lines, and an army of advertisers extolling the virtues of commodity care, 'every man for himself' begins to seem the best available philosophy for survival, both for staff and for patients. The social capital that made the NHS possible in the first place was a shared popular understanding of solidarity. If that understanding becomes replaced by consumerism, the NHS will have lost its foundations.

Though government has at last begun to fund our NHS at a level approaching that reached long ago by other West European governments, this pours into a vessel already so fragmented into competing independent units, and so beset by the bureaucratic demands of accountancy and management, that little cash or goodwill may remain for improved patient care after the management consultants and corporate interests now invited to usurp all the potentially profitable functions of the NHS have taken their share. So long as the NHS remained a socially funded gift economy, independent of business, it was grossly underfunded compared with public health care systems in every other advanced economy.[3] The shift to anything approaching adequate funding was delayed until the previous boundaries between the NHS and business had already been destroyed. The central planning that originally redistributed specialist staff away from London and other university centres, and began to match investment in care services according to their burdens of sickness rather than their wealth, was systematically removed, completing a process already begun by previous Conservative governments. In the name of decentralisation and with a rhetoric of returning hospitals from government to the people, hospitals were driven to adopt Trust status as independent, competing units, each responsible for its own economic viability, encouraged to sell off all assets surplus to basic requirements – mainly building land.[4] Prime Minister Blair has made it clear that, so far as he is concerned, continued funding is conditional on further 'progress' down this road, echoed by his current heir-apparent, Gordon Brown.[5]

Meanwhile, like workers producing for any other commercial market, NHS professionals at every level find themselves compelled to run ever faster, just to stay in the race. This perpetual acceleration has two causes, the first essential and inevitable, the second unnecessary and gratuitous. As they must be and have always been, each week NHS goalposts are shifted by advances in science and technology. The good news that more can be done comes in the *British Medical Journal*, *Journal of the American Medical Association*, the *Lancet*, the *British Journal of General Practice* and the *New England Journal of Medicine*, but staff already know without being told that to transform what *can* be done into what actually *is* done needs more people, and these new people must be educated and paid for. No wonder most doctors do not keep up with these journals, because they tell them only of new tasks added to their already heavy burdens, without any assurance of resources to support them. Now to this necessary uphill struggle are added the rising demands of managers desperate to keep their units solvent in the contrived competition between hospitals imposed since the early 1980s,[6] and now also being imposed on English Primary Care Trusts.

Who wants or needs market choice?

Patients have been encouraged to believe that as market consumers they have a right to state-of-the-art care for any health problem, without regard to material realities limiting any public service, including good evidence that apparent new advances are real and effective, before they have been adequately researched in large whole populations rather than small experimental subsets. Ignoring the huge pitfalls entailed in comparing different hospitals serving different populations with differing levels of illness and differing social resources for coping with them, league tables claiming to measure the quality and quantity of outputs from competing hospitals have been made available, so that patients can search the Internet for their 'best buy', with actual costs still, for the time being, met by the state.[7]

In 2002 government presented its plan for 'e-booking' referrals from primary care to hospital specialists, called 'Choose and book'. Using an NHS information technology programme still under development, this required all patients in England (but not Wales or Scotland) to be offered four or five choices between hospitals – which must include at least one in the private sector – by December 2005. Hospital Trusts in England were instructed to set aside 15% of their funds to pay for these private sector referrals.[8]

'Choose and book' implies about 9.4 million online hospital appointments each year when it comes fully into operation, presently forecast for 2006. According to the 2002 public service agreement numbers of such online appointments should have reached 205,000 by the end of December 2004. In fact, only 63 such appointments had been made by that date. At present this programme has an anticipated total cost of around £30 billion, though the talk among people involved in its development is of £60bn. This could become yet another IT disaster, on a scale large enough to bring down a government.[9] This is not just a technical problem to be solved by IT programmers, nor does the problem centre on the reluctance of staff to use computer technology rather than traditional written records.[10] It concerns a fundamental error of political judgement and economic philosophy, imposing a market on a service where it was neither asked for by the public nor needed by staff. There is no evidence of any mass popular demand for such choice in referrals, either from patients,[11] GPs or specialists. The programme fails to recognise the nature of clinical decisions as fundamentally different from business decisions. Even in focus groups used in research initiated by Prime Minister Blair to test New Labour policies among representative groups of undecided voters, participants did not regard choices of this kind as important to their personal lives. Like most of the more committed electorate, most undecided voters just wanted their local schools, health centres and hospitals to be available and efficient.[12] The question patients actually ask is: 'Who would you choose, doctor, for yourself, your spouse, or your child?' They expect to hear the truth, unbent by material conflicts of interest, because at least until recently, such conflicts did not exist in a cash-free service without fees. In the 'reformed' NHS applying economic incentives and penalties at every possible point of judgement in order to push professional behaviour in preferred directions, such trust comes increasingly into question.[13]

If patients were not in fact demanding market choice, what about GPs? In this 'Choose and book' scheme, the National Audit Office feared yet another costly failure, so it surveyed GP opinion. Of 1,500 NHS GPs sampled in 2004, 61% viewed market choice negatively, only 3% thought it could be useful. The Health Secretary's response has not been to question the government's assumptions, but to initiate a campaign in 2005 to educate GPs on this issue, hoping this will persuade them to want what neither they nor their patients now believe to be useful or necessary.[14]

In 2003, celebrating the 55th birthday of the NHS, then Secretary for Health John Reid described his programme for consumer choice, now being implemented following the general election in 2005:

> For the last 60 years there has been a two-tier health service in this country. One tier has been the NHS, where people traditionally have not been given the choice, and the other has been for those people with money who can buy the privilege and jump the waiting lists. I want to make sure those two tiers do not operate for the next 60 years…. Wherever possible we will empower patients by giving them genuine individual choices – about where, when, how and by whom they are treated.[15]

Since then Patricia Hewitt has taken over the health ministry, with the same message. In a key speech to the Social Market Foundation, her junior Minister John Hutton argued that only by introducing competition and choice could Britain secure the values on which the welfare state was founded. Paying tribute to Clement Attlee's postwar government, he warned that inequalities remained in health and education: 'It is these stark facts alone that make the case for public service reform', he said. 'They are the powerful arguments against accepting the old model of top-down, monolithic public services run from the centre … the model of public service delivery we have inherited has simply not been responsive enough to tackle some of the social divisions that still scar our society.'[16]

To prove that this is becoming a new consensus for all parties aspiring to power, in the same issue of the *Guardian* appeared an opinion piece by Stephen Pollard under the title 'Tories need a Clause 4', arguing that their only hope of recovery is to remake the

Conservative Party into a standard bearer for the poor, through two measures: consumer choice in marketised public services, and flat rate taxes, so that everyone would pay the same tax, rich or poor. His audience will understand that, as always, the best way to enrich the poor is first to make the rich richer still, by giving them public services to run as profitable business, and by abolishing income tax. This will create a wealthier society, in which with enough at the top, something must eventually spill over to reach the bottom.

Now the New Labour message is private care for everyone who wants it in a consumer-led service. Concealed within this offer is continued expansion of care agencies financed by investors aiming to maximise profit, until the public and private sectors reach a balance between the profitable problems suited to care as a traded commodity, and the unprofitable problems left to whatever remains of the NHS as default provider. Reid presented an offer nobody could refuse, except the thoughtful but probably dwindling minority who still suspected that NHS care was usually safer and more effective than private care, because the profit motive could never be trusted to give higher priority to other ends.

Where's the catch? Granted a return to progressive taxation at pre-1979 levels (which even then were about average for the EU and much lower than in Scandinavia), the NHS could meet all *needs* for effective health care.[17] However, there is no way it could ever meet all *demands* for health care conceivable in a consumer market, driven not by needs but by wants, promoted in turn by providers with an economic interest in larger sales.[18] The central theme of this book is that rational and effective health care cannot follow the pattern of market competition for profit. Plausible health care could certainly be distributed as a profitable commodity, but not in a National Health Service worthy of the name, caring for all citizens, promoting and maintaining health and caring for the sick, curing when it can, and without substantial direct charges to patients. Charges for commoditised care might initially be small, as Bosanquet and Pollard and other advocates for 'reform' have advised,[19] but once through the 'free at time of use' barrier, we can be sure that charges would escalate. So long as health care is distributed as a social gift, it can have limits set by a combination of public expectations and scientific knowledge (further discussed in Chapter Three), but as soon as it becomes regarded as a commodity, demand will rise to whatever the public can be worried into demanding.

If we take the analogy of feeding a population, the food supplies needed to maintain a healthy, varied and generous national diet for all of the people are calculable, and, for sufficient time ahead to allow rational planning, they are finite. With measured supply we could meet measured need. The nation could be fed, and fed generously and diversely, with much less capital-intensive, more creative production and distribution networks than we now have, if investment were determined by needs rather than profits. As commodities, however, food supplies must continue to expand in variety, complexity and ever more ingenious presentation, simply to keep ahead of the competition and find new sources of profit. As there are limits to what even obese people can eat, an increasing proportion of this expansion must lie not in needs but in fancies, otherwise the entire business would collapse. The market for food supplies expands not by feeding more hungry people, but by meeting consumer demands actively promoted in every possible way by corporate food industries, and by the public brainwashers they employ – and we accept as the price for cheap broadcasting.

If the NHS follows this path, it will lose all real connection with its original purpose: but this is the direction in which not only New Labour but almost all governments are now dragging their national care systems, set not by voters but by the World Trade Organisation (WTO) and the World Bank (WB),[20] legally enforced by the General Agreement on Tariffs and Trade (GATT) and its subset, the General Agreement on Trade in Services (GATS), which governments of virtually all trading nations have signed, either willingly or under duress, but always behind the backs of their voters.[21] In the name of ever-widening consumer choice, political parties compete not over policy, but over presentation. They are all heading in the same direction, their differences concern only presentation, speed and the catch-phrases required to deceive different sections of public opinion.

Nine characteristics of the NHS as a distinct economy

Until the early 1980s, when Margaret Thatcher began to draw profit-seeking business into the NHS economy, the pre-'reform' NHS had nine distinctive features:

1. It was a single, unified national service[22] including all staff grades devoted directly or indirectly to care, freely available to all citizens according to their need, and almost entirely free from personal charges.

2. It was a gift economy including everyone, funded from general taxation (of which the largest component was income tax),[23] neither a contributory insurance scheme nor a commodity economy funded by consumers in an open market.

3. Its most important inputs and processes were personal interactions between lay and professional people. These interactions in fact (though originally not in professional theory) depended on conjoined evidence and judgements from both. Professionals, patients and populations could therefore begin to develop as co-producers of health, not as providers of health care with interests potentially adversarial to their patients.[24]

4. Its products were potentially measurable as health gain for the whole population, not as processes acquired by individual consumers.

5. Its staff and component units were not expected to compete for market share, but to cooperate to maximise useful service. Commercial secrecy had no function and became unthinkable.[25]

6. Continuity was central to its efficiency and effectiveness, and discontinuity and fragmentation were its most important sources of inefficiency and error.

7. Its local staff and populations intuitively believed they had moral ownership of, and loyalty to, neighbourhood NHS units. Consumer choice between competing providers was to most people meaningless. Everybody knew of GPs or hospital units they did not want to use, but the remedy for this was generally seen to lie not in alternative market choices, but through steps to educate staff, raise their morale and improve resources at these points of weakness.

8. None of its decisions and few of its procedures could be fully standardised, all of its decisions entailed some uncertainty and doubt, and all these processes operated within a continuously shifting context of expanding knowledge. They were therefore unsuited to commodity form either for personal sale, or for long-term contracts.

9. The NHS was, and despite attempts to industrialise it still remains, a labour-intensive economy. Every new diagnostic or therapeutic machine generates new needs for more skilled staff, able to control and interpret the work of machines, and translate them into human terms so that patients can participate in decisions, and in health creation and maintenance. Though machines create need for new technical skills they also create need for new more specialised human skills, particularly educational skills, applied

through personal interactions to exceptionally vulnerable people, not episodically, but throughout their lives.

These nine features define the fundamental differences between the socialising path set for the NHS by Bevan in 1948, and the commercialising path down which governments have driven it since 1983. The central thrust of industrial efficiency is to produce more of a cheaper product of higher perceived quality, faster and at lower cost. It achieves this, first by mechanising human labour (making people work more like machines and less like creative thinkers), then by replacing human labour with machines operated by a smaller workforce. By forcing NHS staff into this industrial mould, and by fragmenting what was originally a proud and unified national service into competing units and outsourcing supportive functions to for-profit franchises, managed care is destroying its most valuable potential assets: the morale, unity, social commitment and imagination of its workforce, and the goodwill of its public. It is also degrading the people the NHS serves, from citizens moving steadily toward co-producer status, to consumers concerned only with their own wants.

So far this process seems to either to have more or less paralysed resistance, or met only defensive trade union responses, in virtually every country subjected to it, even though no government has yet won positive support from a majority of its population for such 'reform'.[26] As a more general global crisis of disintegrating and unsustainable society becomes daily more obvious, governments are blocking their most readily available path for escape, as well as betraying their electors. So why do they do it?

Henry Ford: nothing succeeds like success

Capitalism may not be beautiful, but it delivers the goods. *Things* get better, even if *people* are thereby made worse. Henry Ford achieved colossal increases in productivity by replacing human labour by machines wherever this was possible. Where it was not, he divided human skills into elementary units, perfecting each single necessary function but eliminating all others, so that human activity came to resemble the work of machines, losing individuality and locality, but achieving huge reductions in costs, and gains in precision and in productivity. Once this step taken, the next is obvious: to replace those human functions that still remain by even more sophisticated machines, now including elements of intelligence. So far as I know, a car produced from start to finish entirely without human labour does not yet exist, but we can be sure that it will, some time in the foreseeable future.

Fascinated though Ford was by cars, they were not his ultimate product. He was not a dilettante aristocrat funding production from his own pocket, he had to attract investors by making more money for them than they could get elsewhere in a competitive market for capital. Making cars was just his particular way of making money for shareholders. The cars he made became the single most devastating weapon of world capitalism. US society's most potent icon became cars owned by working men, almost unthinkable in any other country until after the Second World War, except in Hitler's Germany, where the same principles were vigorously applied. At the depths of the post-1929 depression, starving refugees from the Oklahoma dustbowl fled to California in their model-Ts, and in Ohio today the new US unemployed use drive-in soup kitchens. Compared with the wheeled rustboxes produced at even greater human cost by countries that tried to develop socialist economies on the Soviet model, there was no contest. Capitalism has won the war of commodity production hands down.

But it has won at a price. It works by squeezing all that is human and creative out of the production process, eventually excluding labour itself. People lose their significance as creators and producers. They become valued, and may even come to value themselves and each other, chiefly by how much they acquire and consume, not by what they produce. In the economically developed world, this has been the common experience over two centuries. Craft skills that gave people the dignity and self-respect acquired from useful labour and creative work, was first subordinated to the requirements of factories and machine production and distribution, and then eliminated. Doctors and nurses are the last major occupational groups to be forced into that pipeline. They don't like it, but nor did the handloom weavers, engravers, cabinet makers and other skilled craftsmen of the 18th century, when their skills became valueless and they had to seek work in the mines and mills. Nor do subsistence farmers and peasants the world over, who can starve more cheaply on tinned baked beans than on what they can grow but no longer sell. Descendants of 18th-century British craftsmen are, undeniably, by orders of magnitude better off today, and on virtually every material measure. On all other measures, gains are less obvious.

For medical or nursing practice to justify exemption from this apparently inevitable and universal historical process demands a powerful body of evidence, and this must be expressible in material economic terms. If industrialisation and commercialisation of health care can raise its productivity and reduce its costs to anything like the extent achieved by Henry Ford for his cars, then these policies will win the contest. No amount of hand-wringing by more sensitive consciences, nor machine-breaking by skilled craftsmen facing ruin, could stop the pioneering industrialists in the early 19th century, nor will similar pleas on behalf of humane personal care resist industrialisation of health care in the 21st.

Marketeers insist that competition and more aggressive management will raise productivity in health care as surely as they did for production of cars, without any decline in quality – indeed, they promise that quality will improve. We shall see. There is as yet little convincing evidence that industrialisation of health care can deliver this promise, and a great many reasons as well as mounting evidence that it cannot.

Henry Ford's social and economic thought was crude. No economist today seriously suggests that health care should be produced in ways resembling production of cars. The foundation of modern macroeconomics developed by J.M. Keynes and Joan Robinson at Cambridge understood that public services produced value, and that government intervention, government spending and existence of a public goods sector outside the market in health and education were essential because of market failure to provide these social functions for the whole population. No contemporary health economist openly supports the few who argue in favour of total marketisation of health care,[27] nor do any for-profit health care corporations wish to take over all the current functions of the NHS. They would just like to help out with those functions they feel most appropriate to the skills and resources they offer – which happen also to be the potentially most profitable, most readily industrialised to commodity form, and entailing least risk for investors. All this is true; and yet these economists also give profound respect to Professor Milton Friedman, doyen of the Chicago school of economics, which everyone admits has dominated economic thought ever since the idea of shifting public service back to the marketplace returned to respectability in the 1980s. Here is what Friedman had to say on this subject: 'Few trends could so thoroughly undermine the very foundations of our free society as the acceptance by corporate officials of a social responsibility other than to make as much money for their stockholders as possible.'[28]

This was included in the set of ideas for which Friedman was honoured by a Nobel prize, so it has some authority. All of us, including even health economists who still support continued commercialisation of the NHS, need to face the fact that for the past three decades, the foundations for their thought have largely returned to the same simple, brutal but effective ideas used by Henry Ford and his successors, expressed with equal crudity by United States presidents, and used by news media and politicians as the basis of the simplistic assumptions they present to the general public as indisputable fact.

Eclipse of Keynesian economics

It was not always so. From 1945 to the late 1970s or early 1980s, economists could argue that their ideas provided a more sophisticated, more civilised, and more hopeful alternative, and that Friedman and his mentor Hayek belonged irreversibly to the past.[29] Ever since 1948, there has been a powerful lobby against the NHS as a free public service, trying to return medical care so far as possible to the marketplace, but until the early 1980s this was a barely significant political force. Up to the late 1970s, all political parties in or close to power accepted J.M. Keynes' modification of classical economic theory, recognising that sustainable operation of the capitalist system required some socially necessary expenditures and investments that no market could deliver, simply in order to maintain a stable society within which wealth could be created by workers, be accumulated by capitalists and, it was hoped, be invested in socially useful progress.

Unlike Joan Robinson, Keynes was no socialist. His *General Theory* published in 1936 was written to modify classical economics in ways that could deflect Marx's fundamental criticism, and re-establish faith in capitalist economy after the Wall Street crash of 1929 and consequent global crisis – a global crisis of ideology as well as economy. Keynes and Robinson pioneered the concept of gross national product (GNP), a huge step forward toward regulated national economies.[30] Within this they incorporated a fundamental error. Because no figures were then available to measure gains from public health, educational or social services (nor are they now) they made a consciously false assumption, simply to get on with their larger task; they estimated the output contribution of these services to GNP as equal to the sum of their costs to government. Obviously this failed to take into account value added by these public services, even though Keynes and Robinson both recognised that they did in fact create added value. The values the services produced were not marketed commodities, so they would have to be measured in new ways, which nobody then tried to develop. There are now some attempts to do this, which could open up important new possibilities, but for the most part this fundamental error persists.

International failure to make social investments after the First World War was one of the main underlying causes of a train of events culminating in the Second World War, and eventual popular rejection of the Conservative Party in the British general election of 1945, despite all the apparent advantages of Winston Churchill as its leader. In 1945, to have any hope of re-election to government, pre-war conservative parties throughout Europe, almost all of which had eagerly participated in Hitler's empire, had to reinvent, rename and reorganise themselves around state welfare systems and regulated markets.[31] For the next three decades, conservative parties competed with socialist, social democrat and communist parties in commitment to full employment, social housing, mass education, social welfare and national health care services. The US was an exception,[32] because socialist ideas had never sunk deep roots there except in a few industrial areas, isolated and intimidated to vanishing point by the early 1950s, because the war had enriched rather than impoverished its economy, and because Nazi occupation had not identified its most conservative politicians as collaborators.[33] Even there, however, industrial workers needed to see with their own eyes a steadily rising standard of living to establish that capitalism was their best option, and so they did.

The foundations for this social consensus began to change in the early 1970s, a shift usually attributed entirely to the economic crisis when oil-producing countries began to set prices that were profitable to their own rulers, rather than to oil companies in the US, Britain, France and the Netherlands. Though this did indeed cause major difficulties for western economies, giving them less latitude for diversion of profits to tax-funded social welfare, a more potent factor was the by then obviously dwindling ideological competition offered by the USSR and its satellite economies. This competition had been serious. In 1913 the Tsarist Empire, with 9.4% of the global population, produced 3.6% of world industrial output. By 1986 the USSR, with less than 6% of the global population, produced 14.6% of world industrial output. Though the USSR had suffered 27 million deaths (including over 80% of the male age group 18-25), loss of 50% of its industry, and relocation of the other half over thousands of miles in the midst of war, up to the 1970s this economy grew faster than a US economy that had been doubled rather than halved by war, had never been bombed or invaded, and had total wartime manpower losses around 300,000.[34]

Up to the 1970s, this faced developed capitalist economies with powerful ideological competition, countered in large part by sustained rises in working-class living standards, and investments in education, social welfare and health care. Both these advantages were substantial. As all industrial economies began to shift from relatively crude basic outputs to more sophisticated, knowledge-based products requiring great mobility of information and thought, the crudity of the Soviet economy became increasingly visible to everyone, including ordinary Russians themselves. A rising proportion of the new Soviet ruling class established in the 1930s recognised opportunities to appropriate public investments to their own personal ownership, shifting bloodlessly from the state capitalism created by the USSR to the bandit capitalism prevailing in Russia since 1991.[35] Though the final collapse of Soviet communism came only in 1990, Conservative politicians without personal experience of the worldwide rout of their parties in 1945 recognised much sooner that socialism (as they understood it) was no longer a serious political force. Keynesian policies had always been essentially political rather than economic. The important reasons for adopting them had disappeared, so out they went. In Britain, the funeral was first announced not by Margaret Thatcher (who usually gets the credit) but by Jim Callaghan, the Labour Prime Minister she replaced.[36] Having already lost belief in its own message, old Labour opened the door for a return to deregulated capitalism, invading every corner of society in search of new markets. Margaret Thatcher saw and took her opportunity, and set the agenda followed ever since by every party within reach of power.

A new and limitless market

To governments, the appeal of commercialisation lies not only in the promise of higher productivity, real or illusory, but also in the wealth this might create for investors, and relief from their own responsibilities to fulfil the promises made by Bevan in 1948, which they can neither implement without upsetting their sponsors, nor openly repudiate without losing their activists and voters.

The shift of NHS care from public service to an industrial model is generally referred to as managed care. This international development was well described by Richard Smith when he was editor of the *British Medical Journal*, and was still resisting industrialisation of care:

> In September 1996 leaders of US managed health care plans met in Mexico City to discuss opportunities for extending their business internationally. The meeting was organised by the American Association of Health Plans and the Academy for International Health Studies. Workshops looked at market opportunities in Israel, Korea, Venezuela, Canada, Mexico, Russia, France, Singapore, Brazil, New Zealand, Australia, Puerto Rico, South Africa and Argentina...The businessmen who run the for-profit managed health care plans in the United States see no reason why they should not follow the path of their colleagues in other businesses and compete globally. Indeed, they may have to. Wall Street expects them to keep growing, which means signing up more people to their plans. And, as one chief executive of a health plan put it, 'We are soon going to run out of people in the United States.' Managed care plans already cover 100 million Americans.... Solid evidence that schemes do reduce costs and raise quality is lacking, and academic study of the health plans is difficult because they are changing so fast. But the assumption in the United States seems to be that the proliferation of managed care plans has stopped American health care costs from rising for the first time in two decades.... So perhaps managed health care – which has emerged from a country with one of the world's most irrational health care systems – will end up being exported around the world. Just as more and more of us are fed by American fast food chains, so many of us may receive our health care in some way through American managed health care plans.[37]

Though investors in US managed care plans saw themselves as 'running out of people', 40 million US citizens had no health insurance, and this number is still rising. New markets seek not people who need, but customers who demand. Managed care in the US did indeed interrupt a previously terrifying escalation of costs, but did so essentially by wresting control of care processes from the hands of physicians and surgeons with an economic interest in promoting them, and handing that control to larger, more remote, more powerful and far more ruthless health care corporations. These were closely linked to insurance companies, which in turn invested enough millions of dollars in both main political parties to guarantee both their immunity from state ownership, and whatever state subsidies they needed to stay profitably in business with minimal risk. After decades of steadily rising costs, managed care has held total US spending on health care to just under 15% of GDP, compared with around 8-9% in West European care systems that, unlike the US, include all citizens.[38] The costs of pharmaceuticals and all clinical interventions are both still much higher in the US than in Canada or the UK, and despite managed care, are now again rising, but this time to enrich health care corporations rather than entrepreneur physicians and surgeons.

Because UK doctors had already lost control of all but a small top slice of medical trade, managed care here could not make substantial savings by eliminating superfluous but profitable interventions, as health management organisations (HMOs) have now largely managed to do in the US. The NHS had already secured huge savings by using its power as a single purchaser to reduce prices for pharmaceuticals, which even today remain far below US prices.[39] The UK now spends around 6% of its GDP on health care, and plans to increase this to the West European average, around 9%, by 2006. In cost terms, from 1948 to the present day, no other developed economy has ever got so much for so little. In the UK, verified gains in productivity in terms of health outcome will depend on evidence that managed care in a competitive market works more efficiently than already long-established socially inclusive, cooperative public service.

As yet, advocates for market-oriented managed care have based their public arguments on faith, not evidence, but investors have more dependable motives. If its potentially profitable components (mainly routine body repairs and maintenance) could be separated from those that have so far tended to generate loss (mainly emergencies and continuing care for complex chronic disorders), this reduced vision of health care could become extremely profitable, in an infinitely expansible market. Health care now promises added life, a promise backed for the first time with convincing evidence that it is real. With its mind-modifying and body-repairing treatments and procedures, life can be made longer, less painful and at least apparently more beautiful, in whatever terms may currently be fashionable. Such promises are now not only plausible, their results are measurable, and failure to deliver can end in the courts. Coming at a time when the rate of profit for virtually every other commodity is in continued long-term decline, added life could be the ultimate product in the ultimate market. The prospect is intoxicating; so many investors are intoxicated, a state easily conveyed to their attendant journalists and politicians.

Separating cure from care

Though the first few years of managed care plans in the US were indeed very profitable, they soon ran into trouble when they had to provide continuing care for sick people, rather than episodic repairs for otherwise well people in whom some particular body part had either failed, or seemed at risk of doing so. By 1998, more than four out of five US doctors practised in HMOs operating managed care plans. HMOs found in practice that their business ceased to be profitable if more than 65% of insured consumers submitted a significant claim for care in any one-year period.[40] Superfluous care for the worried well was profitable because its processes and results were predictable and costs could be reduced through volume production of fragmented, specialised interventions by competing agencies. At the opposite end lay the extremely complex, scarcely predictable needs of patients with multiple chronic disorders, usually containable or even reversible by assiduous, sustained and imaginative care by generalists, occasionally supported by referral. This required imaginative community-based generalists with local, personal knowledge, as well as hospital-based specialists. In their customary annual renegotiations of what traditional family doctoring had accustomed people to consider a lifetime contract, US managed care plans now compete to recruit profitable well people and to discard unprofitable sick people.[41]

Investors in corporate health care now see few lucrative opportunities in continuing care for sick or disabled people. This is a new development. In the 1980s, NHS responsibilities for care for sick older people were effectively abdicated, and without any electoral mandate or serious prior public discussion, handed over to privately run nursing homes.[42] Very sick people in NHS hospitals were discharged, often against their will and the wishes of their relatives, to find whatever care they could afford in either local authority homes (which, unlike the NHS, had to charge for care) or privately operated care homes.[43] Responsibility for institutional care for the chronic sick and dependent older people was almost completely transferred from the NHS to local government authorities, and these were compelled by law to make at least 80% of provision through private nursing homes, so that many local authority homes closed. Over half of all UK health care beds are now in private nursing homes outside the NHS, though this process of attrition is hard to track because government no longer collects these data centrally.[44]

As in the case of HMOs, these homes could be profitable so long as their clients were old and infirm but essentially healthy, but they soon became unprofitable if they had to provide the staff levels and professional skills needed for people with incontinence, unable to feed themselves, or with progressing dementia. Their natural response has been either to refuse such patients in the first place, transfer them to NHS hospitals as acute cases and then refuse to take them back, or sink into the demoralisation found all too often by local authority regulators, where necessary staffing levels and skills have simply not been maintained. Inflation in house prices took off in the 1990s, so that selling large houses became more profitable than running them as nursing homes. Unlike the NHS, for-profit providers had no statutory duty to provide a service if they did not find it profitable. Thousands of nursing homes, particularly in the South-East of England, were closed simply because their profitability as real estate had come greatly to exceed their profitability as care homes. If this was an experiment in how privatisation affects a huge public service, the lesson was clear: private investors cannot be relied on to provide public service. If the market had ever done the job better as well as profitably, public services would never have been invented.

A lesson of more interest to investors was to steer clear of continuing care for complex chronic problems. The presently approved agenda for public discussion is separation of the curative functions of the NHS (essentially perceived as episodic human repairs and simple maintenance, technology-intensive and potentially profitable) from its caring functions (where processes are labour-intensive, profits are low and unpredictable risks are high). Most continuing care functions will probably stay with what remains of the NHS, after corporate contractors have taken what they want.[45]

Concepts of disease

A more subtle but equally damaging consequence of separating cure from care is that it may set back for several generations the rational application of new knowledge in human biology to health problems as they exist in reality rather than in textbooks. The way we, both staff and patients, think about disease and how to treat and prevent it, was broadly established in the 19th century, when the dominant paradigm for personal care had already been set by provider–consumer transactions in a professional market, and by the contemporary state of biological thought, dominated by description and taxonomy. This strongly favoured reification of disease – separation of diseases from the people who had them, as though they were some sort of invading parasite that could be attacked as a target separable from the patient (an important and transiently fruitful idea discussed more fully in Chapter Three). In the 1960s, doctors began to appreciate that most of the diseases seen in advanced economies were not invasions. Cancers, diabetes, coronary heart disease and most mental illness, for example, were more or less inseparable from their human hosts. These processes entailed either premature senescence in cells, or behavioural responses to their environments, or most commonly both. Such problems could not be targeted without very detailed and complex biological and social knowledge of unique individual people, as well as their diseases. Their effective treatment required sustained hard work from patients as co-producers of their own treatment and health maintenance, which in turn depended on an at least elementary understanding of what was happening to them – personal health literacy.

Where care could develop as a cooperative task sustained over time, protected from economic pressures, and made available to whole populations rather than self-selected customers, this transition to a more sophisticated view of health care made steady progress. It seemed to provide a paradigm able to use new medical knowledge that required intelligent and informed participation by patients in decisions about their present and future health, and integrated with public health policy. This is now threatened by regression to a primitive political and media culture almost exclusively concerned with episodic body repairs, where patients may become critical and demanding consumers, but lose whatever progress we have made toward shared understanding of the complex causes of disease, whose rational treatment is equally complex, entailing changes in personal and social behaviour beyond simply accepting surgery or taking tablets.

Steps needed to transform NHS care into profitable business

Colin Leys[46] identified four essential steps necessary for transition of public service processes to market transactions, the essence of 'reform':

1. Services must be divided and reconfigured as saleable commodity units, packaged and more or less standardised – commodification of services.
2. The public must somehow be induced to prefer services in this new commodity form.
3. The existing workforce must be reconfigured and somehow remotivated to produce these commodities for employers operating for profit.
4. Public services have to be maintained even if they are not profitable. Risks to private investors must therefore be limited by continued guarantees from the state.

In other words, all the nine features of the NHS already listed, which made it a distinct, unified, nationwide economy independent of business, designed to meet social needs rather than to maximise profit, must be minimised or eliminated. Despite all the advantages claimed by industrialisers and commercialisers, these four steps have proved difficult and politically hazardous for all the politicians who have so far dared to initiate them, because those nine positive features were and still are precisely what made the NHS loved by the nation like no other institution.

Of the four steps listed by Colin Leys as essential for internal competition, only the first has any substantial appeal to voters, and this only because it has provided quick and credible means to shorten the queue for elective surgical and diagnostic procedures.[47] Corporate contractors can provide these services profitably because they are already delivered episodically in more or less standardised form; a competitive market already exists to set prices, and tight monitoring is already in place to protect quality against price competition. The private sector has substantial unused capacity (at least 50% overcapacity before NHS 'reforms'), to expand its business into a flexible space provided by the state. Experienced staff can be recruited from the NHS.[48] With government support, the private sector has therefore been able to sell its spare capacity at marginal cost, though in fact NHS purchasers have been compelled to pay higher prices to private contractors than to their own in-house units for the same work.

Contrary to most expectations, new providers so far preferred by government have not included established private companies such as BUPA, Capio or HCA, nor has it preferred British to multinational companies. Of seven successful bidders for NHS contracts in 2004, five were based mainly in North America and one in South Africa. Only one was based wholly in Britain.[49] British private care has traditionally aimed at consumers in the top 5% of income, who only used the NHS for super-specialist services that the private sector was unable to provide. Its consumers were rich, so they could afford high fees. Private care was never seriously interested in the mass market in the lower two-thirds of income distribution. On the contrary, it suited these companies, and the part-time consultants who served both them and the NHS with little regard for conflicts of interest, for a two-tier, private–public service to continue indefinitely.

However, since 1948, the only way most people in the UK were ever driven to consider private care was not because they thought it was better, but because NHS care was not available when and where it was needed: not persuasion, but coercion. In the 1970s, every patient and every GP knew that any patient referred, say, for planned orthopaedic surgery, could jump an 18-month to three year waiting list and see the same consultant next week, simply by paying a fee for a private consultation. Urgent hospital admission would soon follow, because such consultants could find reasons to justify urgent priority, which lay in their hands, without any agreed criteria.[50] This could have been stopped by any government with enough courage to create a substantial difference between the earnings of whole-time and part-time consultants, but no such government ever materialised.

As for Leys' third point, reconfiguration of the workforce, hospital workers other than doctors and nurses underwent this destructive process long ago. In the 1980s, all staff below nursing grades were compelled to bid against private contractors for their own jobs, and either continue with even lower wages and worse conditions than they had before, or accept a new employer primarily dedicated to profit rather than service. Virtually all possible gains in efficiency from this process have already been made. According to Duncan

Nicholl, one-time chief executive of the NHS, output per capita in the NHS rose almost 30% between 1982 and 1991, compared with 16.5% for the economy as a whole, before commercialisation of the NHS had got into its stride.[51] Between 1982 and 1995 there was a 32% rise in inpatients across all acute specialties despite a 25% fall in beds, a 250% rise in day cases, and an 81% rise in throughput per acute bed. There was a 58% rise in cases per 1,000 population for all specialties, and a 54% rise for acute specialties. Inpatient activity rose overall by over two-thirds.[52]

These productivity gains were obtained at a colossal price in staff demoralisation and demotivation, with dirty hospitals a predictable consequence.[53] Twenty years ago there were about 100,000 NHS hospital cleaning staff. By 2003-04, so-called efficiency policies pursued by first Conservative and then New Labour governments had almost halved this number to 55,000.[54] If corporate contractors try to squeeze the workers they recruit from the NHS even further to compete with their former colleagues, effects on morale will be catastrophic, but to satisfy their shareholders, they will have few other options. With 80% or more of costs of production attributable to labour, profits from health care mainly depend on reducing this figure, and transferring productivity gains to top management salaries and profit. Zealots exist for whom no staff ever work hard enough. According to Eric Caines, NHS personnel director from 1990 to 1993, the NHS still needed to reduce its staff (including doctors and nurses) by 20% across the board,[55] but systematic exploitation of staff and industrialisation of their work has eventual consequences that limit the policies of any government that has to get itself re-elected. A systematic review by US researchers (including 15 different studies of 26,000 hospitals and 38 million patients from 1982 to 1995) showed that patients in for-profit hospitals were 2% more likely to die than those in public service hospitals, after standardising for relevant variables such as age and case-mix.[56] Profit is an inefficient motivator for quality health care.

First nurses, then doctors, will be next in line for similar industrialisation if the policy of competitive out-sourcing continues, steadily reducing the NHS in England[57] from a virtually monopoly provider of services, to a commissioner of services by a variety of enterprises competing for profit; a virtual organisation simply holding the ring for contending market-led providers. There has always been a minority of both doctors and nurses apparently indifferent to whether they serve all of the people in the NHS, or some of the people in private care, but I know of no evidence that rapid growth of the private sector has increased this minority. Obviously, if the private sector grows, so will the job opportunities it offers, but in my experience most of its workers are at best apologetic about their new employment, if not ashamed that they have abandoned what they once saw as a noble ship, which they now believe to be sinking. There was honour associated with NHS employment that no health care corporation will ever achieve, whatever its public relations mouthpieces may claim. The glossier their brochures and the smoother their tongues, the less anyone believes them.

Corporate providers exist to make profits for their shareholders and colossal salaries for their senior managers.[58] Everybody knows this; it cannot be concealed. These profits have to come from somewhere. Within the pre-'reform' NHS economy profits did not exist. That was the foundation for trust between caring professionals and their patients, guaranteeing that clinical decisions were virtually free from economic pressures in any direction. Apart from fraud (a substantial and predictable factor as soon as commerce penetrates any public service),[59] the only new sources of profit remaining for corporate providers are faster throughput with additional pressures on staff,[60] redefinition of their tasks toward those that are profitable and away from those associated with financial loss, and sales promotion to increase demand.

Medical tasks previously reserved for hospital-based specialists are being returned to primary generalists, nurses are taking over routine technical responsibilities formerly reserved for doctors, and new grades of nursing aide are being created to take over the less technical aspects of nursing care. This is a minefield of conflicting interests, with managements hoping to reduce costs by dilution of skilled labour, and staff hoping to see more of their real potential realised in practice. Because most patients can, with sufficient training, learn to apply even complex decisions and many technical procedures to themselves (for example, people with diabetes, epilepsy, or on continuous anticoagulants) it follows that, with sufficient training, virtually all health workers at all levels could do the same: but 'with sufficient training' is the critical phrase. Training is labour-intensive, costs time and money, and should thereafter be reflected in higher wages. Business styles of management have dissipated much of the mutual trust on which such change depends, but because of staff shortages at every level for at least the foreseeable future, the workforce is in a relatively powerful position and, within the NHS, present auguries look good.[61] If corporate bidders for

NHS work share the costs of this upgrading, job substitution may offer little scope for more profit. More likely, corporate providers will continue to recruit staff already trained by the NHS. Early moves toward local wage bargaining have tended to create more problems for management than they have solved. They have weakened national union negotiators, but encouraged the rebirth of the local militancy that transformed NHS unions in the 1970s from passive backwaters to militant flood tides. Corporate investors expecting easy profits from commercialised NHS services could soon be disappointed.

Leys' last point, shared risk between government and private investors, was already agreed in principle long ago, but never frankly admitted. For public discussion, the whole point of the Private Finance Initiative (PFI), Public–Private Partnerships (PPPs), and other government responsibilities sold or hired out to for-profit investors, was that these investors provided the money and took the risks, while taxpayers received the better service supposedly assured by an all-private rather than public enterprise. In practice, investors have taken the profits[62] and left taxpayers with most of the risks, locked into 30- to 40-year contracts protected indefinitely from detailed public scrutiny by commercial secrecy, and often barely comprehensible even to the lawyers who draft them.[63]

The PFI idea was first developed by John Major's Conservative government. Speaking in Parliament in 1996 as the Labour Party's shadow Minister for Health, Harriet Harman described it as privatisation: 'When the private sector is building, owning, managing and running a hospital it has been privatised.' Before they could get it off the ground, the Conservative government fell, whereupon New Labour adopted PFI (later renamed PPP – Public-Private Partnership) as 'the only show in town' – a way to fund NHS capital programmes without public borrowing, and opening new opportunities for profitable investment. It was therefore approved by the World Bank, International Monetary Fund, and World Trade Organisation, sufficient reason for this to become Labour policy even though not a single organisation within the party's membership or affiliated unions had ever suggested it, and most have opposed it ever since.

Costs to the NHS of PFI schemes were between 9.1% and 18% of initial construction costs, whereas government could, under traditional Treasury rules, borrow at interest rates of between 3.0% and 3.5%.[64] PFI hospitals have systematically reduced staff and beds below predicted requirements to ensure profitability.[65] Competition for patients as consumers between hospitals functioning as independent business units means winners and losers, but no essential public service can be allowed to fail, without endangering re-election of the government in power. A bankrupt hospital will be named, shamed and humiliated, but finally must somehow be saved, possibly with a new set of investors as owners, but always supplemented by whatever state funds are needed to keep it afloat. For NHS hospitals commercial risks stay with the public, just as they have for railways, the Channel Tunnel, weapons development and every other venture too big and of too much social importance to be allowed to fail.

Ever since Thatcher's launch of NHS marketisation in the 1980s, we have had varying sorts of quasi-market with quasi-competition, with rules set by government in collaboration with top multinational industrialists, bankers and the expert brains at their command. More and more people outside the NHS get richer, while NHS staff run ever faster to stave off bankruptcy of their competing units.

The pre-'reform' NHS economy

Medical care being in constant and universal demand, and commanding high prices from those able to pay, at zero price demand must reach infinity, and soon bankrupt the service. So claimed Ffrangcon Roberts[66] in 1952, on behalf of classical economic theory. He was echoed in cabinet first by Stafford Cripps, then by Hugh Gaitskell,[67] Attlee's chancellors of the exchequer. His view was reinforced by Conservative Minister for Health Enoch Powell,[68] and finally set in stone by Alan Williams as the foundation for his York school of health economics.[69]

Despite the apparently self-evident logic of theory, the hard fact remained that for more than three decades the NHS not only existed, but seemed to deliver a service comparable with or better than any other developed economy, at lower cost than most of them, and at less than half the per capita cost of care in the US, where the system was least socially inclusive and most exposed to market choice and competition. Evidently, classical economic theory did not explain or predict behaviour in the real world of health care.

Economists cannot point to a single real example of any nation that has depended entirely on a competitive market economy for health care of its entire population. Nor can they find a single example of demand for medical care actually approaching infinity. Putting oneself in the hands of doctors, entering the pipeline of any care system, is never a simple or easy decision, even if cash charges are eliminated. There were, and still are, all sorts of reasons why people who needed medical care in 1948 did not choose to receive it. Only one of these reasons changed in 1948, when doctors' fees were effectively abolished.[70] Of course, there was a huge rise in demand, because costs of care had deterred many people from seeking treatment, most notably working-class mothers who had borne and reared many children, and could only now afford to be ill or to contemplate surgery. For the first 20 years of the NHS, there were huge waiting lists for gynaecological repairs, cholecystectomies for gallstones, hernia repairs and cataract surgery. Millions of women who had previously consulted doctors only for their children (and even then, only for potential emergencies) began to consult for their own problems. There was a huge rise in demand, in GP workload and in hospital referrals,[71] resulting in long waiting lists for admission; but this was anticipated, calculable, and in the course of time it was coped with, despite always-inadequate funding and resources. Nowhere did demand approach infinity, whatever that means.[72]

Direct charges to patients (initially, token prescription charges) were first applied to the NHS in June 1952, not because demand was approaching infinity or NHS spending was out of control, but because the beginning of the Cold War in 1948 initiated an immensely expensive nuclear arms race unsustainable by the UK budget as a whole, for which the Labour government paid by retreating throughout its social programme. Nye Bevan resigned from government over this issue.[73] The rest of the cabinet, then as now, accepted press campaigns describing the NHS as a bottomless pit for the taxpayer, with direct charges the only way to restore sanity. This was typical of the defeatism that led to Labour's replacement by the first postwar Conservative government in 1951. Confident that its evidence would confirm these assumptions, the Conservative government set up a royal commission to study spending in the NHS.[74] This, the famous Guillebaud Report, found not only no wasteful spending, but that the NHS was underfunded for all its essential functions. As it was now hugely popular, Health Minister Ian Macleod recommended a large rise in NHS budget allocations; which, to be fair, Macmillan's Conservative government, still seeking consensus, eventually accepted.

From July 1948 to June 1952 there were no direct charges to patients of any kind – neither for GPs, nor specialists, nor dentists, nor opticians, nor for any prescribed medicines nor appliances.

How was this possible? First, of course, because demand was not infinite, but more or less reflected burdens of ill health and public expectations of what could be done to relieve it. Second, bulk central purchasing greatly reduced the cost of many NHS consumptions, most obviously of pharmaceutical products. The cost of drugs to the NHS was, and still is, much lower in Britain than in the US, for precisely this reason. A state monopoly made a lot of practical sense. Third, because the NHS was an internally cash-free, gift economy, it was spared huge bureaucratic burdens weighing on all commercial undertakings. For its first two decades, NHS administrative costs chugged along at about 2% of total costs, rising to around 6% in 1974 when the NHS underwent its first transition to tighter management. There it stayed until 1983, when Conservative government began to push market competition into the NHS internal economy. Administration costs gradually rose to around 12%, where they remain today. Each step further into the market has raised administrative costs and increased bureaucracy; repeated Conservative calls for money to be spent on care rather than paper have been purest humbug. How does this compare with the US, where managed care has had a free hand to demonstrate the natural superiority claimed by its advocates? In the US, average administration costs for health care run at an average 20% overall on lowest estimates, with most estimates over 30%. US for-profit hospitals spend 23% more on administration than comparable US not-for-profit hospitals, and 34% more than hospitals run by state or Federal government, but still the for-profit market share continues to expand at the expense of traditional service.[75] Administration costs in France and Germany both lie above 20% of total spending, though their insurance-based systems have repeatedly been proclaimed as the only conceivable alternative to Americanisation for NHS 'reform'.

The higher costs of care organised as business rather than public service have three main causes. First, when the incentive to work is to maximise personal earnings, and when the incentive to manage or invest is to maximise corporate profit, administrative controls are necessary to at least try to contain biased or perverse decisions and fraud. Trust cuts costs, commerce promotes mistrust. Second, when care becomes a bought and sold commodity, it must be fragmented into precisely costed units; such costing is a major continuing overhead expense. Finally, profit has to come from somewhere, to satisfy shareholders, retain their investments and evade takeover by other corporations promising higher profit. Though for-profit care tends to reduce labour costs, mainly by employing fewer and less skilled staff either casually or on short contracts, this cannot reduce costs overall while maintaining high rates of profit.

Experience of cash-free economy

By the 1970s, the NHS had developed a largely cash-free internal economy, in which staff time became the effective currency. Within always-inadequate global budgets, different hospital departments got for themselves as much as they could justify to managements operating by consensus, relying partly on professional prestige (heavily weighted in favour of surgeons and physicians, and against geriatricians and psychiatrists) and partly on advancing scientific evidence (the main weapon for new or neglected specialties). Senior consultants were inside these deals, everyone else – nurses, other hospital staff, GPs, and above all patients and catchment populations, were kept outside. However, this semi-feudal culture contained within itself an embryonic economy geared to human needs rather than profit, always seeking expression, and continually reinforced by the generally humane and socially intelligent orientation of advances in knowledge.

In the early 1980s, I became interested in how this theoretically 'impossible' economy actually worked. I hoped to use my own primary care unit in Glyncorrwg, and its relations with specialist facilities at local hospitals, as material for a pilot case study. We already had a huge amount of recorded data from 1965 onwards on patient consultation rates,[76] referral rates, prescribing rates and prescribing costs in relation both to other South Wales practices and to practices throughout the UK, certification rates, accident and injury rates, and social data about our accurately defined local population, including updated occupations and rates for unemployment (actual worklessness, not claims for benefit). Ours was then probably the best-documented practice in Britain, from our own studies, from participation in nationwide surveys, and from small projects by visiting students.[77] I was naively optimistic that when our local consultants and hospital administrators knew what we needed data for, they would allow us access to my patients' hospital records. So to develop at least an elementary economic theory from concrete reality rather than abstract surmise, we seemed to have all we needed, except for a properly trained economist.

I knew personally two of the biggest names in UK health economics. One was not interested. The other came down to the practice, looked and listened around, but again – nothing doing. It seemed that I would have to embark on what we then called the Unit Costs Project on my own, without expert help. The project seemed simple. Our clinical decisions at Glyncorrwg Health Centre could easily be related to a defined population of users, a limited range of diagnostic and treatment interventions, and a small number of secondary and tertiary (super-specialist) referral units. We would identify costs for each decision, and see how clinical behaviour translated into economic quantities.

In fact, it proved extremely complex. The senior consultant at our main referral hospital refused me access to any of my patients' hospital records, which immediately shrank the scope of any study (he seems to have feared evidence of possible malpractice, and consequent litigation). To my surprise, nobody in our local X-ray departments or pathology laboratories knew the cost of anything they did. Unit directors of radiography and pathology knew about their global budgets, and necessarily worked within them, but costs per item of service varied enormously according to throughput and how close to maximum capacity staff and machines were working, needing reserve capacity for workload varying between wide limits from time to time. They were concerned to balance their books – not to spend more than they got from hospital administration – but they had no interest in making a profit, only in providing a service. As both departments had hugely improved their service to GP users over the previous 20 years, motivation was evidently good, but was not prompted by hopes of profit.

'But', I explained, 'I need to know unit costs, for example the consequences of ordering a chest X-ray or full blood count; can't you give me an estimate?' No, they could not give a meaningful answer, because in their terms, this was not a meaningful question. They suggested that I ask BUPA (Britain's then largest provider of private care). BUPA charged its patients, so it must have price lists. So I did, and BUPA, who were very helpful, sent full price lists straight away. Where did their prices come from? Were they based on costs of production, plus a bit for administration and a reasonable profit? No, they said, they had no way of calculating costs of production. They just looked at equivalent price lists in the US, where everything had a price. But as soon as they saw US prices, they knew there was no way even private patients in Britain could afford them. So they reduced them by about two-thirds, and these were the prices they now used and prospered on.

My project stopped at that point, and hardly any of this work was ever published. Still, I had made what seemed an important discovery. If you were not trading, no prices were necessary. If you insisted on trading, you could charge whatever the market would stand – which in competition with a free public service, was a lot less than in the US. Accurate competitive pricing had a high administrative cost, which if you were not competing, you had no need to incur.

In 1983 Margaret Thatcher redeployed Sir Roy Griffiths from commanding supermarkets to reviewing management of the entire NHS workforce.[78] After visiting hospitals all over the UK, he concluded that had Florence Nightingale still been carrying her lamp through the corridors in 1983, she would probably have been trying to find out who was in charge. Management decisions were taken by consensus, and therefore often not taken at all; clinicians ruled themselves. Units of service in health care were not traded, so nobody knew the price of anything except labour. At the top of the hierarchy, private practice plus merit awards plus high salaries sustained earnings resembling minor royalty. At the bottom, the national Whitley Council tied hospital porters' earnings to those of unskilled workers in local government waste disposal – barely a living wage. In return for abysmal earnings, lower NHS staff had job security, and the social status accorded to anyone working in the NHS by a public appreciative of its gift economy. Since 1948, the aim of NHS management had been to sustain agreement between all levels of staff that their traditional rankings be maintained, only allowing such progress as suited senior consultants. Until the industrial disputes of the early 1970s, the NHS sustained traditions of deference reaching back to the 18th century.

Coming from senior business management, Sir Roy Griffiths saw only anachronism. Rightly, he recognised the NHS as a productive system: not a religious institution for hoping, imagining or pretending, but a production system with measurable inputs, outputs and efficiency. He assumed that its products resembled market commodities sufficiently, that hospitals could be made to combine the functions of a factory and a hypermarket, taking referred trade from primary care organised as a chain of small shops handling initial consumer inputs through an NHS franchise.

Griffiths said the similarities between NHS and industrial management were much greater than the differences. Though profit motives did not operate in the NHS, and – for the time being at least – were unwanted, with more aggressive management the NHS could, he thought, be made businesslike yet still be something beyond a business. Inevitably, as in private industry, effective management would be management of conflict; consensus management was a contradiction in terms.[79] This idea appealed to many previously staunch opponents of for-profit care. Having long experience of resistance by their own profession to any progress in social organisation of care, liberal medical intellectuals were not averse to some tough management of their conservative colleagues. They knew the territory better than Margaret Thatcher, and by participating in her programme of counter-reform, they hoped to rationalise care, making it more effective and efficient, while kidding themselves that she would not subordinate medical gentlemen to vulgar commerce. Using sophisticated variants of this theme, many of the intellectual army defending the NHS from 1948 to 1979 reshaped their ideas over the next 20 years, leaving their more steadfast colleagues marginalised and close to despair. A key event in this process of reorientation was their discovery after the New Labour landslide victory in 1997 that, far from reversing commercialisation of the NHS, Prime Minister Blair would soon accelerate it.

A return to progress

This general sense of professional powerlessness was never justified. We are many, they are few. A large majority of opinion, among both health professionals and the people, still longs for a return to a socially inclusive service for citizens rather than customers, based on principles of solidarity and shared risk. We should be looking forward to the better world that growing knowledge makes possible. The NHS should again become a practical expression of a continued and growing popular consensus, that our entire society shares responsibility for misfortunes that could strike anyone at any time, and the cost of doing so should be borne by all, according to the ability of each to pay. The NHS is a necessary institution that we should all pay for throughout our lives, which all of us hope to use as little as possible. If we do not have to use what we have paid for, we have wasted nothing, but can count ourselves lucky. This is the exact opposite of the acquisitive society perpetually thrust upon us as our only possible future. We already know that as soon as anticipated profit affects either decisions about investment in health care, or clinical decisions about personal illness, trust between caring professionals and patients becomes questionable. Whether doctors function as personal salesmen, as they did before the NHS, or as providers in health care hypermarkets, these transactional concepts of health care shrink the NHS to a small and distorted fragment of its real potential, valuing chiefly those elements of body maintenance and repair that seem suited to trade in human engineering, relegating necessary but unprofitable care to minimal public service, and ignoring public health issues altogether.

To get this noble show back on the road, the whole range of health workers, and all the patients, informal carers and potential patients they serve (which means everyone) need to regain, or for the first time acquire, confidence in themselves – in their own ability to understand what the NHS was, is, and could become, and how it relates to the rest of our rapidly changing society. We have to stop waiting for somebody else, with more expertise or more power, to do this for us, because no such leaders will ever arrive. Such confidence depends on having a clear framework within which all of us can fit our own experience, so that reality becomes a source of understanding rather than confusion. The following chapters try to provide this.

Notes

[1] Pre-'reform' health service expenditures 1980-92 in OECD countries as % of GDP:

	1980	*1985*	*1990*	*1992*
US	9.3	10.5	12.3	13.5
Japan	6.7	6.5	6.9	7.1
Germany	8.7	8.5	8.6	9.1
France	7.7	8.2	8.9	9.2
Italy	7.1	6.9	8.2	8.4
UK	**5.9**	**5.8**	**6.3**	**6.7**
Canada	7.4	8.4	9.3	9.9
Australia	7.8	8.3	8.2	8.4
Austria	8.2	8.0	8.6	8.9
Belgium	6.7	7.1	7.7	7.9
Denmark	6.8	6.4	6.2	6.4
Finland	6.7	7.4	8.4	8.5
Greece	4.4	4.9	5.3	5.5
Ireland	9.3	7.9	7.0	7.1
Netherlands	8.1	7.7	8.3	8.7
Norway	6.6	6.6	7.3	7.9
Portugal	6.2	6.6	6.6	6.5
Spain	5.8	5.5	6.9	7.1

	1980	1985	1990	1992
Sweden	9.6	9.1	9.1	8.6
All EEC	7.0	6.9	7.3	7.5
All OECD	7.3	7.4	7.9	8.2
(OECD, 1994)				

The insurance-based care system in France is in many ways a unique case, of exceptional importance because of the vigorous resistance mounted by both medical professionals, trade unions and community organisations to 'reform' on the neoliberal model during the past year, culminating in the rejection of the new EU constitution. This has been excellently explained for English readers by Paul Clay Sorum (2005). Together with rejection of the new EU constitution in the Netherlands and the rise of the Linkspartei in the recent German election, there now seems to be mounting resistance throughout at least Western Europe to the global tide of neoliberalism, and to Tony Blair as its European prophet.

[2] A recent UK public opinion poll showed 89% opposed to commercial provision of health care (Lister, 2005).

[3] In 1971 the Wanless Report, commissioned by government and chaired by a banker, estimated a £267 billion shortfall in NHS investment compared with average EU investment over the previous 26 years (*Lancet* 2001, vol 358, p 1971).

[4] Independence from central control of Trusts, Foundation Hospitals, and other units of the 'reformed' NHS entails abandoning all central planning, and total dependence on competing providers in the market, finally made clear by a statement from Sir Nigel Crisp, NHS chief executive, in January 2005. This could be reversed only by a fundamental change in government policy, restoring the NHS as an independent economy based on cooperation rather than competition. New Labour government claims that its policy transfers power to the people, but this power resembles the power of customers over supermarkets, compelled to choose between competing providers because neither public service nor corner shops in the community are available. A Nuffield Trust study of how policy decisions in English NHS Hospital Foundation Trusts and Primary Care Trusts are taken in practice by executive managers concluded that local accountability existed in name only. Elections to Trust boards of governors were based on so few electors that

they would be considered disgraceful if they occurred in local government (Nuffield Trust, 2005).

[5] Tony Blair's credibility to the electorate, and therefore to his political colleagues whose careers depend on re-election, is now falling. Gordon Brown, his heir-apparent, is no less committed than Blair to making a success of capitalism, to rubbishing any prospect of a socialist alternative, and to subordinating UK policy to whatever any US president requires, but there is one significant difference between them. Brown was born into and emerged from the Labour movement, and is the natural heir to the perpetually delayed and disappointed hopes of its social base. His reconciliation in maturity with established wealth and power follows the traditional career pattern of social democrats, to which voters are accustomed. Blair, on the other hand, was born into the Norman Tebbitt (Right populist) subset of the Conservative Party tradition, has seldom even pretended to respect the Labour tradition on which he chose to build his career (with Thatcher approaching eclipse, Labour was becoming the only credible vehicle for him), and has repeatedly insulted his traditional voters and activists to reassure his preferred conservative audience. Brown has more room for manoeuvre, and could move back to Keynesian policies without loss of face if majority public and Labour Party opinion were to close other options. As the full consequences of oil imperialism and sale of state assets become obvious, this becomes a possibility.

[6] Pollock (2004) gives a full and excellent account of this process from its beginning to the more or less completed plan embodied in current New Labour policies for 'patient choice'. Though the plan may be complete, its imposition on the NHS workforce and communities they serve is not.

[7] McKee (2004). Experience of league tables for state schools, another favoured theme for both Conservatives and New Labour, confirms fears that competing hospital Trusts are likely to concentrate on measured targets rather than improved patient care. A study of random samples of English and Scottish primary schools, with and without league tables respectively, showed that English schools were more likely to concentrate on meeting targets at the expense of other objectives, had narrower curricula, concentrated more resources on 'borderline' achievers, and reported more 'blame

culture'. Differences were large and statistically significant (Tymms and Wiggins, 2000).

[8] Kassem, 2004. The New Labour government has imposed this regulation on all referrals in England, both from primary care to specialists, and from one specialty to another. Though it created Foundation Hospital Trusts to promote competition between NHS hospitals, the 15% guarantee to private sector providers tilts the market deliberately away from NHS provision and further threatens the solvency of its hospitals, of which one in three is now in substantial deficit. This policy has not been applied by Wales Labour in the Welsh Assembly or by the Labour–Liberal Democrat coalition in the Scottish Parliament, reflecting the general hostility to privatisation throughout the Labour Party membership. When Primary Care Trusts in South Oxfordshire, Southampton and Greater Manchester all failed to place any contracts with private sector providers of some specialties, because there were no waiting lists for them and therefore no demand, they were ordered to do so by the government minister. When private sector providers in Trent and South Yorkshire complained that they were getting too few NHS referrals, their Primary Care Trusts were ordered to pay for advisers to go round convincing GPs to make more private sector referrals. Nigel Crisp, current chief executive of the NHS, has said that Foundation Hospital Trusts 'should adopt the same marketing techniques as Tesco in their bids to win customers in the new choice-based NHS market' (Davis, 2005). According to his recent directive to NHS staff, 'the direction of travel is clear: Primary Care Trusts will become patient-led or "patient- and commissioning-led" organisations with their role in provision reduced to a minimum. We would expect all changes to be completed by the end of 2008' (internal NHS memo dated 28 July 2005, gateway reference 5312). In the same week the consumer organisation Which? reported results of a public opinion survey showing that 89% of people thought having a good local hospital was more important than choice of hospitals, and 85% thought having a good local GP was more important than choosing from GPs elsewhere.

[9] Of 254 current government IT development projects reviewed recently by the House of Commons Public Accounts Committee, over one third (70) seemed headed for failure. No details of its reports are available because the Office of Government Commerce says they are constrained by commercial secrecy (Mathieson, 2005).

In England, a new NHS IT clinical software system is being developed by British Telecom and IDX, a large US company experienced in hospital management systems. It aims to develop online records for 50 million citizens, with connections between all NHS doctors and hospitals by 2010, described by the US health technology advocacy group eHealth Initiative as 'the largest scale initiative under way in any country worldwide'. Development costs were first estimated at £6.2 billion, but estimates now vary from £18 billion to £31 billion (Bristol, 2005) and people involved in the programme are talking about £60 billion. It has been described by a UK GP experienced in software development as 'a third rate computer program lifted from the existing system of US hospital administrators' (deKare-Silver, 2005). 'Choose and book' is supposed to be applied universally in England by 31 December 2005. In theory, all patients will, at the point of referral, be given options of time, place and date. The referral can either be booked there and then, or the patient will be given a reference number and phone numbers to confirm an appointment later. GPs are promised this will take them 20-30 seconds, but at a demonstration session in summer 2004 three experienced GP trainers struggled with it for half an hour. The new system is not integrated with any of the existing GP systems now used in well over 90% of all UK practices, or with Microsoft Outlook. It is intended also to be used to obtain specialist advice without formal referral, but this informal advice once received cannot be filed in patients' records, and will be automatically deleted. The whole enterprise reeks of indifference to the experience and opinions of staff actually responsible for patient care.

Scotland and Wales lie outside this development, with their own plans for electronic patient records, integrated vertically through all levels of the NHS, and horizontally with other public service social agencies. The Welsh Assembly plans for IT development were published in June 2005 in *Informing Healthcare: the National Case*. Though these appear to be free from English assumptions that IT must serve a competitive market with a large for-profit sector, it recognises that any Welsh system must function across a long border with England where citizens on both sides use each others' NHS systems, and it also hopes to contain development costs by using the English system where possible. NHS 'reforms' have entailed a relative reduction in NHS funding for Wales compared with England, possibly because so much of new funding now goes to promote competition and private sector contracts, which the Welsh Assembly has rejected. For the financial year 2005/06 NHS funding for Wales rose 5.5%, compared with 9.3% for England. For health care Wales is often compared with the North-East of England, with similar populations and levels of income. Based on planned spending for 2004/05, North-Eastern England will get 5% more NHS per capita funding than Wales, and by 2007/08 present trends would bring its per capita NHS funding at least 20% ahead of Wales (*Western Mail*, 2 July 2005). These economic constraints make it extremely difficult for Wales to pursue the independent policies for the NHS that its voters obviously want, and to which all opposition parties except the Conservatives claim loyalty.

[10] Quality of primary care records is a good indicator of maturity in the system as a whole. Slowly and erratically, handwritten GP records worth reading began to appear in a few UK practices in the 1960s, became commonplace in the 1970s, and became almost universal by the 1980s. Today well over 90% of all NHS GPs use electronic computer-held records for at least some aspects of patient care, including entire registered populations, and since 2004 GPs' contracts have been virtually unworkable without them.

[11] In 2004, only 15% of respondents to a MORI poll wanted to choose referrals themselves, 62% wanted to choose together with their health care professionals, and 23% still wanted to leave such decisions entirely to professionals (Page, 2004a). Though patients are now encouraged to scan league tables for performance of competing hospitals, notably by that custodian of liberal enlightenment the *Guardian*, researchers have found no correlation between measures of consumer satisfaction with different hospitals and their standardised mortality ratios (Page, 2004b).

[12] Wintour, 2004.

[13] Before the 1980s, NHS GPs could, and did, refer patients occasionally to very distant consultants, if an exceptional problem required this. Unnoticed by politicians or the media, this choice was abolished at precisely the time when the NHS began to be reorganised on market lines.

[14] Godfrey, 2005. Discussing choice of referral with a patient takes time, a scarce resource for all clinicians. Faced with pressure to tick the right boxes to please administration, their obvious tactic will be

first to identify that minority of patients who actually want to discuss five choices (at least one of them private) but they will refer the rest through their customary preferred pathways according to their own experience and clinical judgement, which is still what a large majority of patients wants. If that does not produce the 15% proportion of private referrals that the New Labour government wants, clinicians may learn to raise a collective two fingers, and continue to exert their own best judgement. This would probably be supported by most patients, most voters and most members of the Labour Party, few of whom are yet aware of what is being imposed on the NHS in their name. The key is collective action, with media publicity. This obvious weapon has not yet been used, but it probably will be.

[15] Carvel, 2003.

[16] Branigan and Glover, 2005.

[17] Frankel et al, 2000.

[18] The Department of Health has now set up an NHS Marketing Intelligence Unit to teach NHS Trusts how to promote their reputations and compete with each other successfully for patients. This will be led by Stephen O'Brien, former marketing director of Kingfisher, an international home-improvement retail company (*Health Services Journal*, 24 February 2005, p 5).

[19] Nick Bosanquet and Stephen Pollard (1997, pp 98-103), speak frankly to their intended audience of policy formers about how to get the public to accept piecemeal destruction of the NHS, giving a recipe apparently followed by both Conservative and New Labour governments ever since. They undertook their own survey of public opinion, from which they drew the following conclusions:

> The most striking general finding … is the gap between expectations and wants. Broadly, the public wants the NHS to offer everything, and to offer it free; 65% say, for instance, that NHS services should always be free. But, crucially, a mere 13% expect that they *will* be free in ten years' time. Some 67% think that the NHS will provide fewer services and those no longer covered will only be available privately, even though 80% do not like such a

prospect. It is on this expectations gap that modernisers should focus. With expectations so clearly dampened, the battle is already half won ... ideas for reform based on a wholesale switch to non-state insurance schemes are politically fanciful. Even when presented with today's reality of often long waits for non-emergency treatments ... 74% still cling to the NHS rather than paying for private speed. The message is clear. Modernisers need to approach the task of reform not through grand plans involving large lump sum payments or a sudden and widespread switch to private provision, but through sums of money that are easy to contemplate, and that chime with other services.... This survey simply shows what the public will stomach today. It is now up to the politicians and opinion formers to move the argument on.

Politicians and opinion formers have done just that, and it's always the same argument: away from solidarity with its roots in the past, forwards to the future of consumerism, universal competition, and the war of every man against every man.

[20] Succinctly summarised as: '... largely a matter of poor people in rich countries giving money to rich people in poor countries' (Caulfield, 1996). The story has been brought up to the end of the Wolfensohn era by Sebastian Mellanby (2005).

[21] We were warned of this six years ago, but few listened and even fewer really believed this could be happening:

> ... governments are deregulating and privatising public-service funding and delivery ... through policy initiatives such as New Public Management, contracting out of services, compulsory competitive tendering (best value), and public infrastructure privatisation through public-private partnerships known variously as the Private Finance Initiative (PFI), build-own transfer (BOT, or build, own, operate and transfer (BOOT). These policies are generally presented as technical, and therefore neutral, adjustments. [They are] linked to the global trade expansion policies of international institutions, such as the WTO, the International Monetary Fund, and the

World Bank.... WTO talks in Seattle [focused] on revision of the General Agreement on Trade in Services (GATS), a system of international law intended to expand private-enterprise involvement in the increasingly important service sector. GATS includes health care, social services, education, houses and all other services run by government agencies, including telecoms, transport, distribution, postal, insurance, environment, tourism, entertainment, and leisure services. According to the European Commission, services account for two thirds of the EU economy and jobs, almost a quarter of EU total exports, and half of all EU investment abroad. In the US, more than one third of economic growth in the past five years was in service exports. (Price et al, 1999)

[22] In 1948 when the NHS began, care was deeply divided in three wholly uncoordinated parts – the NHS proper (hospitals and GPs), public health as an impersonal sanitary function of local government, and some personal care functions (mainly maternity and child welfare, case-finding and follow-up of tuberculosis and venereal disease, and school medical services) also provided by local government. The NHS began not as a health service, but as a health care service, its activities overwhelmingly determined by illness and consequent demand, rather than by health needs. This essentially irrational division reflected the then much greater power of local government in the Labour Party, which had expected to run the NHS as a whole, for whom loss of public health functions would certainly have been a step too far in 1948. It also reflected weaknesses in GPs, who were generally incapable of either performing these functions themselves, or employing staff to provide them on their behalf. More fundamentally, it reflected the consensus view of virtually all public opinion, which equated health care with treatment of disease. Retrospective critics of this decision should consider the scant support given to Welsh Assembly Minister Jane Hutt when she tried to give priority to coordinated plans for health gain through action on all fronts, rather than to waiting lists for elective surgery. Scarcely a voice was raised in her support. We have to start from where people *think* they are. Leadership concerns not our points of departure, over which we have little choice, but lasting commitment to a more intelligent destination. Within contemporary

consensus views, the NHS in 1948 was a unified service, and became the largest single employer anywhere in Europe.

[23] This also was not wholly true. At the insistence of his Cabinet colleagues, Bevan was compelled to include a small contributory element from National Insurance, as a concession to the Cabinet's conventional view that everything must have a price. Bevan greatly resented this as an unnecessary complication of what was otherwise an extremely simple, and therefore economical, way to fund the service. National Insurance contributions were a considerable personal burden, and a large majority of contributors imagined that most of this was spent on the NHS, though in fact almost all of it went to sickness and unemployment benefits. The NHS remained accessible to everyone, whether or not they contributed to National Insurance.

[24] Hart, 1995a.

[25] In the 1980s, when ideological battles raged to establish the first footholds for business ethics in the NHS, a favourite subtitle for conferences was 'Thinking the unthinkable'. With pride in their own readiness to abandon every achievement of solidarity in the past, we heard a growing parade of managerial and academic careerists proclaim their discovery of the bright side of Thatcherism. This process still continues under the banner of 'reform'.

[26] Saltman (2003) and de Vos et al (2004). There have been examples of successful mass resistance, first in Spain, then in France, the Netherlands and Germany, where threats to their insurance-based services have led to unexpected setbacks for governments trying to implement neoliberal 'reforms', but so far these have lacked any clear picture of their alternative policies.

[27] Marketing of care cannot be dismissed a priori. When, despite its third-world mortality statistics in Harlem, New York was found to have more doctors than its medical market could support, this 'doctor surplus' was solved by paying hospitals not to train doctors. In 1997 hospitals began reducing junior staff by 20-25% over the following six years, and were paid $400m (£250m) for not training this proportion. Savings were redeployed to employ more lower-level staff. Commenting on this, Dr Alan Hillman, professor of health policy at the University of Pennsylvania, said: 'It's amazing to treat

health care like a commodity like grain or milk or meat.... But I really can't find any fault with it. Maybe it is one of the first rational collaborations between hospitals and the government' (J. Roberts, 1997). If and when any medical marketplace succeeds in delivering care to any whole, unselected population appropriately to both collective and individual needs at affordable cost, Dr Hillman and many others similarly inclined may have a case.

[28] Friedman and Friedman, 1962, p 133.

[29] The fascinating story of how Hayek and Friedman first organised resistance following the worldwide defeat of their ideas in 1945, and then re-established 19th-century classical economics as orthodoxy, has been splendidly told by John Kenneth Galbraith (1987).

[30] According to Galbraith, Hitler's economists never developed even the concept of GNP, let alone the data collection and regulatory system required to apply it in practice. Unrestricted power for big business can be self-destructive.

[31] Throughout the 1930s, first Stanley Baldwin, then Neville Chamberlain led a Conservative Party sympathetic to fascism in Italy and Spain, and tolerant of it in Germany, albeit with some apprehension, as a useful opponent of communism. The composition of parliament supporting Churchill's coalition government from June 1940 to June 1945 was determined by the election of 1935, when the policies of appeasement of fascism were reaching take-off speed.

[32] In the later years of Franklin Roosevelt's New Deal, medical cooperatives were developed throughout the rural areas of the US, from 1936 to 1945. In 1938 the *Saturday Evening Post* described the Federal Security Administration (FSA) scheme as a 'gigantic rehearsal for health insurance. It has brought together some 3,000 doctors and more than 100,000 families in twenty-odd states. It has given them a chance to show what would happen if a health insurance law were enacted for them tomorrow.' At its peak in 1942, the FSA had about 650,000 farming people covered by comprehensive health care in 1,200 plans in 42 states, with group prepayments organised jointly between farmers' associations and physicians' county or state associations. Group prepayment had been

proposed by the LaFollette Congressional Committee on Costs of Medical Care, founded in 1927 and reporting in 1932 in *Medical care for the American people: The final report of the committee on costs of medical care*. This noted that medical resources were not 'distributed according to needs, but rather according to real or supposed ability of patients to pay for services'. The American Medical Association described the report as an 'incitement to revolution'. In 1945 the FSA would have been extended to a national health insurance plan similar to those in other developed economies, through the Wagner–Murray–Dingell Bill, supported by President Truman, but in 1946 Congress ended all New Deal legislation supporting the programme. Drs Fred Mott and Milton Roemer, who had headed the FSA programme, moved to Canada to develop the comprehensive health insurance programme in Saskatchewan, which eventually provided the single-payer model for all Canadian health care (Grey, 1999). By the time of the Clinton administration, all that remained of Roosevelt's New Deal was the Social Security Act of 1935. Clinton started the process of eliminating dignified welfare rights for the poor, and George W. Bush is completing it. Tony Blair adopted the same strategy for New Labour, aiming to make the Labour Party a party preferred by big business, with a citizenry no longer committed to solidarity or collective action of any kind.

[33] Britain had its own experiment in Nazi occupation, still largely ignored. When Germany occupied the Channel Islands in 1940, they took over a uniquely conservative, almost feudal area of Britain. The ruling class in the Channel Islands collaborated no less abjectly than the Vichy government in France, including the rounding up and deportation of Jews to the gas chambers. There was active internal resistance, but as in the rest of Europe, it was mostly led by communists. This important and complex story has been told by Madeleine Bunting (1995) with fairness to all sides. It was on a scale small enough to be entirely suppressed by the government in 1945, on the grounds that the truth would damage public morale. The collaborators were honoured with knighthoods and OBEs; the resisters were ignored.

[34] Few people today recall that the allied landing force on D-day 1944 faced only one-sixth of German manpower, together with its allies. From 1941 to 1945, the greatest impact of the war and Nazi occupation fell on the USSR, which made the greatest contribution to victory in human terms. The Soviet economy seemed to have

passed this sternest possible test with flying colours. This, and the extent to which UK and US economies had been compelled to adopt similarly successful policies of state planning, underlay both the popularity of communist ideas throughout liberated Europe in 1945, and the defensive alarm of postwar welfare states in the West.

[35] Kotz and Weir, 1997.

[36] Who famously explained to a BBC interviewer in 1976 that you can't spend your way out of a recession.

[37] R. Smith, 1996. In 2004 Richard Smith embraced precisely the process he here describes, resigning as *BMJ* editor to become chief executive of United Health Europe, European arm of United Health Group, the largest US health care corporation. Under the name Evercare this is now contending for a large share of NHS business, and has been running nine pilot projects in UK primary care since 2003. By contrast, Canada has so far resisted all attempts by US companies to penetrate its health care services (Deber, 2003). Perhaps Canadian politicians and their electorates, closer to the US, are more aware of the risks to their institutions.

[38] OECD, 2003.

[39] The first British Minister for Health to use his full power as a monopoly negotiator was Enoch Powell, whose no-nonsense approach flabbergasted a pharmaceutical industry that had paid the Conservative Party well to serve its interest. Runner-up was Kenneth Clarke, again a Conservative minister, but apparently less frightened of squeezing his fellow capitalists than Labour ministers. George W. Bush, on the other hand, has shown more gratitude, albeit for a much larger reward. His Medicare Reform Bill, recently passed by Congress, includes a provision prohibiting negotiation by Federal government of lower costs for prescribed medication. This clause was prepared by Congressman Billy Tanzin, who has now retired to take up his new post as president of the Pharmaceutical Research & Manufacturers of America, the industry's main lobbying organisation (Dyer, 2005). The main immediate reason why the US pays twice as much per capita for health care as Europeans, and still has no universal coverage, is that all its prices are higher, because they have to include a margin for profit, and because purchasers negotiate in a divided market (Anderson et al, 2003).

[40] Glasser, 1998.

[41] Since 1999, HMOs have dropped more than 1.6 million Medicare beneficiaries, so that only 14% of a total 40 million Medicare beneficiaries are now in HMOs (Charatan, 2001b).

[42] In the 20 years since 1979, when Margaret Thatcher came to power, over 100,000 long-term care beds were lost from the NHS to the private sector; the latter rose from 18% share in 1979 to 70% by 1998. The Department of Health now keeps no record of long-term care beds available in either the NHS or the private sector, having abandoned all strategic planning in this field. Profits came from reductions in costs of staffing, by reducing skills and raising workload. Average annual wages for NHS community and mental health staff in 1999 were £20,000 and £21,000 respectively, but in private long-term care average annual staff wages were less than £8,000 a year. In 1997 the top ten long-term care companies had operating profits at 28% of gross income (Gaffney, Pollock, Price, and Shaoul, 1999a).

[43] In 1990 a 55-year-old man was admitted to a Leeds NHS hospital with a severe stroke, leaving him incontinent of urine and faeces, unable to communicate, walk, or feed himself. The hospital discharged him to a private nursing home in 1991, on the grounds that it had done all that was possible to cure him, and had no continuing obligation to care for him. Like most other health authorities, Leeds no longer had any long-stay beds, nor had it any contract with private nursing homes to provide them. The man's family had to meet the difference between Social Security benefits and the cost of the private nursing home, which came to £6,000 a year. The case went to the NHS ombudsman, who ruled the Leeds Health Authority's decision illegal, but the law was soon changed accordingly (Brindle, 1994). When Labour was in opposition and its MPs imagined their leaders would behave differently, Conservative junior Health Minister John Bowis was asked whether the NHS would now have responsibility for the hypothetical case of a patient on a drip, doubly incontinent, and confined to bed 24 hours a day. He refused to answer (House of Commons Health Committee, 1995). So much for care from the cradle to the grave.

[44] Kerrison and Pollock, 2001.

[45] Despite this unbalanced media discussion, continuing primary care of chronic conditions has had a high priority in the new NHS contract for GPs, with high demands for data recording and high rewards for performance. A recent report from an East London centre serving a population around 10,000 showed staff were recording 158 items of data relating to ten categories of chronic disorder (coronary heart disease, stroke, hypertension, diabetes, chronic obstructive pulmonary disease, epilepsy, thyroid function, cancer, psychotic mental illness and asthma) and 65 achievement targets. These are now a major determinant of practice income.

[46] Leys, 2001a, p 84.

[47] 'Elective' in this context is standard medical jargon for planned and anticipated procedures, as opposed to unexpected, emergency procedures.

[48] As New Labour Health Minister, both Alan Milburn and John Reid promised that NHS staff would never be either recruited or compulsorily transferred to private sector providers. Like all other promises required to secure acceptance of the privatisation programme from Labour MPs, these were broken by the next Health Minister, Patricia Hewitt, when she embarked on the government's procurement programme, described in the quotation at the opening of this book, though she recently retreated from this.

[49] Dash, 2004.

[50] Though this was common knowledge, it was always denied by the BMA, hiding behind the roughly 50% of consultants who always worked full time, and the substantial minority even of part-time consultants who did not take advantage of their conflict of interest (in control of waiting lists, on whose length their private trade depended). The case against this was overwhelming, damningly made by John Yates (1995), but his data refer to the private trade of consultants, not the collective contracts of the new corporate private sector that New Labour now promotes. Media comment rarely makes this important distinction. Newly discovered indignation at the greed of consultants now serves as a generally effective screen for collusion with health care companies to take over potentially profitable NHS functions not marginally, but in entire units.

[51] Rayner, 1997.

[52] Hensher and Edwards, 1999. In 1991 the British Ministry of Health stopped recording hospital resources centrally, making accurate assessment of productivity difficult (Torgerson and Raftery, 1999). Presumably by then policy makers were so sure that market competition always raised productivity that they no longer needed evidence.

[53] Pollock and Whitty, 1990.

[54] www.unison.org.uk/news, reported in *Bevan Foundation News* summer 2005. This sits badly with the Conservative Party's election campaign on MRSA infection as evidence of inefficiency inherent in public service. Both the government and the Conservative Party deny any causal connection between out-sourcing and infection rates, claiming that there is no significant difference between hospitals where cleaning has been out-sourced, and those where it remains in house. This ignores both a 50% reduction in the total cleaning workforce, and the fact that competitive tendering, without tight regulation for quality, has intensified and degraded this work for all cleaners. The correct comparison is between then, when cleaners were part of the NHS workforce and working for patients, and now, when they have become sources of profit.

[55] Caines, 1993.

[56] Devereux et al, 2002. Unfortunately survival was not a measured output in the earlier studies on which assessments of productivity were based. Their priced lists of defined products not only excluded survival, but also diagnostic services, teaching and research (Appleby, 1996).

[57] The Welsh Assembly has used its still meagre powers devolved since 1997 to create what Rhodri Morgan, leader of Wales Labour in the Welsh Assembly government, has called 'clear red water' between NHS Wales and Westminster. The PFI, internal competition, Foundation Hospitals, preferential private sector referral, and almost exclusive emphasis on episodic body repairs as measures of output have all been rejected in Wales, and all prescription charges are planned eventually to be eliminated. There has been relatively greater investment in primary care, and a real effort to develop a

public health approach across customary boundaries between health care and other social agencies, including free swimming for children and pensioners, and free breakfasts for primary school children in the poorest areas. One result of this emphasis on prevention and primary care has been longer waits in Wales for planned surgery, for which in England everything else seems to have been sacrificed. NHS policy in Scotland seems dangerously close to handing all power back to the medical profession, particularly to its ancient stronghold in Edinburgh, but as in Wales, private sector expansion has so far been resisted, and there is a similar emphasis on expanding primary care, shifting much monitoring of chronic disorders away from hospitals and, unlike Wales, promoting the Glyncorrwg model (Scottish Executive, 2005). Northern Ireland, though potentially independent after a good start with its first Sinn Fein Minister, is now too paralysed by sectarian conflict to develop any independent policy.

[58] In both the UK and the US, patterns of managerial income in public service increasingly resemble patterns in the for-profit sector, but still have some way to go. According to Incomes Data Services' review of NHS Trust annual reports and accounts, NHS top management salaries passed £200,000 in 2005, when chief executive (CE) of Hammersmith Hospitals Trust Derek Smith earned £210,000, 35% more than in the previous financial year. Between 1994 and 2004, average earnings for NHS CEs rose by 73%, compared with 50% for nurses (*LRD Fact Service,* 24 February 2005). In the US, pay scales are less unequal in government and not-for-profit institutions than in commercial undertakings, with typical gradients between chief executive officers and cleaners around 20:1. In US corporations, on the other hand, this gradient rises to an average around 180:1(Belsen, 2002). Even today, top management salaries in the NHS can't compare with the top of the private sector.

[59] It has been estimated that of $1,300 billion spent on US health care in 2000, at least $100 billion was stolen by fraud, probably $300 billion – 23% of total spending (Sparrow, 2000). One health care company, HCA (previously Columbia HCA), admitted submission of inflated bills and expenses to government, exaggerating the seriousness of diagnoses to increase claims on Medicare, illegally structured business deals shifting corporate expenses to Medicare, and offering cash incentives, free rentals and HCA hospital investments to doctors for patient referrals to other

HCA providers, all continuing to 1997. Total agreed damages in 2000 were $840m (£560m). HCA operates some health care units in the UK (Charatan, 2001a). Once any public service opens its doors to for-profit contractors, the stage is set for large-scale corporate fraud, which merges almost imperceptibly into whatever skilled accountants and company lawyers can get away with. They are just doing their job.

[60] Day surgery is often quoted as an opportunity for rationalisation of care and gains in efficiency, as indeed it is. There seems to be no obvious reason why this should expand more appropriately in a cooperative public service than in a commercial service, but every reason why it might expand faster for profit, because it more closely resembles the industrial production on which corporate health care is modelled. Patients who want decisions to be based on their own interests rather than those of shareholders will need to consider the risks as well as the benefits of profit motivation.

[61] A new NHS pay system 'Agenda for change' has been pioneered at 12 NHS Trusts in England since 2003, and was agreed by all NHS unions in November 2004 (except for some minor reservations by the radiographers' union SOR and construction workers' union UCATT). All staff without exception will earn a minimum £5.16 an hour and work not more than 37.5 hours a week. This could mean pay rises of up to 40% for NHS trades that have fallen behind, including 27-35% for laundry, domestic and catering, 31-56% for security, 22-46% for porters and 20% for health care assistants. There will be training and career development for all grades, with biggest impact on lowest grades (*Labour Research*, July 2003, pp 14-15 and February 2005, pp 15-16).

[62] The National Audit Office has reviewed one of the first PFI schemes, now in its fifth year. Norfolk and Norwich University Hospital opened in 2001 as one of the first PFI schemes, contracted to Octagon Healthcare, a consortium of banks and property developers, for a minimum of 30 years. Following changes in interest rates, it was refinanced by Octagon in 2003 at a windfall profit of £115m, of which it returned £34m to the NHS Trust, keeping £81m. The rate of return for shareholders rose from 16% to 60% of their original investment, and the contract period rose from 30 years to 39 years ('The Refinancing of the Norfolk & Norwich PFI

Hospital: how the deal can be viewed in the light of the refinancing', at www.nao.org.uk).

[63] Their complexity is inflated by the need to strike legally binding contracts with private sector firms. For example, the contract for Coventry Walsgrave Hospital ran to 17,000 pages. Consequently consultancy fees and negotiation costs vary between 2.8% and 8.7% of capital costs. Another factor is the effect 25 to 30-year PFI contracts have had on small schemes that could have been bought at lower cost through traditional government funding. For example, the catering contract at Birmingham Queen's Medical Centre, valued at £1m, will cost £23m under PFI, and the North Bristol Rehabilitation Unit, valued at £4.9m, will cost £42m (General Municipal and Boilermakers' Union, 2001).

[64] R. Smith, 1999.

[65] Gaffney et al, 1999; and Gaffney et al, 1999b.

[66] Ff. Roberts, 1952.

[67] Foot, 1973, p 290 et seq.

[68] J.E. Powell, 1966.

[69] A. Williams, 1989.

[70] Except as a positive choice by about 2% of the population who for one reason or another stayed with private providers.

[71] Unlike US family doctors since the shift to managed care, NHS GPs have never had any economic incentive to care for their patients themselves rather than refer them to specialists, and their patients pay no fees for referral. Despite this absence of economic motivation, referral rates from primary to specialist care are three times higher in the US than in the NHS, both for adults (Forrest et al, 2002) and for children (Forrest et al, 2003).

[72] This experience was repeated in French Canada, when free care was first made available in the early 1970s (Enterline et al, 1973). It was repeated in Oregon in 1994 when access to public health care services was greatly expanded by new legislation. Planners expected

13,100 new registrations in the first two months of the new scheme, but actually received 25,000. Costs originally estimated at $65m had to be revised to $200m (J. Roberts, 1994). All of these, including NHS experience, were used by conservative critics to denounce free care as illusory and ultimately unrealisable in their 'real world'.

[73] I am aware that this conflicts with conventional wisdom, which contends that Bevan accepted prescription charges in principle in 1950, as necessary to stem the flow of cascades of medicine down the nation's throats. Those who accept this fairy story should do their homework. The issue is dealt with fully by Charles Webster in his official history of the NHS (1988), which is in general conformity with my account. He deals also with parallel retreats in social housing and construction of schools.

[74] Committee of Inquiry, 1956.

[75] Woolhandler et al, 2003.

[76] In British terminology, a 'consultation' is a meaningful contact between a health professional and a patient. A 'visit' is a consultation in a patient's own home. In North American terminology, a 'consultation' is a discussion about a patient between two different health professionals, with the patient usually not present. What we call 'consultations', North Americans call 'visits' – almost always in the health professional's office, hardly ever in a patient's own home.

[77] By 2005, there had been well over 100 publications in peer-reviewed journals and five books, derived mainly from these data.

[78] If 'reform' of the NHS on business lines can be traced to any principal author, credit or blame should go not to Roy Griffiths, but to Alain Enthoven, chief economist at General Motors, who moved with Robert Macnamara to the US War Department in 1966, to try to get control of spending on the Vietnam War. He first applied business competition theory to military decision-making, believing that the main problem was lack of managerial control over senior generals. After Vietnam he moved into the economics of US health care, which, he believed, presented surprisingly similar problems (Waitzkin, 1994). He was invited repeatedly to advise on NHS policy by Margaret Thatcher and Kenneth Clarke in the 1980s, and became the main advocate for market competition in the rest of Europe

(Saltman, 1994). He readily conceded that European public systems were more inclusive and efficient than the US care system when it was dominated by medical ownership (Enthoven, 1990), but insists that with corporate ownership, managed care will assure substantial gains in productivity and control of costs. Where this has so far failed to occur, he attributes failure to insufficiently ruthless application of his principles: hospitals must be allowed to fail (Enthoven, 1993). In his Vietnam incarnation he was a friend and contemporary colleague of Daniel Ellsberg at the Rand Corporation, where he was chief of the office of systems analysis (OSA) in 1966, and was responsible for the promotion of John Vann as coordinator of all US regional civilian activities and pacification (N. Sheehan, 1989/90). Though probably not personally responsible for introducing body counts as a measure of output, Enthoven was a main advocate of quantified evidence as a basis for decisions: by 1967 average monthly body counts had risen to 7,315. Perverse effects of using proxy measures for output efficiency and incentive payments both in wars and in health care deserve more attention than they have received.

[79] Nominated by government rather than elected, hospital management committees before Thatcher were composed of local Great and Good, plus a few token elected councillors from local government. They were usually delighted to agree with their senior consultant surgeons and physicians on how always-insufficient resources should be deployed. With Griffiths came a huge influx of commercially trained managers without health service experience and therefore prepared to challenge the assumptions of health professionals. More than half the members of Trust boards had experience as company directors, three-quarters were male and 98% were white (Hunter and Harrison, 1997). For the first five years or so, there was an active purge of doubters and potential whistle-blowers. Survival depended on loyal collaboration with the new order (R. Smith, 1994).

TWO

What does the NHS create?

The desired product of health care systems is health gain. This can be measured as healthier births, healthier lives and healthier deaths.[1] Care systems have other byproducts, the most important of which are legitimisation of the state and stabilisation of society, but all depend on this central promise, real or illusory. Though this may seem obvious, it is not how the NHS is discussed by leading politicians or news media, for whom the chief measure of success has become the waiting time between seeing a GP and having an operation. Unremarked by politicians or media, there has been rapid progress in the past ten years toward more rational use of surgery, but we are still far from the point where we can assume that just because an operation has been performed, a patient's health has improved, or its further deterioration has been delayed.[2]

The aims of prescribing, giving injections, turning an unconscious patient every 30 minutes, removing a uterus or a gallbladder, or organising a programme for protecting old people with pneumococcal vaccine, are not just to perform these tasks competently, but to produce health gain or delay its loss, and to do so with maximal assurance of doing more good than harm. Health includes happiness. Unhappy people are not in optimal health, but everything short of this need not be regarded as disease.

If we assume that a familiar procedure will be productive in these terms we are flying on autopilot (which, it should be remembered, works well enough most of the time). Meaning well cannot assure doing well.[3] Intervention processes can never completely assure their outcomes. Paradoxically, to intervene safely we must learn procedures so thoroughly and repeat them so often that they become second nature, like walking or driving, but this autopilot state bypasses conscience. Here is what George Bernard Shaw, an Irishman, had to say about English medical conscience: 'Doctors are just like other Englishmen: most of them have no honor and no conscience: what they commonly mistake for these is sentimentality, and an intense dread of doing anything that everybody else does not do, or omitting to do anything that everyone else does.'[4]

In my experience this applies to all nationalities and all professions. Without conscious effort to think critically about what they are doing, sentimentality plus doing what everyone else does is the way most people work most of the time, unless actively encouraged to think critically[5] – most effectively through participation in teaching, or other forms of innovation and discovery. I had hands-on responsibility for patients for more than 40 years, but the time when I would feel completely competent, a totally safe pair of hands for other people's lives, never arrived. Right up to my last week in practice I was still making potentially serious mistakes.[6] Any attempt to apply knowledge from human biology to real lives entails a significant margin of error. Though my mistakes rarely had lethal consequences, that was just good luck. Clinical processes are in fact increasingly well (or decreasingly badly) selected and performed, but suggestions that any more than a few technical procedures can reach the virtual certainty we take for granted in, for example, air travel, are unrealistic.

The chief source of error in medicine is not the quality of performance of processes (though this can never be taken for granted), but with the quality of decisions to initiate those processes, taking into account their full personal, social, economic and historical context. Recognition of error is the foundation of science, but has yet to become a foundation for medical practice, and for nursing such recognition seems even more remote. Aggressive NHS managers and contingency lawyers make this transition even more difficult.

Does health care produce net health gain?

Even assuming full technical competence, we have to keep worrying about whether decisions we take and procedures we perform actually lead to net health gain.[7] We need evidence that the probable good we do exceeds probable harm by a substantial margin, justifiable in simple terms to our patients: or, if evidence is lacking, to remember the often surprising capacity of bodies and minds to recover health through their own capacities, neither assisted nor impeded by clinical tinkering.

Why worry? Is it not self-evident that, on the whole, we have done pretty well? In Britain, average expected lifetimes have increased by 40 years since 1840. They still show no sign of reaching a finite span, assuming that any such limit will ever be reached, which seems increasingly doubtful. Globally, expected lifetimes have doubled over the past two centuries.[8] In Britain, average lifetimes expected at birth have risen from under 50 years in 1901 to about 80 for women and 75 for men by 2001, and on present trends will continue to rise steadily. One reason for this gain is health care. It is not the only or even the main reason, but because availability of care is closely associated with quality and availability of education, food, shelter, regulated labour, rising personal incomes, and other social factors supporting health, it is hard to separate these causes and measure their independent contributions to health.

How can we measure an independent effect if all relevant social factors are in fact always interdependent? For example, better-educated people make more effective and efficient use of health care and, at least in the US, are richer and have better access to it.[9] It is hard to conceive of any real situation in which availability of health care could actually be independent of other categories like income, nutrition, education or housing, on a sufficient scale to reach any useful conclusion. If so, this is not a scientific question, since it can be neither confirmed nor refuted either experimentally, or by continued observation of statistical trends.

There are a few examples suggesting that once basic levels of material subsistence are assured, availability of health care may become a major determinant of health. After its revolution in 1959, Cuba soon attained infant and adult mortality rates at roughly the same levels as the United States, despite vastly lower average income and health care spending per head of population. The annual cost of health care in the year 2000 in the British NHS was £750 per head, less than half that in the US despite similar mortality rates. This compared with £7 per head in Cuba, where 45% even of this small sum was spent on primary care, compared with 16-18% in the NHS.[10] Low personal incomes in Cuba were combined with high social incomes (facilities of many kinds available free and shared by the whole population). As a consequence of this high shared social income, Cuban rates for literacy were probably better than those in either Britain or the US,[11] and health indices reached West European levels.[12]

The Cuban experience confirms that a well-organised health care system including the whole population can help to sustain good mortality indices despite a low GNP, low average personal incomes per head and disgracefully low professional incomes, providing society as a whole remains stable and cohesive, with a strong and shared sense of social and historical direction.[13] At least until the US economic blockade forced it to accept a dual economy (a burgeoning dollar economy of hotels and revived prostitution, alongside an increasingly austere socialised economy of rationing) Cuban society had achieved many other features known to favour good population health: high literacy, vigorous traditions of local solidarity and community, virtually no unemployment, high average energy expenditure and participation in sport, low indices of social inequality, and very low levels of crime, alcohol and narcotic dependence and sexually transmitted disease. The state of siege imposed upon Cuba ever since it dared to take this independent path, and consequent intolerance of dissent, have damaged Cuban society and limited its development, but its positive achievements provide almost unique evidence that if care systems are planned to maximise whole-population health gain, they can achieve high productivity and make a huge contribution to public health.[14]

Can we measure health gain?

Counting interventions, such as doctor-visits, operations, or hospital admissions is easy, but these do not measure health gain. Measures of health do exist, most of them complicated and impractical to use except as research tools on small samples of people. An underused alternative is simply to ask people to rate their own health, and to do so repeatedly over time. Even a simple one item self-report of health status ('Would you say your health is excellent, very good, good, fair, or poor?') is as powerful a predictor of mortality over the next four to nine years as more detailed clinical indicators for middle-aged men, confirmed by the NHANES-I study of 6,440 adults age 25-74 over 12 years, though it was less useful for older people or women.[15] Validated instruments of this kind have been developed and should be more widely used, not as aids to personal care, but as measurement tools to assess NHS productivity.[16]

The alternative, instinctively preferred by management and most professionals, is to measure intervention processes as surrogates for health gain. These are always presented with caveats, warning that they do not necessarily represent health gain or loss accurately, but these caveats seem usually to be ignored when it comes to policy decisions and news media. Policy makers like to have some information to justify their decisions, even if in fact these decisions usually precede the information, so the quality of information may seem to them less important than just having some. Don Berwick has drawn attention to a report from the UK Office for National Statistics concluding that between 1995 and 2003 overall NHS productivity declined by from 3% to 8%, depending on different methods of calculation.[17] As he says, 'Production of what?' It turns out that in this case the 'product' was a weighted average of 16 different NHS activities, all processes rather than outcomes. The weighting was supposed to reflect the relative burden incurred to the NHS by each activity so that, for example, episodes of inpatient treatment weighed 14 times as much as episodes of outpatient treatment. This could lead to the absurd conclusion that a general shift away from hospital admissions for hernia repairs or varicose vein stripping to day care – which everyone agrees would be a more efficient use of both staff and patient time and hospital resources – represented a fall in efficiency.

With 96% coverage and completeness of coding for inpatient episodes in NHS hospitals and little less for consultations in primary care, outcome measurements that truly reflect health gain attributable to clinical decisions are certainly possible,[18] but their design will entail critically important decisions on weighting, which will in turn depend on understanding the nature of care processes, and evaluation of outcomes in terms of long-term health gain. Such understanding is not just a technical matter, at every point it entails social judgements.[19] The general shift away from clinical judgements toward potentially rigid guidelines is an extremely diverse bag of both dangers and opportunities, for which neither conservatism nor radicalism can provide general answers.[20] There may be a potential clinical and scientific consensus to back up such measurement systems, but even if this is so, it almost certainly differs fundamentally from the present managerial consensus.

Health care defeatists

Despite this evidence, confirmed by most people's daily experience, that health care systems can and mostly do contribute significantly and essentially to net health gain, there have been repeated attempts to deny the real value of clinical interventions as a whole. Paradoxically, these seem to have had more influence on political and academic thought in the last quarter of the 20th century (when there was more convincing evidence of net benefit than ever before in history) than in previous centuries (when there was little evidence that more than two or three clinical interventions did more good than harm). Starting in the 1970s, extreme scepticism got intellectual support from a new literature of professional defeatism and populist nihilism, best exemplified by McKeown[21] and Illich[22] respectively, who both denied that clinical interventions as a whole made any significant net contribution to health gain. That this nihilist trend is alive and well, despite even larger recent advances in effective applications of medical science, is shown by re-publication of Illich's *Medical Nemesis* by the *BMJ*, with enthusiastic editorial endorsement,[23] and by McKeown's continued influence on orthodox public health teaching and thought, despite the damaging expert criticism of his original demographic evidence,[24] and despite questions raised by other expert critics to which he gave no answer in the second edition of his book.[25]

Health care systems can themselves become engines of social change on a much broader front than their official agenda implies. They can promote professional and public hopes of social progress, and may then be resisted by people who believe such hopes to be false and misleading. Up to the 1970s, public respect for the power of health care seemed generally reassuring to governments. It was easier and cheaper to concede demands for health care than demands for higher wages or more socially regulated pursuit of profit. Social progress was still conventionally conceived in the frame of the 18th-century enlightenment, a beneficent state supplementing and containing the otherwise universal competition pervading society. McKeown, Illich and (to a greater extent than he liked to imagine) my mentor Archie Cochrane fanned the first flames of a scepticism that prepared the ground for retreat. However, Cochrane's seminal book *Effectiveness and efficiency* also cleared away a lot of rubbish obstructing progress toward more humane and effective care, which certainly needed to be done.[26]

All three of these influential authors implicitly accepted that health care systems must be judged by their health product. McKeown's and Illich's arguments were almost wholly negative. Essentially, they claimed that all systematic attempts to prevent or change the course of illness, other than through less specific social measures, had an aggregate net product of zero or less.

Cochrane's critique of care systems was more constructive, and opened possibilities in two entirely different and ultimately opposed directions.[27] Influenced by Alan Williams and other pioneers of the York University school of health economics, he looked at the NHS as a productive system. Cochrane found it gravely deficient in effectiveness, efficiency and humanity, an item he unfortunately omitted from his title but developed as an important theme. His book appeared in the right place at the right time. It persuaded an entire generation of senior clinicians and health policy experts to accept health economics as essential to policy formation.

Cochrane was mischievously attracted to the idea that doctors not only might do more harm than good, but on balance normally did so. In informal discussion he was not seriously interested in the many other possible explanations for his finding that after standardising data for differences in GNP per head, countries with more doctors (or paediatricians) per head of population had higher infant mortality rates.[28] Though never biased in statistical handling of data, in discussion he was systematically biased against the effectiveness of clinical medicine, perhaps because he was irritated by the arrogant and opposite assumptions of clinicians.

Legitimation of the state as a product of care services

Cochrane did not take account of the legitimation of the state, which had for centuries been at least as important a product of public care systems as health gain. He wanted the NHS to become more rational, entirely in terms of its contribution to health gain. He rightly conceived health gain in the broadest possible terms to include happiness, even though this was hard to measure. He drew particular attention to disgracefully low NHS spending on 'hotel' functions for care of sick older people (feeding, housing and generally looking after them as guests rather than inmates or prisoners). Encouraged by the York school economists, he analysed (not very systematically, as his subtitle admitted) the NHS as an industry, with inputs, processes of manufacture and products. But he paid scant attention to what we might lose by evaluating health care only as production of proven health gain.

Writing in 1867, a few years after Benjamin Disraeli had launched his bold gamble to extend the vote to men who had no property except the houses they lived in, the conservative journalist Walter Bagehot gave the following useful advice to rulers, then and for the foreseeable future: 'As yet, the few rule by their hold, not over the reason of the multitude, but over their imagination and habits; over their fancies as to distant things they do not know at all, over their customs as to near things which they know very well.'[29]

To governments of, by, and for the rich, continuing to rule in their own interest but now compelled to obtain consent from a newly enfranchised electorate in parliamentary democracies, Bagehot taught three fundamental principles still relevant today. First, such rulers must learn to respect the brains of their voters.

The poor could reason just as well as the rich. The old adage of the advertising industry is apt: never underestimate public intelligence, never overestimate public knowledge. Second, rulers must so far as possible control the imagination of the multitude about 'distant things they do not know at all', meaning the whole world outside what was familiar in their daily lives. The billionaire owners of newspapers and broadcast media still see to it that multitudes at home fear and remain ignorant of multitudes abroad. Finally, the rich should prudently respect the people's 'customs as to near things which they know very well', and wherever possible, make themselves seen as their sponsors. These customs now include free access to doctors, nurses, hospitals and the NHS, which rich people naturally assume to be a state charity.

Health economists adapting to neoliberal[30] agendas welcomed *Effectiveness and efficiency* as an important step toward more rational care. Had they not accepted this, had they stayed loyal to the new path on which Bevan had set their feet, *Effectiveness and efficiency* could have served progress. Instead, economists assumed that as a production system, health care must function in essentially the same way as the industrial commodity production and trade with which they were familiar and comfortable, albeit with numerous qualifications. I fear Cochrane would have shared that view, had he lived longer. Despite his fondness for mischief, he was ultimately an Establishment man.

Analysis of health care as a production system

Historically, analysis of health care as a production system reaches back to the first birth of health economics and its companion science, epidemiology, through the work of Sir William Petty in the wake of the English revolution in the 17th century,[31] followed by Pierre Louis after the series of French revolutions after 1789.[32] Since then, objective analysis of social health and health care has endured repeated births, declines and rediscoveries, always related to political climates.

Every rebirth of health care economics met majority professional resistance because it endangered trade in a then extremely questionable product. In 1914, Codman presented an objective analysis of measured inputs and outputs of surgery in a Boston hospital, and was consequently scorned by his professional colleagues for the rest of his life.[33] In the first months of the NHS, Ferguson and McPhail[34] analysed the consequences of hospital medical care: two years after discharge from hospital 56.6% of patients were either no better, or dead – a shocking statistic at that time, and therefore generally ignored. Few professionals had enough faith in their work to welcome the challenge to measure their outputs, and in those days this was not a message the media wanted to hear.

Withdrawals of medical labour in trade disputes or strikes created natural experiments. In 1976 a slowdown of medical labour in protest at high malpractice insurance rates in Los Angeles County was convincingly associated with reduced population death rates, probably because of a reduction in planned surgery.[35] Most of this surgery was probably done not to prolong life, but to improve its quality, but it inevitably entailed a small operative risk. In 1983 a GPs' strike in Jerusalem lasting 27 weeks, which stopped all public sector care except emergency hospital admissions (which rose by over 20%) showed exactly the same mortality both during the strike weeks and during the two weeks preceding the strike, as in the previous year when there was no strike.[36] Evidently the nihilists had a case good enough to deserve an answer.

This raises the huge issue of whether shifts in life expectancy are in any case a valid measure of NHS production. If most NHS processes concern not saving life, but making it happier and less painful, then gains in happiness and reductions in pain should be better measures of output. They are much harder to measure, but certainly not impossible, each having its own substantial research literature. On the other hand, reliable data on deaths and ages at which they occur are far easier to obtain and interpret, and they have an immediate intuitive meaning to everybody. Moreover, the most serious negative byproducts of medical and surgical interventions designed to improve life rather than extend it are fatal events. Though almost all surgery is now associated with less than 1% consequent mortality except in very old people, this still means that more surgery implies more deaths. Mass medication also implies negative as well as positive outputs. As even positive gains are usually small, positive balance of quality-of-life gains against length-of-life losses should still begin from comparisons between treated and untreated people in terms of all-causes mortality. Mortality is a crude measure, but still provides the most convincing foundation for argument and action. We also need measures of morbidity, and perhaps even more their opposite – measures of self-rated well-being – but these almost always follow the same patterns as mortality, and lessons from them are usually much the same.

Gap between possibilities and realities

John Bunker's classic review *Costs, risks and benefits of surgery*[37] renewed Codman's work in a more critical but also more confident and therefore less defensive era. Later, in 2001 he estimated the overall contribution of medical and surgical care to prolonging life over the 50 years since the Second World War, when he had entered practice as an anaesthetist. He concluded that possibly half our added years of life gained in the second half of the 20th century might be attributable to medical intervention.[38] Reviewing Bunker's evidence in a masterly review of the entire English language literature on the actual and potential contribution of medicine to reduction of mortality, Nolte and McKee[39] found his assumptions too optimistic, mainly because of the gap between what had proved possible in research trials, and what was actually achieved in practice – because routine care does not match research practice, and even more, because routine practice simply does not reach a high proportion of people who need it, even with universal free access through NHS primary care.

Until very recently most research trials took place in contrived worlds where the population and professional carers differed profoundly from those in ordinary practice. Most trials excluded older people with complex problems, though most real problems occurred in precisely this group. For most common chronic disorders, single, uncomplicated problems are rare. Usually single disorders represent a much-simplified perception of reality by doctors who have to use narrow disease labels in order to choose effective treatment or referral aimed at what they hope will be a vulnerable link in the causation of illness; they are not aiming at a realistic description of all the health problems actually borne by patients.[40] Shortage of time, narrowly specialised skills and limited imagination all encourage health professionals to limit the problems they recognise to those they feel able to cope with – either to solve, or at least to contain.[41] Specialists are by definition encouraged to limit their responsibility in this way, even though many of the disorders in which they specialise tend to be closely linked, with interdependent causes (and therefore interdependent solutions).[42] Though solutions for many specific health problems have been developed precisely by ignoring other problems, and this deliberate simplification can be useful, it is easy to forget that this is usually a falsification of reality, convenient for professionals, but often leading to absurd inefficiencies for patients.

As Barbara Starfield has said, rediscovery of the complexity of reality is now the most important field for research in primary care,[43] which could eventually lead to a major reorientation of the whole NHS, if it resumes progress as a unified service. On the other hand, if it continues to fragment into competing units, it will be much more difficult to bring services together to deal with complex health and social problems rationally and in a coordinated way.

Can we close the gap between what present knowledge makes possible, and what present resources can achieve?

Nolte and McKee compared mortality rates for disorders amenable to treatment in 19 developed economies in 1998. The US ranked 15th for disability-adjusted life expectancy and 16th for premature mortality from treatable causes. The UK ranked 10th for disability-adjusted life expectancy, and 18th for premature mortality from treatable causes.[44] Neither had much to boast about.

Ever since pioneers began a proactive search for treatable chronic ill health in whole populations, we have known that roughly half of most common chronic disorders in the English-speaking world are undetected, half those detected are not treated, and half those treated are not controlled; the 'Rule of halves'.[45] This approximation was originally derived from community studies of high blood pressure,[46] but similar whole-population studies of many other problems have indicated a similar order of magnitude for under-diagnosis, under-treatment and loss from follow-up. These have included type 2 diabetes,[47] deafness,[48] visual impairment[49] and incontinence in older people,[50] glaucoma,[51] coeliac disease,[52] asthma in children[53] and adults,[54] kidney failure,[55] vertebral fractures from osteoporosis,[56] suicidal depression,[57] domestic violence,[58] prostatic obstruction,[59] heart failure,[60] atrial fibrillation,[61] schizophrenia,[62] follow-up after strokes[63] and coronary heart attacks,[64] and psychosocial problems in children.[65] Institutionalised patients, nominally under skilled supervision, fare no better, with roughly half of all their treatable needs not recognised.[66] This list is incomplete, just evidence that I have come across while reading a few journals of general medicine over the past decade or so. 'Halves' is only an order of magnitude, but in many of these studies the proportion of people with unmet needs is much higher. In Britain during the past three decades, presented, identified and treated health problems together represent about half the real problems of which they are a part, often less. For whole populations, US figures seem similar: higher rates of ascertainment, more aggressive attitudes to treatment and higher expectations from patients with access to personal care; all combine to reduce unmet need, but the 15-20% with access only to emergency care often have gross unmet needs that are now rarely seen in the NHS.

Eliminating the rule of halves

Where health care is free, and primary care teams have registered patients whose names, addresses, telephone numbers (and soon e-mail addresses) are known, we don't have to wait for people to feel ill to search for important risks to their health systematically.

In Glyncorrwg we decided in 1968 to screen the whole population for important, treatable health risks, so that current knowledge could be, so far as possible, fully applied. Because even very high arterial pressures rarely cause symptoms until they have already caused serious organ damage, this important health-related variable needs to be measured in every adult, at intervals of about five years throughout life. This was therefore our first subject for screening, beginning in 1968 and completed by 1970.[67] Of those aged 20-65,[68] we reached 100% of men and 98% of the women, creating what was, so far as I know, the first community in the world in which everybody's blood pressure was known, and everyone likely (on contemporary evidence) to benefit substantially from treatment was able to receive it.[69] Between 1968 and 1987 we then searched systematically for other common treatable causes of ill health in everyone over 20, mainly using ordinary consultations to collect data beyond that required for the usually minor complaint in hand. At review in 1989 of all 1,207 adults in this age group, 44% had chronic chest problems, 36% were current smokers, 19% were obese, 16% needed treatment for high blood pressure, 11% had serious alcohol problems and 3.5% had diabetes, all using defined diagnostic criteria. Most of these problems overlapped with each other.[70] Not only were there too many health problems for referral to specialist care to be feasible, but their problems were also too complex. They all needed skilled community generalists, only a few needed hospital-based specialists.[71]

Was all this case finding[72] and anticipatory care justified by evidence of eventual health gain?[73] It certainly was. In 1987 we compared death rates under 65 for the five years 1981-86 in Glyncorrwg (which had developed this cumulative proactive programme since 1968) and in the socially similar community of Blaengwynfi[74] (which had received only traditional demand-led care from three successive doctors between 1968 and 1985).[75] Age-standardised death rates under 65 were 28% lower in the community receiving planned proactive care over the five-year period. Differences were mainly in deaths in the first year of life and for cardiorespiratory causes of death, the pattern expected when medical interventions are more effective.[76]

Our techniques were based on very high customary use rates typical of all coal-mining communities with long traditions of free care and heavy burdens of sickness and injury; on very high response rates to our research studies, secured through the trust generated by experience of continuing and emergency care readily provided;[77] on staff embedded in the local community, with all the efficiencies inherent in caring for people already well known; on well-kept personal medical records, always available, used at every clinical contact, and reinforced by frequent informal contacts in non-medical settings; and above all, on a registered, accurately defined population, so that every audit numerator had a population denominator – the absolute precondition for any sort of research relevant to health care policy.[78]

Repealing the Inverse Care Law

The world over, the more any community needs good medical care, the less likely it is to receive it – a banal truism I summarised in 1971 as the Inverse Care Law.[79] High objective scores for social deprivation,[80] low average community incomes per head, high morbidity and premature death rates and high primary care workload[81] are all consistently associated with low average consultation time.[82] Poor people get more and earlier illness than rich people, but their communities are least attractive to doctors.[83] Far more potentially clinical time has to be wasted on the legitimation of entitlements to the host of miserly benefits required to keep poor people going, above all on certification of fitness for work.[84] Experience of mass unemployment, with devastating and lasting consequences for social and biological health, is the most important common factor shared by all these communities.[85]

The Inverse Care Law is mainly an effect of the market, that relentlessly subordinates human values to the pursuit of profit. It is a human construct, not a law of nature. By taking health care out of the marketplace, this can and should eventually be eliminated. By forcing socialised health care back into the market, it will be reinforced, a crime for which politicians who drive this policy should be held fully responsible.

The pre-'reform' NHS provided a framework within which it was possible for GPs, at high personal cost in the form of lower net income, to initiate systematic proactive care as well as good traditional reactive care.[86] We eventually got some evidence that we were succeeding. In 1981–89, ranking all 55 electoral wards in the County of West Glamorgan for deprivation by the Townsend Index, both Glyncorrwg and Blaengwynfi lay in the five most deprived wards. Ranking the same 55 wards for age-standardised mortality under 65, Glyncorrwg lay in third place (alongside the most affluent areas of Swansea), and Blaengwynfi ranked 32nd. Good demand-led care in Blaengwynfi had obviously made a difference, but it probably could have been substantially more effective if it had been supplemented by systematic search, recall and planned clinical policies applied to the entire population. This evidence is limited by the small numbers and 'natural experiment' design, but on this policy issue, it's still virtually all the evidence there is, at least for the UK.[87]

Productivity in primary care

This experience attracted attention from government and the medical civil service, apparently providing an initial model for what eventually became the GP contract in 2004.[88] When I was working in NHS primary care, GPs were contracted to provide 'the services normally provided by a general practitioner'[89] – in other words, GPs were required to do what other GPs did, a resounding tautology that satisfied all governments from 1912 to 1990. Since the 1987 White Paper and ensuing 1990 contract, there have been successive revisions designed to encourage proactive work considered by government likely to raise outputs of health care, and to shift responsibilities for ambulant care from hospital outpatient departments back to primary care, particularly for continuing care of chronic health problems.

A speech in 1989 by Conservative Secretary of State for Health Kenneth Clarke set an entirely new agenda for primary care, followed by every government since, Labour or Conservative.[90] Before Clarke, no minister for health (including Nye Bevan) had ever taken the clinical product of primary care seriously. They had been concerned almost exclusively with satisfying users rather than verifiably improving either their health, the health of their communities or their efficiency as gatekeepers to hospital-based specialists. The task of GPs had been to do whatever was either not yet possible for hospital-based specialists, or seemed to them too trivial to deserve their attention. Hospital specialists provided the engine, primary care provided the clutch, connecting hospitals to popular needs but defending them from the full impact of undifferentiated, unprioritised public wants.[91] Unlike hospitals in the US or most other West European countries, NHS hospitals could concentrate on work appropriate to them, because access to specialists in the NHS was obtainable only through referral from GPs. Everyone had free access to a GP functioning as a personal doctor,[92] acting also as gatekeeper, both in the interests of government concerned to contain costs of hospital care, and in the interests of patients concerned to avoid iatrogenic risks disproportionate to probable benefits. In the mid-1960s, British government began to recognise the value of this function when they saw the economic consequences of its loss in the US, where family doctors were becoming a nostalgic memory, and in Western Europe, where they were becoming marginalised by direct access to specialists.

More than any other single factor, this gatekeeper function had made the NHS more cost-effective than any other western care system, but governments saw mainly what they wanted to see – that primary care was much cheaper than hospital care. They also saw that primary care was often slipshod, poorly organised, understaffed and poorly equipped, but as GPs were independent contractors, this could be seen as a failure of GPs rather than a failure of government. GPs acting only as signposts and selectors for referral of about 5% of their consultations to 'real' doctors (hospital-based specialists) were cheap for the other 95% of consultations they dealt with themselves. However, accurate choices for referral depended on generalist skills of high quality and sophistication, and sufficient consultation time to exert them. All these raised the real costs of primary care. Patients' acceptance of gatekeeping depended on confidence that primary care was appropriate and effective, so investment in primary care had to rise.[93]

Patients, then and now, trusted doctors and nurses more than any other occupational group. Despite several decades of hostile media criticism, 91% of the British public still generally trusts doctors to tell them the truth, compared with 88% for teachers, 77% for university professors, 76% for judges – and, at the bottom, 20% for politicians and 16% for journalists.[94] But though they trusted GPs to tell them the truth, rising expectations and declining deference ensured that to retain public trust in their effectiveness as well as their truthfulness, GPs would have to apply advancing knowledge in primary care, as specialists were assumed to be doing in hospitals. Contrary to government, media and general popular assumptions, as prevalent today as they were in 1989, generalist skills demand at least as much knowledge, education and commitment as specialist skills. They also require material resources and much larger and more diverse teams than they had in the past, implying a huge shift in the proportion of investment in primary care relative to hospital care, for both to reach comparable standards. Public investment on the scale required cannot be routed through GPs if they are seen as independent contractors, assumed to be running a small business in which profit depends on how much of the money gets spent on themselves and how much goes into the service. In terms of human investment, though not technical investment, primary care is not a cheaper alternative. It probably cannot develop to its full potential in either the corner shops of the past or the supermarkets of our currently anticipated future. Neither primary care nor hospitals can develop optimally in a marketplace. These truths have not yet been accepted by any government or major political party. They do seem to be dawning slowly on the BMA, which has quietly come to recognise that in areas where NHS workload and social needs are high and resources are scarce, a salaried primary care service may be the only way to recruit committed staff.

All governments have now taken the first step toward rational understanding of health care. They all recognise it as a production system, with measurable inputs, outputs and efficiency, and that it can no longer be a quasi-religious institution exempt from criticism.[95] The Clarke agenda set out in 1989 saw nothing beyond that. It assumed that the internal economy of the NHS in essence resembled the external economy of capitalism, susceptible to similar measures of input and output, similar fragmentation of work and responsibilities, similar relations between providers and consumers, similar motivations to maximise profit rather than service, and similar destabilisation of traditional customs and loyalties. Led by ruling opinion in the world's most wasteful and socially inefficient medical economy, the US, Thatcher's and Clarke's successors in government, including New Labour, have accepted its agenda. Continuity of personal care, which provided the foundation for our successful work in Glyncorrwg, was the first casualty of the drive to industrialisation, and the next was the gatekeeper function.

The recent contract finally agreed with GPs in 2004 is designed around primary care as a production process, aiming to raise process efficiency by an extremely complex and administratively costly and demanding combination of rewards for attaining targets and penalties for failure. This encourages an industrial approach to care processes, maximising GP incomes where all specified boxes can be ticked, but ignoring huge areas of practice that have as yet no specified box for ticking. When GPs were paid extra money for home visits after 10.00 pm, calls coming in at 9.30 tended to be kept waiting for an extra 30 minutes. This is called gaming – playing the system, essential to realistic business planning. Sticks and carrots certainly provoke movement, but in very complex systems requiring frequent judgements between often-conflicting priorities, it is unwise to apply to intelligent men and women methods developed for donkeys. It depresses morale, destroys imagination and eliminates conscience.[96]

Byproducts of the NHS

Health problems are all partly social in nature, because humans are social animals. Health care is conventionally separated from social care, but is in fact a particular subset of social care. This conventional separation has in many ways been useful for understanding problems in isolation, but as soon as we look closely at any particular problem in its full biological and social context, we have to recognise that these divisions are arbitrary.

Just as health and social problems are ultimately so interdependent that neither can be fully understood on its own, so are their solutions. If the NHS has a measurable product, much of this must be a social product rather than a personal gain for individual patients. Because the foremost aim and claim of the NHS is to produce personal health gain, its authority rests on this. All other social products are usually considered as byproducts, if they are considered at all. Again, the distinction is arbitrary. It reflects a society that crowns individual consumers as kings, and then wonders why there is no longer a kingdom.

We have already considered the NHS as the legitimiser of the state. As well as treating and preventing illness, the pre-'reform' NHS produced social stability and consensus. It served as an important brake on the socially destabilising effects of market society. It helped to stabilise society sufficiently for wealth to accumulate in an increasingly unequal and therefore unstable distribution,[97] but also for workers to organise under substantial legal protection (now largely swept away). Being itself a successful product of solidarity, the NHS also reinforced solidarity, gave it new social forms and provided a protected site within which it could grow. To the extent to which the NHS can develop its own distinct internal economy and culture, it can serve the interests both of people who live from what they own (whose interests lie in undisturbed accumulation of apparently self-replicating wealth), and of people who live from what they do (whose interests lie in solidarity, to defend what they have, and to develop customs and institutions on which a cooperative society may eventually be built).

The NHS can serve both of these fundamentally conflicting interests only if it regains economic and cultural independence, re-established by a firm central political will.[98] Once the NHS becomes drawn into the production of health care as a marketed commodity, once the authority of the NHS becomes a brand for longer and better life as a traded commodity, both these functions will inevitably decline. Why are doctors and nurses trusted more – at least four times more – than politicians and journalists? Because still, in general, their livings do not depend on selling to people what they don't need but can somehow be induced to want through fear, fashion or vanity. They still provide real solutions for real problems, according to generally agreed priorities determined by objective evidence rather than the needs of trade. If the NHS becomes merely a branded franchise for business contractors, its social authority will disappear as fast as in any other privatised public service.

On 10 May 2002 a headline dominated the front page of the *Guardian* newspaper,[99] the paper that now represents British Left-Liberal opinion in the absence of any socialist newspaper with large circulation:

'HEALTH CRISIS LOOMS AS LIFE EXPECTANCY SOARS'

So, the NHS faces the prospect of people living longer – but surely this was what the NHS is trying to do? The achievement was perceived as a problem only because the NHS was at the time of this headline still a public service, not a business – and therefore a consumer rather than a producer of wealth, in the insane economic terminology accepted as much by the *Guardian* as by the *Daily Mail*. Why should we not devote ever more of our growing social product to education and health, if this investment broadens and lengthens opportunities for our descendants? Because wealth is not seen as a social product, but as a reward for personal cleverness by someone in charge.

The NHS as an expanding field for new employment

Another byproduct of the NHS is jobs. As machines replace human skills, and as subsistence wages in Asia replace dignified wages in Europe and North America, jobs are in dwindling supply. If we ask how government can justify the huge subsidies from public money it gives to the export of weapons for destroying life, press and politicians remind us of the jobs that depend on the arms industry. The NHS also creates jobs. Unlike the weapons industry, it not only saves lives but is also increasingly labour-intensive rather than capital-intensive, and its expansion depends in large part on further developing the skills of its workforce. In expanding health care, everyone wins.

In 1993 US economist William Baumol predicted huge changes in the composition of the US economy in the 50 years 1990-2040.[100] To simplify his argument he assumed that existing productivity growth rates in each of three sectors, health care, education and manufacture/agriculture, would remain roughly constant. By 2040 total output of the US economy would thus have increased by about 350% in value. Materially, the nation as a whole would become three and a half times richer.

With the same assumptions, he then considered expected changes in total spending (public and private) on health care, education and manufacture/agriculture, each as percentage shares of their combined total. Because of rapidly rising productivity in manufacturing and agriculture through replacement of human labour by machines, their share of total spending would fall from 81.7% to 36%. In contrast, productivity of labour in education and health would still depend on increasingly sophisticated human skills and interactions with students and patients acting as co-producers rather than consumers. This sector would therefore grow much more slowly. Spending on education would rise from 8.7% of total spending in 1990 to 29% by 2040, and spending on health care would rise from 11.6% to 35%.[101] While industry and agriculture would become ever less labour-intensive, quality health care and education would become ever more labour-intensive, both relatively and absolutely. Health and education professionals would become relatively more costly to employ. Assuming this divergence continued at the same rate, by 2040 proportional spending on education and health care would rise more than three-fold, while proportional spending on commodity production would be halved.

Over 80% of costs for both education and health care are attributable to wages. A predicted three-fold rise in spending therefore implies something not far short of a three-fold rise in employment in these two fields – close to the three-and-a-half-fold rise anticipated for output of commodities. Baumol concluded that because total output of wealth (as traditionally understood) would rise by three-and-a-half times, there would be plenty of this to fund higher spending on education and health care (and on high culture – orchestras and opera were his own principal interest). It would just depend on social and political choices.[102] The wealth would certainly exist, and 'society' (whoever that was) could choose how to use it.[103]

Baumol's ideas about how political choices are actually made seem naive,[104] but there are other reasons for believing that continued expansion of health care and education as public services will eventually have to be resumed. First, only as public services, wholly separated from pursuit of profit, can they work efficiently to maximise their product as health and educational gain, rather than a rising torrent of commoditised procedures to chase consumer demand. The contrast between pre-'reform' NHS administration costs at 6% of total spending and US administration costs averaging 34% in for-profit hospitals speaks for itself. Other gross inefficiencies flow from fragmentation of care and misdirection of investment, explored in later chapters. Second, only as public services, wholly separated from pursuit of profit, can the NHS and education provide a stabilising frame for an evolving society, given rising conflicts of interest between people who live from what they own, and people who live from what they do (and conflicts within those who do both – see Chapter 5). When either of these public services becomes seen as a business, they lose this stabilising function.[105] Realisation that these two factors operate could make a return to an independent NHS economy feasible. Whether such a return will actually happen depends on shifts in British and world politics of which there is now little sign, but with independence for public services as the only available exit from rising instability, such shifts will certainly occur, creating new opportunities for change.

Summary and conclusions

The NHS is a production system with health gain as its main product. Gains in life expectancy are easy to measure but hard to interpret. Gains in happiness and relief of pain have been substantial. They are harder to measure, but that is no excuse for not trying. Assessments of the contribution of care to health gain have swung from naive optimism, when doctors enjoyed a special relationship with the rulers of society, to equally naive pessimism, since they became a costly embarrassment. Though medical care is of less importance to health than material and intellectual nutrition, it has been applied very incompletely to whole populations, even in care systems outside the market. The aim should be to bring everyone within the scope of effective anticipatory care.

As an independent gift economy, the pre-'reform' NHS had social authority and public trust. As a principal byproduct, it helped to provide a robust social framework both for accumulation of wealth, and for development of new social customs and institutions for a future sharing society. Policy makers ignore this stabilising effect at their peril.

Notes

[1] The concept of healthy death, not just its timing but the nature of terminal experience, has been familiar to experienced clinicians for generations, but until recently has not been articulated, and has therefore been grossly underfunded (Murray et al, 2004).

[2] The extent of potential error in decisions to operate is seldom appreciated, even by doctors. For example, judging from their prevalence at routine autopsy, from 9% to 21% of British adults have gallstones (Barker et al, 1979). Only about 18% of these people are likely to get pain or any other harmful consequence over 15 years' follow-up (Gracie and Ranschoff, 1982). Cholecystectomy is now an almost completely safe procedure, with an intrinsic mortality risk of only 0.17% (Roslyn et al, 1993), and with rapid recovery if modern endoscopic methods are used; so rapid that since endoscopic methods largely replaced open surgery, the total NHS cholecystectomy rate has risen 25%, and spending on cholecystectomies has risen 11.4%, despite a 25% fall in cost per operation (Lam et al, 1995).

So upper abdominal pain is common, gallstones are common, and (excluding patients with acute cholecystitis, duct stones or obstructive jaundice, as all studies here quoted have done) their association may be causal or fortuitous. Cholecystectomy therefore may or may not be a rational intervention, though it is safe, seldom painful and has a diminishing unit cost.

Most follow-up studies show persistent pain in 20-30% of patients after cholecystectomy for gallstones thought to be causal (Jess et al, 1998). In a controlled prospective study, 233 consecutive patients seen by 75 Rotterdam GPs complaining of recurrent upper abdominal pain, and suspected of symptomatic gallstones, all had ultrasound scans. Of those with confirmed gallstones, 61% were in pain, compared with 45% of patients without gallstones. Those with confirmed gallstones were offered cholecystectomy. Of those who had the operation, 87% ceased to have pain, compared with 63% of those with confirmed gallstones who declined operation, and 83% of patients with abdominal pain but without gallstones who had no operation. These differences were not statistically significant (Berger et al, 2004). In another study, case histories of 252 patients who had undergone cholecystectomy were shown to a panel of physicians and a panel of surgeons. The physicians agreed operations were appropriate in 41% of cases, inappropriate in 30% and could not agree in 29%. The surgeons agreed operations were appropriate in 52% of cases, inappropriate in 2% and could not agree in 46% (Scott and Black, 1992).

Despite this chaos, experts have agreed on consensus criteria that are supposed to make rational choices possible. Using such criteria, a one-year prospective study of all 960 patients on waiting lists of six Spanish hospitals for cholecystectomy concluded the operation was inappropriate in only 0.7% and uncertain in 7.9% (Quintana et al, 2004), a wonderful advance if it is true. We shall know that only after these patients have finished waiting, have had their cholecystectomies and either lost or retained their pre-operative symptoms. Cholecystectomy rates for different populations in Britain still show huge variability without any rational explanation (Aylin et al, 2005).

[3] Eisenberg, 1988.

[4] G.B. Shaw, 1907, Preface.

[5] This was demonstrated dramatically by Stanley Milgram's experiments in 1961-62, showing that most ordinary citizens of New

Haven, Connecticut, were willing to administer painful and even life-threatening electric shocks if instructed to do so by someone in apparently established authority (Blass, 2004/05).

[6] In the Glyncorrwg practice, in 1986 we reviewed 500 consecutive deaths from 1964 to 1985, all those occurring in a total population varying between 1,600 and 1,800, almost two-thirds of them at home. We had routine information about deaths in hospital, but inquiries about unexpected deaths in which errors seemed possible were generally treated with hostility, and access to hospital records was refused. Of all these deaths, 45% were preceded by avoidable causal factors of some kind, almost half of them attributable to my own errors (Hart and Humphreys, 1987).

[7] That is, health gains exceed health losses. All medical interventions necessarily entail some possibility of health loss, so the outcome of care must always be a net product.

[8] Cambridge Group for the History of Population and Social Structure and Max Planck Institute for Demographic Research in Oeppen and Vaupel, 2002.

[9] The most powerful single contributor to health gain on a mass scale is maternal literacy. Mothers who can read and write, and therefore begin to understand and criticise and make their own decisions about child care and relationships with their partners, live longer and healthier lives, and so do their families (Briggs, 1993).

[10] Boseley, 2000.

[11] MacDonald, 1997.

[12] Ochoa, 2003.

[13] Cuban experience has a historical parallel in Sweden. Though it was one of the poorest European countries in the late 19th century, it then attained, and has maintained ever since, the world's best public health indices in virtually all dimensions. This was achieved through universally accessible and inclusive health care and education systems used by all of the people, together with a high social wage. This development preceded, and to some extent

enabled, development of a modern industrial economy (Agdestein and Roemer, 1994).

[14] Though education remains Cuba's highest national priority, its budget having risen from 6.3% of spending in 1998 to 9.1% in 2003, there is growing social polarisation, with 20% of Cubans living in urban fringes mainly from black economy. The political elite and a new generation of Cuban businessmen seem fascinated by developments in China. By decreeing that socialism was irrevocable, Cubans ended a debate they had never completed. The Cuban Communist Party remains the backbone of state and administration, but is atrophied as a political party, with its national congress two years overdue in 2004 and still without a scheduled date. Democratic freedoms are a functional necessity for high productivity, but this remains a forbidden topic. The Cuban writer Abilio Estvez has written that his generation looks at society 'with a gaze full of bitterness, full of scepticism'. He explains that the Cuban revolution now looks like Catholicism 'which sacrifices the present in the name of heaven and paradise; the revolution sacrifices the present in the name of the future, which doesn't interest me. What interests me is how I live today' (in *Encuentro de la cultura cubana*, vol 26/7, winter 2002/03. Quoted by Janette Habel, 2004).

[15] Idler and Angel, 1990. See also Idler, 1992.

[16] For example, Garratt et al, 1993, and Paterson, 1996.

[17] Berwick, 2005.

[18] Lakhani et al, 2005a and 2005b.

[19] For example, evaluation of cost–effectiveness of procedures should entail estimates of varying cascade effects on future risks of health loss from interventions at different points in time or on different pathological processes. The weights attached to these may profoundly affect funding and allocation of resources even where some elements of planning have been retained, at the present state of quasi-privatisation reached by most West European health services (Brouwer et al, 2005). Complete transition to consumer–led services and price competition would have such nonsensical consequences for allocation of resources that it is unlikely to occur anywhere, but

even within planned services there is mounting pressure for short-term estimates of the effects of procedures.

[20] 'We can estimate the cost of a disability or saving a life, but we cannot express the value of the product in economic terms in such a way that we can compare the prevention of mental deficiency in a child with saving the lives of so many men and women in their 60s. Decisions have to be made subjectively, and in practice are usually the result of a judicious balance of competing pressures. It is a field in which gardening is real and botany is bogus' (Doll, 1973). Clinical gardeners must now somehow survive through an era managed by industrialists advised by often over-confident botanists.

[21] McKeown, 1979.

[22] Illich, 1976.

[23] R. Smith, 2002.

[24] Johansson, 1994.

[25] Godber, 1980.

[26] Cochrane, 1971.

[27] Hart, 1973.

[28] Cochrane et al, 1978.

[29] Bagehot, [1867] 1963, pp 250-1. His own position was frankly stated: 'I can venture to say, what no elected member of parliament, Conservative or Liberal, can venture to say, that I am exceedingly afraid of the ignorant multitude of the new constituencies. I wish to have as great and as compact a power as possible to resist it' (p 281).

[30] The term 'liberal' is ambiguous. In the US it has now lost all precision in usual speech, joining 'communist' and 'socialist' as a term of abuse and demonisation. Everywhere else, this word rightly retains two meanings: freedom of thought and tolerance of dissent on the one hand, and freedom of property and trade on the other.

This dual meaning was originally opposed to then conservative ideas of monarchy, aristocracy and inherited ownership of land as foundations for stratified and immobile societies.

Global industrialisation of all social processes is now understood everywhere, even by academics in the US, as a neoliberal offensive, even though its most reckless advocates are described as neoconservatives. Most obviously, the neoliberal offensive seeks to extend commodity production horizontally by free trade, displacing weaker domestic and subsistence economies through price competition. Less obviously, it seeks to extend commodity production to include what used to be the shared infrastructure of society, including activities hitherto more or less protected from commerce, such as schools, universities, high art, policing and prisons, and popular sports. The state, hitherto clothed by these social institutions as a socially neutral force holding society together, is now selling these off cheaply to anyone willing to buy and operate them for profit. Ideas generated by ideological total war against socialism have been confirmed by victory in the cold war, becoming ideas of total business. This now threatens the still only partially realised social promise of the 18th-century Enlightenment, the central strand of liberal thought for more than two centuries.

Liberalism has always had a dual character, two equally necessary and inevitable sides of the same coin. It began by liberating thought through subordinating everything else to the market. It approaches its end by transforming thought itself into a commodity, and thus subordinating it to the market – an unsustainable position for human imagination.

[31] Hull, 1963. The English revolution provides one of the first examples of innovative thinking and administrative action on public health. As Charles Webster has written,

> ... The collective evidence tends to support Bowden's view that the period 1620-1650 'witnessed extreme hardship in England, and were probably the most terrible years through which the country has ever passed.... The social planners of the Puritan Revolution proved to have a correct appraisal of the crisis of health facing the nation. Their first priorities – economic diversification and agricultural improvement – were measures particularly designed to insulate the lower classes against dearth and economic fluctuation. It was anticipated that

improvements in diet and general well-being introduced by personal initiative would radically alleviate the problem of disease.' (Webster, 1976)

This anticipated similar developments in France after 1789.

[32] Foucault,1973; Lilienfeld and Lilienfeld, 1982; Morabia, 1996.

[33] Codman, 1914/1992.

[34] Ferguson and McPhail, 1954.

[35] James, 1979; Roemer and Schwartz, 1979.

[36] Slater and Ever-Hadani, 1983.

[37] Bunker et al, 1977.

[38] Bunker, 2001.

[39] Nolte and McKee, 2004.

[40] After 20 years of systematic proactive case-finding covering the whole adult population in Glyncorrwg, we had 154 men and women with treated high blood pressure, meeting our strict and conservative criteria for intervention; in other words, we had defined virtually the whole hypertensive population. Searching these for evidence of 12 other common clinical problems, only 3% of the men and 7% of the women had high blood pressure as a single disorder (Hart, 1993, tables 18.1 and 18.2).

[41] GPs who have studied their own consultation patterns report proportions of consultations dealing with two or more different health problems varying from less than 1% to over 50% (van den Acker et al, 1996). Obviously this reflects neither social nor biological reality, but different ways of relating to patients and perceiving their problems. European people asked to list their own health problems report much higher prevalence of multiple problems. In the age group 55-79, 27% report no major health problems, 73% report at least one problem, and 60% report more than one (van den Bos, 1995). Similar rates to these self-reported rates have been found by primary care teams when they have actively sought problems in

whole registered populations, and not relied only on presented demand to indicate their existence (Abramson et al, 1982; Stewart et al, 1989).

[42] High blood pressure, diabetes and coronary heart disease are all associated, in that if you have one of them you more likely to have another. Around 1% of people with high blood pressure have entirely different causes, which need to be remembered and looked for. For the other 99%, people with any one of these problems are much more likely than the general population to get any or all of the others in this bundle. Most of the solutions for all of them are the same, and so are the steps to prevent them. Most people in all three groups share one underlying feature, insulin resistance. The educational, career and service structures of medical and nursing care are just beginning to recognise this truth, though it was suspected by thoughtful clinicians in the early 1970s, and well established as a dominant new idea by the 1980s (Reaven, 1988). However, to reintroduce confusion into this wonderfully simplifying argument, all of these health risks are worsened by cigarette smoking, and in terms of net risk reduction, stopping smoking is the single most effective treatment for all of them, even though smoking has little effect on insulin resistance. Alas, the real world is rarely simple.

[43] Starfield, 2001. This will require a paradigm shift in either attitudes or composition of those now leading British biomedical research. As Iain Chalmers has said, 'the smaller the thing you study in biomedical research the higher your status. So prions have a higher status and people who study whole societies have a very low status' (Cole, 2005).

[44] Nolte and McKee, 2003.

[45] Hart, 1992a.

[46] Wilber and Barrow, 1972.

[47] Kinmonth et al, 1989.

[48] Stephens, 1988.

[49] Wormald et al, 1992.

[50] Prosser and Dobbs,1997.

[51] Fraser et al, 2001.

[52] Hin et al, 1999.

[53] A. Jones, 1994.

[54] K. Jones et al, 1991.

[55] Chandna et al, 1999.

[56] Cooper and Melton, 1992.

[57] Isometsä et al, 1994.

[58] Richardson and Feder, 1996.

[59] Cunningham-Burley et al, 1996.

[60] Mair et al, 1996.

[61] Sudlow et al,1998.

[62] King and Nazareth, 1996.

[63] Young, 2001.

[64] Eagle et al, 2002.

[65] Bernal et al, 2000.

[66] Moore and Molyneux, 1997.

[67] Hart, 1970.

[68] We soon realised that for blood pressure control, we needed to screen people over 65 as well as younger adults, and did so, though we never published on this. Using ultrasound sensors and following a strict research protocol, we also screened a five-year cohort of newborn children and followed them up for ten years, initially at

three-month intervals to age one, and annually thereafter. Even under apparently standard conditions and using research quality measurements, we found these measurements so unstable that for clinical decisions they were clearly useless. In the light of this experience, the American Hypertension Society's encouragement of their paediatric specialoids to screen children for hypertension and treat those in the top 5% or so of the distribution with antihypertensive drugs seemed to us another unjustifiable example of a search for markets in a market-driven health care economy. Our other screening measures in childhood, most notably an active search for childhood asthma and urinary tract infections, were very successful. In general, we found that effective anticipatory care for adults needed to start in childhood, and effective anticipatory care for older people needed to start in middle age. This meant that a large proportion of care needed to become proactive, initiated not by patients' symptoms but by objective assessment of avoidable risks.

[69] Hart, 1974.

[70] When 'Well Men's Clinics' became fashionable in the 1980s, we did not have enough well men to create one; we were too busy dealing with the problems turned up by proactive search. By UK standards this was an unusually sick population, but it was typical of those to be found wherever people were still employed in heavy industry, or had become unemployed by its collapse, or transferred to lower-wage employment. Poor people everywhere have poor health, and the potential workload for proactive primary care is colossal.

[71] Horder, 1977.

[72] Battles raged in the 1970s between GP pioneers of whole-community screening for high blood pressure, and epidemiologists who opposed it. The issue was eventually resolved by calling continuous whole-population screening by primary care teams 'opportunist case-finding', and reserving the word 'screening' for the more formal procedures of epidemiologists and the burgeoning well-man and well-woman clinics of private health care.

[73] Later work confirms that we had good reason to search for treatable but untreated chronic illness, with opportunity for prevention.

Follow-up analysis of patients admitted to hospital in Australia found that 16.6% of admissions were prompted by acute events occurring within already-established continuing disease. Roughly half of these events were judged readily preventable by continuing anticipatory care in the community – preventable, but not prevented (*Medical Journal of Australia* 1999, vol 170, pp 411-15).

[74] Hart et al, 1991.

[75] The first of these doctors, Dr Cliff Thomas (now deceased) provided care of at least average quality, and the last two, Dr Stan Hill and Dr Brian Gibbons (now Secretary for Health in the Welsh Assembly) provided exceptionally good care, but without planned proactive search or active recall for follow-up.

[76] Kaul, 1991.

[77] Hart and Smith, 1997.

[78] The importance of inclusive population denominators cannot be stressed too much. Countries such as the US whose care systems depend on consumer choice in a market can create such population denominators only in specially contrived situations such as university practices, usually sited in socially deprived areas otherwise lacking any good primary care provision. Though only a few British primary care units used the full potential of this facility for research, it certainly influenced thought at the leading edge of innovation, and dominated ideas from the 1970s onwards, not only among innovative GPs, but also at the British Ministry of Health. The present rush to consumerism and market choice negates this trend.

[79] Hart, 1971. Banal, because one might as well cite the Inverse Shoe Law, stating that barefoot children are least likely to have shoes. The Inverse Care Law shocked people because whereas they customarily regard shoes as a traded commodity (so that it is natural for Imelda Marcos to have 3,000 pairs while many Filipino children have none) health care is still regarded as a human right, unsuited to trade. This view of health care seems to be held more widely and tenaciously in British than in US culture.

[80] Hannay, 1997.

[81] Wilheim and Metcalfe, 1984.

[82] Stirling et al, 2001.

[83] Carlisle and Johnstone, 1996.

[84] Doctors paid by capitation want to keep their patients as customers and therefore to please them. However, if doctors have established friendly relationships with their patients, as most still do, insulting these friends becomes a real problem. Dutch doctors, watching what happened to German doctors employed by Bismarck's *Krankenkassen*, had a large enough private market to defend their status as professional gentlemen. Though they accepted the beginnings of a much less inclusive insurance system for industrial workers in 1914, they refused to accept responsibility for certification of incapacity, so this has been performed ever since by independent doctors salaried by the state. In 1990, the last time I looked at the figures, rates for short- and long-term sickness absence were 2.6% and 3.4% respectively in UK, 5.0% and 3.3% in Germany, and 7.1% and 8.9% in the Netherlands. These relativities had been maintained over many years. If the intention was to support sterner work discipline, it clearly failed. Assessment may have been easier when men had to work hundreds of metres below ground, lying on puddled stone floors to hack as best they could, undercutting coal with a pick, with as little as 50 cm between floor and roof so that even shoulder movement was hardly possible, and all this for coal cut and loaded for less than 2 shillings a ton, but sold at the pit head for 9 shillings and exported for over 12 shillings a ton. Judging from my own experience of certification of miners and steelworkers from 1961 to 1992, the most important factor in judging disability was knowledge of patients' previous work record, and their reputation among their workmates and wives. Mining communities were generally well informed about the many social and personal factors affecting attendance at work, including exhaustion, demoralisation, fear (absence always rose after serious accidents or near-accidents), economic rewards of work and economic penalties for absence. In Glyncorrwg we had huge levels of short-term absence in the 1960s, when wages were disgracefully low. As soon as wages rose after the 1972 and 1974 strikes, morale rose and absence attributed to sickness or injury fell steeply. Though a few doctors always enjoyed acting for management, a large majority tended to give their patients the benefit of the huge doubts surrounding all

such judgements. In my experience and in usual conditions (I exclude international rugby matches) true malingering was and still is a rare (but paradoxically disabling) disease (see Yelin, 1986).

[85] Steinar Westin (1995) cited referenced data on the following effects of unemployment found in controlled prospective studies:

Consultation rates with GPs	+22%
Referrals to specialists	+60%
Length of sickness absence	+50%
Death within 10 years	+50-100%

From 1970, when the last mine in the Afan valley was closed, miners in Glyncorrwg often travelled long distances to mines elsewhere. In 1981, male unemployment in the Afan valley was officially estimated at 38%, based on claims for benefit in our travel-to-work catchment. Workers at two local factories had been working 12-hour shifts, seven days a week for the previous three months to complete urgent orders. A boy leaving our local school had written 55 job application letters without getting a reply. Three vacancies for apprentice electricians at the local steelworks attracted 7,000 applicants from all over Britain. In 1983, just before the year-long miners' strike, we measured unemployment in the Glyncorrwg practice population ourselves, based not on claims for benefit but on whether people had jobs (so that people claiming sickness benefit were included). Of all men aged 16-64, 48% had no work. Of young men aged 16-24, 60% had no work. After the strike, the British coal industry was virtually destroyed. Coal-mining communities entered two decades of appalling demoralisation, with very serious social and health consequences, particularly for young people, which are only beginning to diminish today.

[86] Independent contractor status ensures that GPs fund their practices at least partly from their own pockets; they can choose how much to spend on staff and equipment, and at what point they will take on a partner to share case-load. This, and the small-mindedness that so often follows from it, is the most important reason to support salaried service. Throughout my years in practice, my net income was never more than half the average net income for GPs, even though we were able to use our MRC-funded research staff to assist in some routine care. Much the same applied to other GPs

who tried to provide optimal care in those years. I understand things are a bit better now, I do not know how much.

[87] Of course, the improvements in health we secured in times of full employment would almost certainly not have withstood the effects of defeat and return to pre-war levels of mass unemployment, especially late effects such as drug dependence in teenagers, and I have no later data. Countries that, unlike the UK, sustained socialised health care systems with adequate funding, reduced or eliminated social class differences in mortality (Netherlands Central Bureau for Statistics, 1992; Kunst and Mackenbach, 1994a and 1994b; Kunst et al, 1995). After they embarked on neoliberal 'reform' programmes, social class differences in mortality reappeared. This pattern occurred in both Sweden (Whitehead, 1990; Whitehead et al, 1997; Whitehead, Gustafsson and Diderichsen, 1997) and Finland (Lynch et al, 1994; Kosskinen et al, 1996; Forssas et al, 2003).

[88] Rivett, 1998, p 411.

[89] This definition was provided in the *Red Book* setting out the terms of the GP contract. Apart from one major revision in 1967 to encourage group practice, better buildings, and employment of office and nursing staff, the *Red Book* stood virtually unchanged from 1948 to 1990.

[90] Clarke, 1989.

[91] A second, backup clutch system was provided by hospital accident and emergency (A&E) departments, providing episodic patch-up care for patients either unable to access primary care, or without confidence in it. In decaying urban centres this was a major gap in the NHS care system, causing serious concern in the 1980s, when it was rightly regarded as a sensitive indicator of primary care performance. Self-referrals to A&E departments are now expanding relentlessly, along with an increasing diversity of walk-in clinics and phone-in advice centres, in line with the consumerist policies favoured by both Conservative and New Labour governments, regardless of the damage this does to continuity, or of the inefficiencies inherent in caring for people you do not know. When I worked in the South Wales valleys most GPs still did most of their own suturing, and direct self-referral to A&E was negligible in the Glyncorrwg practice.

[92] Though the NHS presents no legal or economic barriers to access, there can be many administrative barriers in areas of social deprivation and high primary care workload. About half the people sent to prison in Britain are not registered with a GP, often a reflection of drug dependence, psychotic mental illness or both. These patients are very hard work and, as self-employed contractors, many GPs do their best to avoid them. Less businesslike GPs, who believe that these people need and benefit from care more than any other social group, end up with a disproportionate number of this kind of patient.

[93] That such investment was justified is supported by US experience; across the United States mortality fell by 14.4 deaths per 100,000 people during an 11-year period in areas where the number of primary care doctors rose by one per 10,000 people. The effect was greatest on black mortality – that is, on those with highest health care needs (Shi et al, 2005).

[94] MORI poll reported in *bmaNews*, 12 March 2005.

[95] Hart, 1992b.

[96] In line with New Labour and previous Conservative government beliefs that the way to get doctors to do anything is to pay for it, one item in the recent GP contract rewarded them for getting all patients seen within 48 hours of a request. The result, of course, was that all forward booking disappeared in most practices: patients who needed to be seen at regular intervals for monitoring chronic health problems such as high blood pressure or diabetes, instead of being booked three or six months ahead, were told to ring for an appointment within two days of that expected date. And of course, when they did so, lines were blocked with other callers. Told of this by an angry young mother at a live broadcast, Prime Minister Tony Blair was astonished to hear what had become common knowledge for everyone except higher government, and set up an official inquiry.

[97] Both within Britain, and on a global scale, inequality has reached extremes never before known. According to the *Sunday Times*, the number of £ billionaires in Britain rose from nine in 1988 to 26 by 2000. By then the Duke of Westminster had £3.7 billion. In one year in the 1980s, when he was reputed to be the richest man in

Britain, his accountants managed to reduce his income tax liabilities to zero. In the world as a whole, in 1996 there were then 358 US$ billionaires whose total wealth equalled the combined incomes of the poorest 45% of the entire world population, 2.3 billion people (Jolly, 1996).

[98] Such political bravery is not impossible for nations retaining sufficient self-respect to apply principles even in the real world. Canada's National Health Service made all trade in health care illegal. Needless to say, such legally reinforced solidarity is under constant assault. The Canadian Supreme Court recently ruled that federal legislation prohibiting private health care insurance violated Canada's constitutional Charter of Rights and Freedoms, therefore becoming invalid, if public health services were unable to deliver care of reasonable quality in a reasonable time. Like all systems funded mainly from income tax, Canada has a permanent crisis in NHS funding, and therefore waiting lists for elective surgery. According to the court, a patient who had to wait almost a year for hip replacement surgery met these criteria. This probably opens the door to many more legal challenges to the ban on trade in health care (Spurgeon, 2005).

[99] Today's *Guardian* readers may be surprised to know that this 'left' broadsheet newspaper advised its readers to vote for the Conservative Party in 1951, and set the pace for systematic vilification of Aneurin Bevan as a rabble-rousing danger to society from the time he resigned from the cabinet over introduction of prescription charges.

[100] Baumol, 1993.

[101] Between 1978 and 2000, people employed in UK production, construction, transport and utilities fell from 40% to 24% of the total employed workforce, while those employed in education, health care, social work and other public services rose from 13% to 17%, broadly confirming Baumol's trends (MacGregor, 2000/01, table C). Between 2000 and 2004, UK manufacturing lost over 720,000 jobs, 18% of its total workforce. Successful competition requires larger investment in skills, research, development and innovation, for which well-funded universities, schools and health care are necessary foundations. In his paper *China, Europe and UK manufacturing* (2005), TUC chief economist Ian Brinkley shows that

though UK business and its government seem to think the only way to compete with China is to reduce labour costs and deregulate employment, companies in Germany, which they cite as having the highest labour costs and most burdensome regulation in the EU, have almost doubled the value of their exports to China over the past five years, growing five times faster than exports from the UK (*LRD Fact Service* 2005, vol 67, pp 105-6).

[102] Towse, 1997.

[103] This issue has been excellently researched by John Appleby, chief economist at the King's Fund, an establishment think-tank rarely far from government. Chancellor Gordon Brown accepted the 'fully engaged' option proposed by Derek Wanless in his review of UK spending on health care. Wanless comes from the world of business and has never been accused of socialist tendencies. On his estimates of projected spending, NHS spending as a percentage of GDP had risen from about 5.2% in 1977-78 to about 6.8% by 1997 (when New Labour took office) and nearly 8% in 2005 (at the end of New Labour's second term). Assuming 'full engagement', he forecasts this will rise to 9% in 2007-08, 11% in 2012-13, 12% in 2017-18, and 12.5% by 2022-23. Though NHS spending today is seven times higher in real terms than in its infancy in 1950, spending on all other goods and services has also risen three-fold, without any disastrous effects on our economy or culture. If the British economy grows at 2% a year, this allows NHS spending to reach 30% of GDP by 2055, by which time present spending on all other goods and services will have doubled (Appleby, 2005). It would not be difficult to present these figures in ways that would terrify voters, rather than help them to understand the real meaning of rising material productivity. Judging from Conservative and New Labour campaigning in the recent general election, we shall soon see this occur, particularly if, as now seems likely, 2% annual growth rates cannot be sustained in market economies led only by the search for profit.

[104] Baumol's hope that those owning the means of production of wealth would voluntarily invest their growing surplus in higher culture, more thoughtful education, or more humane and effective health care for the whole of society as human rights and an expanding social wage, rather than pocket it for themselves, is not credible. His economic ideas are imaginative, but his politics are

quixotic. Nothing shows this better than his own choice of a name for his discovery: he called the increasingly unaffordable cost of personal labour throughout the arts, education and health care 'Baumol's disease', and economists who have developed this topic have accepted this term. In fact what he had found was not a disease, but an anomalous and threatened fragment of health, somehow surviving within profit-driven societies.

[105] People who already use private agencies for health care or to educate their children cannot see this. Most of these agencies disguise themselves so far as possible as charities, truly devoted to that subset of the population either born to rule, or who have through their own hard work fought their way up the ladder, and thus proved their superiority to demoralised folk, incapable of using either doctors or teachers intelligently. Private sector schools, and perhaps to some extent private health care facilities, have a unifying effect on those who use them, if only to justify their choice to the rest of us. That is solidarity of a kind, but not the sort I am talking about.

THREE

How does the NHS create?

As a production system, the NHS as a whole can be regarded as a black box, with inputs into one end, outputs from the other, and a mystery in the middle. What happens inside this black box we call process – all the extremely complex chains of decision and intervention that somehow transform inputs into outputs. This is a generally agreed metaphor for all modern industries, in which production processes have become too complex for non-specialists to understand in the ways that earlier and simpler processes, for example production of coal, steel or cars, could be understood in the past. I hope to show that the nature of what goes on in the black box producing health gain is qualitatively different from what goes on in black boxes producing commodity goods or services. Health gain is always a value, but it need not, and for optimal productivity of health gain should not, be a commodity.

To analyse this for any theory of political economy, old or new, we have to make some simplifying assumptions. Most health economists assume that within the NHS black box a hierarchy of professionals provides a range of services for patients, first creating, then transferring these services as commodities to patients as consumers, but with the price of sale met in full or in part by the state. Health economists recognise that, unlike other transactions in the ideal world of classical economics, consumers of health care in all state systems, whether based on taxation or insurance, are so hugely less informed than providers, so shielded from immediate cost penalties, and so vulnerable to abuse by providers through fears of illness, that major modifications of classical theory are necessary and inevitable.[1] However, they still retain classical theory as a core. For most health economists, patient-to-professional encounters remain transactions, conveying applied medical science as a commodity from professional producers to patient consumers, with satisfaction of wants as its product, not health gain.

There is not a single example of any developed economy in which medical care for everyone is provided through a normal commodity market, without some component of risk shared by the state. Private medical trade can exist only as a parasitic adjunct to some kind of state-aided system, if only because mass care alone can provide enough experience of uncommon or extreme events to support education and research and to maintain expertise in these fields, and a large enough pool of shared risk to meet the extreme costs of extreme cases. For many centuries, optimal state-of-the-art care for the few rich has been based on the experience of state-of-the-art care for a small minority of the many poor reaching teaching hospitals in large cities. In Britain at least, the modern care system has grown from prepaid care for industrial workers, not from private care for the affluent. Even in the US – the archetypal free medical market[2] – about 42% of all costs of care are met by the state, even though they are transmitted so far as possible through commercial outlets. In other developed economies, for all but a small fringe market, actual purchasers are state agencies, insurance companies or other third parties (or most often combinations of these) buying on behalf of consumer groups, not individual patients. Though this must change market behaviour fundamentally, contacts between health care professionals and patients are still seen by most health economists as essentially provider–consumer transactions, albeit substantially modified.

Empirical study of the actual processes of clinical judgement, decisions and interventions shows that this classical view, however modified, is only one way of looking at care processes, and probably not the most effective or efficient. There are other ways that, if more appropriate to the extremely complex and evolving nature of relationships between patients and professionals, might offer wider and more effective opportunities to increase productivity and create new opportunities for health gain.[3]

The consultation process

In 1960, using contemporary gendered and disease-centred terms, the great paediatrician Sir James Spence defined the consultation as:

> the occasion when, in the intimacy of the consulting room or the sick room, a person who is ill or believes himself to be ill, seeks the advice of a doctor whom he trusts. This is a consultation and *all else in the practice of medicine derives from it*. [my emphasis][4]

If we broaden this to include all other kinds of personal health problem and all other kinds of health professional, and if decisions taken in such consultations define the nature of all consequent processes throughout the health care economy, then any economic theory trying to understand the operation of personal care systems as a whole should start from analysis of how players relate to each other at this initial point of production. This is the elementary particle of health care economy, as atoms and molecules are the elementary particles of physics and chemistry. If you get the shape of this basic block wrong, you will meet the same problems as a builder who tries to create a rectangular structure from elliptical bricks.

Note that though intuitively right for most experienced health professionals, Spence's simplistic view is rarely shared by health economists, journalists or politicians, not for the good reason that it omits all reference to collective public health functions or planning and organisation of care (discussed later on), but because technical interventions are the focal point of their vision, rather than the complex personal (or, for public health, social) interactions that precede and generate these interventions. They tend to assume that whether writing a prescription, performing a surgical operation or interpreting a diagnostic image, all these interventions are commodities sold as items to patients as consumers, even if the ultimate purchaser is some public agency. Because some clinical interventions resemble other less complex forms of commodity transfer, say cars or mortgage services, these (rather than decisions to initiate them) are their preferred focus for analysis.

To this most experienced health professionals will answer that though clinical procedures need to be performed competently and with thrift, the most fundamental issue is not whether they are done well or at best value for money, but whether they are done at all: whether any particular procedure is in fact the optimal solution for a patient's particular problems, yielding maximal health gain at minimal costs in time, pain, unhappiness and added risk. Entry to each level of the care system hierarchy entails at least some creative negotiation, at best a collaboration, between patients and professionals, not just a consumption. The consultation ends with decisions either to do nothing, or to intervene at primary care level, proceed upwards to a higher specialist, sideways to a different specialist or segment of primary care, or out from the care system altogether to some other more appropriate social agency, including a return to patients' and their families' own resources. The appropriateness of these decisions are critical to solution of patients' problems, and thus to productivity, effectiveness and efficiency of the NHS as a whole.

In defining consultations as the elementary particles from which the health care economy is formed, Spence left unanswered three important questions: how do these episodic consultations relate to each other – as isolated choices or linked into a sequential story? Do health professionals and patients relate to each other as providers and consumers, or in some other way? And finally, where are public health and the planning and organisation of care in all this? Spence's view concerned reactive personal tactics, with little to say about health and proactive care strategies. Answers to these three questions are linked. How most professionals, most patients and most governments view them still remains ambiguous.

Episodic and continuing care

With enough money in their pockets, and for such health problems as seem easily separated from the rest of their lives rather than inseparable from them, people today seem to see themselves mostly as episodic consumers. On the other hand, for health problems that seem inseparable from life problems and remain insoluble by body repairs, they still seek continuing care for themselves personally. At local and national government level they seek continuing assurance of a healthy environment in which to live, a socially healthy and biologically safe society. They then see themselves not as consumers, but as participant citizens, using a shared public facility.

When people look at the NHS not as spectators but as experienced participants with real problems, they want much more than a consumer role. Complex, continuing problems, including both biological and social factors, present the most difficult challenges to clinical medicine, and account for a high proportion of overall workload and costs. In the US, over 45% of people outside institutional care have one or more chronic health problems, and these account for 75% of US health care expenditure. In the late 1980s when these studies were done, most of these people with chronic problems were neither old nor disabled.[5] With ageing populations this proportion of people with chronic problems will rise. In 1948, when the NHS was born, it promised care from the cradle to the grave. Though successive governments have never fully accepted this responsibility,[6] and since 1979 have actively sought to repudiate it (but quietly), it endures as a public expectation that has been hard to evade.

Most acute episodic problems arise from these continuing problems, often because they have either not been treated at all, or not been treated effectively. Both medical professional and popular cultures prioritise acute somatic care. A study of GPs in Liverpool showed that they rated acute physical problems as appropriate to their responsibilities twice as often as chronic physical problems, and more than three times as often as psychological problems.[7] Chronic problems require more chronic than acute solutions, requiring emphasis on continuity. Episodic interventions fragment care, tending to keep patients in passive roles and promote professionals to heroic roles. Acute demands are inescapable prompts to professional action in a freely accessible service, whereas chronic needs can always be postponed. Acute crises have therefore dominated GP medical culture, supplemented by hospital emergency departments for episodic crises beyond GPs' competence or capacity, even though many of these crises need never have occurred, had there been efficient continuing anticipatory care.[8]

As primary care has become more rationally organised to control risks and prevent a rising proportion of crises, continuing primary care has become an area susceptible to forward planning, with predictable clinical content (providing numbers are large), and with opportunities to develop work by a wider variety of health workers, at much lower cost than the acute interventions arising when continuing care has not been given. Failure to develop systematic continuing care, doing a few simple things well for all who need them, has costly consequences. Terminal salvage prompted by crises is dramatic and heroic, but almost prohibitively expensive. Analysis of costs in an intensive care unit in Los Angeles showed that 8% of the patients used half the resources, though over 70% of these high-cost patients died while using them.[9] More rational care implies a shift in both professional and patient behaviour back from crisis interventions and body repairs toward continuing care, from concentration on effects to greater attention to causes, and toward greater interest and investment in the uncertain beginnings of disease, where clinical and social care meet the boundaries of public health. All these shifts depend on greater continuity: continuity of care, of experience, of thought, and across interprofessional boundaries.

Studying how errors occur, Cook, Render and Woods at the Veterans' Administration Patient Safety Center of Inquiry of the University of Chicago[10] found that in care systems more complex than the elementary doctor–patient particle considered by Spence, there were inevitably many gaps between people, stages and processes. Analysis of clinical errors usually revealed many gaps, but few of these seemed to produce errors. They concluded that safety was increased by understanding and reinforcing the normal ability of all players (including patients) to bridge these gaps and maintain continuity. This view contradicts the usual industrial management view that systems need to be isolated from their unreliable human element. To maintain continuity despite necessary division of skills, care systems need to become more human, more flexible and more open to judgement, not more tightly controlled.[11] It also contradicts the nostalgic view that continuity can be assured only by discarding teamwork and retreating to single-doctor, single-patient relationships.

Consumer choice?

Think tanks like the King's Fund, with ears prudently ('realistically') tuned to sponsorship, endorse wider consumer choice as a self-evident path toward more participation by patients in their own care. They underestimate and accept as inevitable the damage to continuity that consumer choice between competing providers must necessarily cause, and the piecemeal attrition of mutual support between agencies created by commercial secrecy and rivalry. The general public, and to a lesser extent medical and nursing professionals, now face both ways. People want future technology but dread its apparently inevitable consequence − that human contacts will become ever more infrequent, fragmented, tenuous and potentially adversarial. They want more episodic repairs, but tend fatalistically to accept that the price for these must be less personal, less continuing care, because this association has been their common experience.

Spence's elementary particle ignores the public health context within which personal care must operate to be effective. This indifference is still shared by most patients and most clinicians, but understood (and generally deplored) by health economists and policy makers. Historically, public health functions have always been divided both from repair and from care. If we accept that health care systems should produce health gain, some professional and institutional agency must exist to translate this aim into material, measurable terms across the whole population. This agency must set the strategies for the system as a whole, with latitude for tactical decisions at points of production. Such a system would include both personal care, in which consultations would operate as elementary particles, and collective or population care. This is difficult, perhaps impossible, to achieve in a system decentralised and fragmented into units competing for consumers. If it can be achieved at all in such circumstances, this will be by tight state regulation, compelling entrepreneurs to address public needs rather than profitable wants. Such regulation will then be pilloried as an intrusion on natural pursuit of profit, a burden on business that works best when left alone to do as it wants, by the permanent media claque to be expected when most sources of information and opinion are not only owned by top business people, but are themselves businesses run for profit. Orthodox health economists and policy developers address these problems as they address all failures of the market to meet social needs: by building parallel regulatory and supplementary structures to perform the functions that markets neglect or ignore, but these bolted-on solutions are always liable to attack as parasitic bureaucracy.

In fact, given political will and real respect for participative democracy, Spence's useful perception can easily be expanded to include public health decisions about groups and populations. Public health decisions also should entail consultations, though in a loftier sense than Spence ever intended, in which the same players are collectively rather than individually represented. Most public health doctors have in the past had the same arrogant, paternalistic and condescending attitudes to their public as clinicians had to their patients. Though many were progressive, all were by contemporary social conventions compelled to be despots. To rediscover integrity, both public health and clinical professionals must find ways to democratise their work, and accept their communities and their patients as their equals. If they succeed in this, both collective and individual consultations can still form fundamental units in a productive NHS economy.

Accepting that all sustainable change has to begin from where we are with the people we have, and from below rather than from above, the solution to this hitherto insoluble problem of integrating personal and community care must lie in the redefinition of the nature of personal care. This must include collective responsibilities within communities for the many health problems that are soluble only through collective action, and reconnect collective public health with personal clinical medicine. For most people in Britain (but apparently only a minority in the US), personal care in the health service is still seen intuitively as a collective gift based on shared responsibility. In the pre-'reform' NHS this was already evolving toward a less unequal consultation process, as a natural development from a less deferential public, quite separately from any transformation of citizens into choosy customers responsible only for themselves. And fewer health professionals were entering practice without undergraduate education in the social nature of their work.[12]

The patient–professional interface

When sociologists first started studying medical consultations objectively in the 1950s and 1960s, all were impressed by one most obvious finding: the extraordinary sustained rate of major decision-making, especially in primary care. By 'major' they meant, for example, decisions that patients' problems were or were not appropriate to the care system, that patients were or were not sick, that symptoms did or did not require further investigation or referral to a specialist, that health problems required treatment or were best left alone, that patients needed referral to this rather than that specialist, or to some activity or agency right outside the care system. Each of these decisions concerned next steps on pathways leading either sideways and away from the care system, further and deeper into it, or back to continuing care at primary level. Few of these were what most clinicians thought of as big decisions, but they looked big to sociologists, they felt big to patients, and had huge implications for the rational functioning of the NHS and its costs. These decisions actually *were* big, but most had to be taken within spans of five to ten minutes, many in less.

For clinicians, especially in primary care, the gravity of decisions becomes clear only in retrospect. For example, pneumococcal meningitis is a rare, insidious, frequently lethal disorder, usually in very young children, initially presenting as a slight fever with minimal illness – much like any other minor viral respiratory infection. Early treatment with appropriate antibiotics is effective, but escalation to irreversible brain damage may occur within a few hours if diagnosis and treatment are even briefly delayed.

The problem of handling 10,000 or more minor viral upper respiratory infections in such ways as to prevent one death from late diagnosis of pneumococcal meningitis (occurring at any random point in that sequence of 10,000) depends mainly on how apparently trivial problems are first handled, and what indications worried mothers understand for contacting their professional adviser again, perhaps only hours or even minutes after their first encounter. How such contingencies can be handled safely over the telephone, by nurse-practitioners who can't even see their patients, nobody has yet explained. Of course, the situation is rare, but similar situations precede most of the unexpected deaths in children that still occur, and the care system should be organised to respond to these.

Outcomes of care for exceptional problems depend on the nature of care for routine problems. Early recognition of life-threatening, rapidly progressive, treatable disease of this kind remains one of the most important processes of primary care, though it has rarely been studied prospectively because of the huge numbers that would be needed to find even a few such events. It depends always on delicately balanced relationships between two groups of players, health professionals and patients, merging evidence from both to synthesise effective decisions that create an eventual health product. In this scenario, there are no consumers, only two different kinds of producer.

I have chosen this example because I have experienced real cases, some with happy outcomes, others ending in tragedy. Broken into successive episodes with successive decision points about what to do next, one of these with a fatal outcome was used for a videotape, teaching clinical skills to doctors in primary care training.[13] The retrospectively 'right' and 'wrong' answers appeared to change at each successive decision point, in ways that at first seemed counter-intuitive to most students. The task at first contact with such a mother and child could not include an invasive search for every one of a vast range of possibilities, most of them so unlikely that most doctors would not see more than one or two in a working lifetime. Defensive medicine, diversion of effort from solution of patients' real problems to anticipation of doctors' hypothetical problems if faced later by charges of malpractice, erodes trust, incurs prohibitive cost and paradoxically impedes the clear thinking necessary to recognise exceptional situations before it is too late. At the same time it is vital that whatever the decision at each point in the story, it must not obstruct or exclude some unlikely yet possible later development. Initiative must remain with the parent (usually, but not necessarily the mother), because she is the only observer of her child who can be constantly present, and is familiar with her child's normal behaviour. This means that at each stage in the story she must feel completely confident that any decision she may make to use her time to renew contact will not be dismissed as a waste of professional time. This was the 'right' answer to questions posed by this videotape early in its course, not instant application of a diagnostic or treatment sledgehammer to every presenting peanut.

However hard this may be, professional and lay time must in such situations be equated; to assume that doctors' or nurses' time is more valuable than patients' time has dangerous consequences for these infrequent, unpredictable but (on a whole population scale) calculable outcomes. These cause a large and rising proportion of premature deaths as their frequency diminishes, to become concentrated in fewer and more exceptional events. Between the mother and her doctor, evaluations of risk and consequent decisions needed to be shared so fully that responsibility for their eventual results, whether successful or catastrophic, would also be seen and felt to be shared more equally. This implies a relationship between patients and professionals approaching those within families, not as a virtually unattainable ideal for sentimental reasons, but as an achievable aim for practical reasons. 'Our doctor was almost part of the family' is still a familiar phrase, not quite a folk memory, and represents a powerful weapon we need to retain.

Less than ideal experience

Everyday experience for most patients falls far short of this ideal. The following true story comes from Andrew Herxheimer's DIPEx archive of patients' accounts of their own experiences of illness:[14]

> 'OK, last August one Sunday evening I was reaching over on my desk to get a pen and felt a dreadful pain inside my right breast. Prior to that I had had some itching, my nipple was itching very, very intensely and, er, I didn't think about it, itchy nipple to me didn't mean anything suspicious. But when I felt the pain and the lump, er, I immediately was struck with fear and foreboding and didn't know what to do. My family were away visiting the in-laws and I had a dreadful night, but I had an appointment at the doctor's for the next day for something else, something totally unrelated. When I saw the doctor that day, the next day after finding the lump, er, when we'd finished about the prior consultation I mentioned that I'd found a lump in my breast and I was terribly afraid. He sent me in to see the nurse, the practice nurse, and, er, she basically dismissed it as being hormonal, my age, "80% of breast lumps are nothing, don't worry, go home, keep a diary."
>
> I went home feeling still very anxious and very worried

and, er, kept a diary. That was on the Monday. On the Thursday I hadn't slept for two nights, I felt dreadful and, er, so I phoned the nurse again and told her. And she said "You need an appointment with me and the doctor so can you come in on Tuesday?" That was eight days after the original appointment, which I agreed to. I went to the surgery that day and sat in the nurse's room for 22 minutes, half naked, feeling absolutely ghastly. She came into the room and said that the doctor was too busy to see me. That was like somebody stabbing a knife in me. Er, she took my blood telling me that this was all hormonal and I had nothing to worry about, go home. I went home, I went outside of the practice and broke my heart in the car. It still hurts to talk about this bit of my treatment because I felt as if I wasn't worthy of even seeing a doctor at that point. To be told that the doctor is too busy to see you when you have an appointment, when you're very worried and you've got a breast that won't even fit in your biggest bra was dreadful.

Anyway I went home and my sister, who was a mammographer of all things, was away on holiday. She came back on the Saturday and I confided in her. It was at this point that my life was turned around. She made me promise her that I would go to the doctor's and demand an examination. That I did on the Tuesday. I had the appointment for the results of my blood test and I walked into the doctor's, put my diary on the table, and said "I demand an examination." The doctor said he had examined me and I told him he had not and he said "OK, let's examine you now, I'll go and get the nurse." Prior to this the nurse had told me she wasn't qualified to examine breasts, but that appointment she did examine my breast with the doctor there. Again I felt as if I wasn't worthy of the doctor's attention, that the doctor was shunning me again but at least he did the right thing and he sent me straight to hospital.'

I sat in a largely medical audience listening to this patient's account of her experience, in a presentation about the DIPEx project. It was initially greeted with incredulity. Most of the audience seemed to think it lay outside normal experience of NHS care, in a sphere of criminal rather than clinical behaviour, like Dr Harold Shipman's deliberate slaughter of more than 250 of his patients, discovered a couple of years earlier. I'm afraid it had not surprised me. The range of behaviour of doctors and nurses is as wide as that of their patients.

Effective clinicians learn that no observed human behaviour lies outside our normal experience, even including Shipman. The aim of the DIPEx database is to understand the full range of patients' experience, just as the collected databases used for evidence-based medicine aim to include all clinical research experience. For a GP and a nurse both so obviously to fail even to try to understand their patient's fears, and so recklessly to dismiss the possibility that she was right and they were wrong, was certainly unusual – but cancer of the breast also is unusual, in that a large majority of lumps in the breast are indeed not cancerous, and this was the nurse's justification for dismissing her patient's fears. Even more unusual was my first example, pneumococcal meningitis presenting to me as apparently transient minor illness in early childhood, but professionals have a responsibility never to forget such possibilities.

The Shipman analogy also is apt. The only rational explanation I have seen for his behaviour was addiction to exertion of power – power of life or death over patients he had particularly encouraged to depend on him as their friend. Potential origins for such addiction exist for every student of medicine or nursing, because some use of this power is central to their work. Wherever practice becomes de facto unaccountable except to personal conscience, conditions exist for addiction to power and escalating abuse. Patient-murderers like Dr Harold Shipman and Nurse Beverley Allitt were extreme examples of dysfunctional professional behaviour, just as child torturers and murderers are extreme examples of dysfunctional parenting, but all these crimes lie within the limits of human behaviour, not outside it. These criminals are not monsters from some other species, but extreme versions of our potential selves; they look like us.

As a group, caring professionals have a long way to go before their relationships with patients always reach the quality they would like to receive when they themselves need care. Viewed not as consumers but as fellow-workers in production of health, patients also have much to learn. When these two groups bring their skills together, both learn from each other to become more tolerant, thoughtful, effective, better informed, and therefore more open to doubt. In this as in all social change, speed is less important than direction. The seeds of this change have always been there, in all consultations. We have always had some real, not mythical, examples of close, continuing and productive relationships between caring professionals and their patients, who have shared their evidence and have each respected the expertise of the other. The real problem has been to achieve care systems that promote rather than impede sustained growth of these relationships, which develop naturally in consultations between equals.

Material preconditions for optimal decisions

As I write, average time available for consultations in NHS general practice has risen slowly from about two minutes in the 1950s to about eight minutes by 2000. Many practices now reach averages of around ten minutes, without including a generally new dimension of nurse time, but there are still plenty with booking times of only five minutes per patient. The lowest average consultation times have always been in industrial (now mostly post-industrial) practices whose rates of complex morbidity, particularly psychiatric morbidity, are highest and therefore require most time for appropriate decisions.

Of those NHS patients who have received only five minutes of consulting time or less, only 30% think this is insufficient,[15] a disturbing finding. Doctors of the sort who engaged in objective studies of their own work before managed care policies compelled them to record data routinely (from whom almost all published research on general practice derives) are more aware than many patients that every measurable variable relating to quality improves with more time available, and all deteriorate with less,[16] at least within the fairly short consultation times customary in NHS primary care. With times of around 30 minutes available in Sweden and Finland, differences may be less critical. UK doctors who work faster do less listening, less explaining and transmit less information to their patients. They allow less patient participation,[17] and probably do less critical thinking, though so far as I know we have no evidence on this. Studies of trainee GPs in the late 1970s showed that unless they had special teaching using audiovisual feedback, with increasing experience they learned to work faster but to communicate less.[18] GP and undergraduate training has greatly improved since then in most centres, but under excessive (in most places, usual) workloads this trend soon reappears.

Studies of family doctors in North America, again selective for the minority of doctors willing and able to participate in research, show average consultation times of 22.6 minutes for new patients, and 17.7 minutes for patients already known. Even so, within US medical culture at least 20 minutes is said to be necessary for patients to participate fully in decisions.[19] Despite their more generous time, research in 1984 showed US physicians gave their patients an average of only 18 seconds to tell their story before interrupting and diverting them to their own preferred topics.[20]

The story in Europe is mostly the same.[21] Having enough time in consultations, and having GPs with time and inclination to listen, explain and encourage discussion of problems (which are patients' highest priorities and usually result in substantial clinic over-runs)[22] conflicts with administrators' higher priorities for starting and finishing times required for managed care targets.[23] Only in Sweden and Finland is there good evidence that decisions in primary care really have optimal time, averaging around 14 minutes for somatic problems and 30 minutes for psychological problems.[24] Average consultation times of less than one minute are usual throughout the former colonial world, for those who can afford access to medical care of any kind, now that patient charges have been restored almost everywhere as a precondition for funding by the World Bank.

Even within the consultation times now available for grossly under-resourced health workers in many care systems, a start can be made in helping patients to bring their own full potential to make decisions in primary care more accurate and relevant to the solution of their problems. Much more can be achieved in a short time if good records are created and maintained, with defined story lines and clear, cumulative (preferably graphic) display of tracking variables such as weight or blood pressure, which patients can see and understand, and if patients see professionals whom they know in a stable team. When patients begin to participate in decisions, they may gain confidence as citizens to support staff demands that they are paid for the time and diversity of skills necessary for truly shared decisions.

In a beautifully simple research study in former Yugoslavia, Igor Švab showed that letting patients present their own problems without interruption had virtually no effect on consultation length,[25] but yielded gains in goodwill and consultations more relevant to real problems. Contrary to GP folklore, most patients worry about saving their doctors' time. Most try to use less time themselves to make more available for others with more difficult problems.[26]

Medically unexplained symptoms

For up to about 30% of symptoms presented to GPs, and about 40% of symptoms presented to specialists, no evidence of any somatic cause can be found. Similar proportions of unexplained illness seem to have prevailed ever since the birth of universal public care systems after the Second World War, and were probably even greater in the less accessible but more consumer-oriented medical trade preceding them. Because medically unexplained symptoms more often involve fear of disease than disease itself, greater burdens of real disease also cause greater burdens of fear, and consequently more presentation of medically unexplained symptoms. Somatic morbidity is therefore always positively related to high psychosocial morbidity, and does not displace it.

Of medical outpatients referred to a London hospital in 1952, 39% showed no evidence of somatic disease. This study was repeated the next year, when it was 40%; apparently a constant, at least locally.[27] Studies in the Netherlands in 1994 showed about half of all patients referred to general medical outpatient clinics had no detectable organic abnormalities.[28] Studies of UK primary care in the 1980s and 1990s showed 20-25% of adults consulting GPs had no detectable somatic cause for their symptoms.[29] Though most of these symptoms are minor, transient and self-limiting, over one-third of them persist, causing distress, disability, frequent consultations and ultimately referral to specialists, often followed by cross-referrals between specialists, eventually ending with a psychiatrist.

Many if not most of those initially referred to medical specialists are sent for symptoms suggesting serious but early disease, suspected by patients or primary care staff. When no evidence of disease can be found, this outcome is as positive and necessary as confirmation of disease followed by appropriate treatment. Even so, later progression may reveal that early serious disease was in fact present. There is horrifying evidence of this from practice in the heyday of Cartesian dualism, when hysteria was a common dustbin diagnosis. Eliot Slater managed to follow up 85 out of 99 patients initially diagnosed as suffering hysterical symptoms at London's National Hospital for Nervous Diseases at Queen Square between 1951 and 1955, an average of nine years after this diagnosis.[30] Of these 85 'hysterics', 12 had died (four by suicide), 14 had become totally disabled, and 16 were partially disabled. Only 43 (50%) were still able to live independently, and only 19 were free from symptoms. By the time of follow-up, only 33 (40%) still lacked any sign of somatic disease, but even among, these ten now had good evidence of psychotic mental illness.

Trying to answer the question why these referred patients had been effectively dismissed, he found two features they all had in common. First, they had no physical signs of disease: but this had to be true at an early stage of virtually any disease. Second, they all had a multitude of symptoms. Since it was unlikely that all the complaints of patients with many symptoms could be accounted for by any organic condition, it followed that some of them must be non-organic; but if some of them were non-organic, why not all of them? This convenient and common professional assumption was very dangerous. It ignored the effects of disturbances in function of other organs and systems on brain function, and of disturbances in brain function on function of other organs. Fortunately even the National Hospital at Queen Square, a stronghold of professional conservatism, was capable of learning: a similar study repeated in the late 1990s showed that of 73 patients with medically unexplained motor symptoms, only three were found six years later to have a previously unrecognised neurological disease.[31] Slater not only destroyed hysteria as an acceptable label, he buried the dualist paradigm that gave it birth, at least among neurologists at Queen Square level.

Apart from the risks of misdiagnosing serious organic illness as minor disorders of emotion, thought or behaviour, we have consistent evidence that people with all forms of mental illness have higher mortality from organic disease.[32] The burdens on patients and on society caused by mental illness generally exceed both in volume and distress those caused by somatic illness.[33] A US cohort study of people over 65 showed that depression was associated with a rise in all-causes mortality of about 24% regardless of age, sex, lifestyle or physical illness.[34]

Thought is a function of brains, as ticking is a function of clocks. If you smash brains they stop thinking, just as if you smash clocks they stop ticking. People who believe in consciousness without a brain or souls without bodies can still work effectively in health care, but only by separating the credulity needed for their mystical beliefs from the scepticism necessary for safe practice. Without a distinction between ideas and things, between what we want and what verifiably exists, no useful understanding of health or illness is possible.

There are few tissues and no organs without some ultimate central connection to the brain. Every external input to the brain can modify thought, and every internal thought can modify perceptions, including pain and other common sensations like weakness, fatigue or the sounds of blood flow through the inner ear that are normally suppressed from consciousness. All thoughts can, in some circumstances, induce change of some kind in all those organs or tissues that have some ultimate central connection to the brain cortex.[35] These peripheral changes may in turn be centrally perceived and reinforce thoughts and fears about their cause, and so on in a rising spiral of fear. All disorders therefore have potential psychosomatic components, organic disease is a common and potent cause of mental and emotional illness, and mental or emotional illness (or robustness) may modify the course of organic disease, though evidence of substantial objective effects is much harder to find than the more enthusiastic psychosomatists often claim.

As there can be no such thing as a conscious patient without an active brain, thought modifies the natural history of every human disorder. This has nothing to do with moral strength or weakness. A patient usually disabled by severe pain may still be able to dance, sing or read a book, and may then suffer less pain, or even none at all, while doing so. This is not evidence that the pain or the disorder causing it is not real, it simply demonstrates that pain is a subjective sensation, the perception of which changes in different states of mind. Symptoms that commonly turn out to represent no recognisable underlying disease include chest, back or abdominal pain, tiredness, dizziness, numbness, headache, shortness of breath and sleep difficulties.[36] These presenting symptoms together account for roughly half of all first episodes of illness met in primary care. When followed up a year later only 10-15% are found to have been associated with detectable organic disease.[37]

Do consultations for medically unexplained symptoms represent over-use?

The high proportion of consultations for symptoms that prove in retrospect to have no medical explanation provide the main material evidence for myths of NHS over-use, particularly at primary care level. In industrial and post-industrial areas this myth gets some support from local knowledge (real or imagined) of the extent to which consultations are inflated by claims for benefit. These once formed a high proportion of GP workload in industrial areas, though much less in white-collar residential areas. Administrative reforms over the past 20 years have very greatly reduced this function for

GPs, but it remains a powerful folk memory, reinforced by the mistaken but common belief that costs of social insurance benefits come from the same purse as funding for the NHS.

The myth that consultations for retrospectively diagnosed 'non-illness' represent over-use or abuse is refuted by evidence, but this has not deterred advocates of NHS 'reform' from using it as a weapon in argument. Bosanquet and Pollard confirmed its grip on public opinion in their survey noted in Chapter One. Apparently unconcerned about whether it was true, they identified it as their best entry point for eroding obstinate public support for an inclusive NHS funded through social solidarity:

> ... almost two-thirds say that people visit their GP when there is no real need, simply because the service is free at point of use ... it is the public's readiness to concede over-use ... that points the way forward.... With 64% saying that there is over-use, there is a strong moral as well as practical case for a charge ...[38]

There is no way that any care system can function without the number of people consulting about worries greatly exceeding the number whose worries eventually prove justified. For example, rectal bleeding is an important signal of possible bowel cancer, for which early surgery is life-saving, but it still commonly presents too late. About 20% of adults have some rectal bleeding each year, but less than 1% of them consult a GP, and the proportion referred to a hospital specialist for further investigation is ten times less even than this.[39] For this example alone, and there are many others, there is overwhelming evidence that patients use the NHS too little rather than too much.

A case for systematic over-use can be made for proactive care, screening people for possible presymptomatic disease, where this is not supported by consistent evidence of net benefit. Where this is driven only by concern for public health, and where it is limited by competition for scarce staff time in primary care units responsible for the full range of primary care in whole, socially inclusive populations, we can be reasonably sure that proactive care will be undertaken only where there is good evidence of substantial net benefit. The real risks of over-use begin when we go down precisely that care-as-commodity path that Bosanquet and Pollard and other 'modernisers' want to pursue.

For example, screening for prostate cancer by measuring prostate-specific antigen (PSA) still lacks consensus endorsement by international medical science,[40] but by 2003 PSA screening in the US and Australia was too profitable to accept limiting evidence without a struggle. Autopsy studies of representative samples of men over 50 show that about 30% harbour cancer cells in their prostate glands, but only 8-10% develop clinical cancer during their remaining lifetimes. It is therefore not surprising if some microscopic evidence of cancer is found when six or more biopsy samples are taken.[41] Over 80% of clinical prostate cancers in men under 60 occur at PSA concentrations below the conventional screening threshold at 4 ng/ml.[42] Even with this threshold there is gross over-diagnosis and over-treatment, if the aim is to achieve not normal microscopic appearances, but longer and better lives. Attempts by expert professional groups to draw public attention to this evidence in Australia and the US have led to concerted personal attacks in the media, largely through patients' groups funded and used by the professionals and companies engaged in the private screening trade and consequent inflated surgery.[43] As profit enters, motivation, thrift, caution and scepticism depart. The limits of marketed interventions are set not by evidence, but by what the market will stand: in this case, by the readiness of frightened people to spend money on their own false reassurance.

What evidence is there that user charges, known to health economists as co-payments, have the selective effects on consultation rates required to restrain over-use, even if that were a real problem? Obviously user charges discourage use, but economists have good evidence that consulting behaviour has little elasticity. Poor people will give higher spending priority to consulting a doctor than to food, if they believe medical advice is needed.[44] The effect of user charges is simply to reduce all consultations across the board, regardless of the nature of the problems that prompt them. The effect is selective only for those with lowest incomes, least able to afford them, but most likely to be sick.[45] In the early years of the African AIDS pandemic, user charges were imposed at state-funded sexually transmitted disease (STD) clinics in Kenya on advice from the World Bank and as a precondition for international aid. Consultation rates fell by 60%.[46] Public care systems have collapsed throughout Africa: no money, no treatment.[47] User charges are advocated not to promote more rational behaviour, but to shift public behaviour 'corrupted' by experience of a free public service back to a 'normal' commercial pattern.

Emotional illness

At any one time, about 20% of people are in states of significant emotional distress.[48] About one-third of these consult their GP,[49] and in about 66-75% of these this problem is recognised as such.[50] Many people also fear illness, particularly when a friend or relative has recently suffered some unexpected and catastrophic event. Emotions, particularly fear, create their own symptoms: rapid heartbeat, rapid breathing, difficulty in breathing or swallowing, and perception of internal processes that are normally excluded from consciousness.[51]

The content of primary care is ultimately defined by patients, not doctors. The most powerful predictor of a successful outcome of consultation is agreement on a list of patients' main problems.[52] A Canadian study in the early 1980s showed that both parties agreed the same agenda for 76% of somatic problems, but for only 6% of psychosocial problems.[53] It is not patients' fault that only a minority have any of the diseases that used to dominate the curriculum in teaching hospitals and questions in examinations, and still do so in many. If patients accept the costs in time and loss of independence entailed in going to their doctors, their problems should be taken seriously even if time is short. The possibility of serious early disease is never absent, and cannot be dismissed only on the grounds that it is statistically improbable. However, misdiagnosis of emotional illness as organic disease can be just as destructive. Either way, experienced and effective clinicians give priority to positive evidence of problems (mental as well as physical) that patients probably do have, rather than negative evidence purporting to exclude problems they probably don't have. Mental illness deserves positive diagnosis in its own right, mainly from patients' own stories and opinions as initially presented. It should not appear to be a punishment for not having detectable physical disease.

Who decides what is illness, and why?

The scope of medical diagnosis is defined socially, not biologically. All life is by definition biological, so which aspects of life are regarded as within the scope of health care depends on conventions that in turn depend on whether a problem seems more likely to be soluble by this than by some other route. This judgement must eventually depend on agreement between patient and professional. As care comes to depend less on symptoms, and diagnosis becomes more an anticipation of impending risks, the initiator of this process may increasingly be a proactive professional.

Problems that can be solved quickly and completely by medical treatment, like meningitis or acute intestinal obstruction, are obviously a medical responsibility, but cure of this kind is a small fraction of NHS work. Particularly in mental and behavioural health, the border between what is and is not medical is much less obvious than it may seem within contemporary conventions. Judgements do have to be made. From time to time the idea is resurrected that all mental illness lies only in the eyes of beholders and of ruling social conventions. Experience of treatment has often been worse than experience of disease, and once a disease label has been applied, often on weak evidence, it may be difficult to remove.[54] However, this need not mean that disease is not real (both for patients and their families)[55] or potentially fatal.[56] Mind is a function of a material organ, the brain. Why should the brain, alone among body organs, be immune from disease?

For example, as well as systematic studies of how thought and behaviour in schizophrenia differ from normal in a wide range of cultures,[57] and impressive evidence that it depends little if at all on environmental experience,[58] we now have a huge accumulation of evidence about ways in which the biochemistry of thought in schizophrenia differs consistently from the biochemistry of thought within its very wide normal range. Continued search for better ways to modify this abnormal chemistry is rational and appropriate to the problem. We have good evidence that established treatments are effective,[59] and more so when applied early, in the first presenting episode of the disease.[60] Treatments should include psychosocial interventions,[61] which are very labour-intensive, as well as medications, which are much less so: a difference that often leads to almost exclusive reliance on medication. We need to remember that harmful side effects even of current treatment may be substantial, and to bear in mind at least 200 years of history in which a long list of behavioural, physical and chemical interventions have been imposed, many of them violent, with a ruthless arrogance that is in retrospect breathtaking, on people with schizophrenia.[62] How can we be sure that our present interventions are any less arrogant than those of the past? Only by *not* being sure: by awareness of our own fallibility, even though we know far more now than we did then.

We need to approach management of mental and emotional illness with extreme caution and sensitivity, and recognise that in this field more than any other, every intervention is experimental, and none can ever have a completely predictable result – and also to remember that patients need and want effective treatment, not philosophy.[63]

These judgements are hard enough in adults, but in children they become almost impossible. Starting in the US, professional perception of childhood mental illness justifying medication began to rise slowly in the 1970s, and steeply after 1980. The proportion of children who are unhappy most of the time, and the proportion whose behaviour at home or at school disrupts family life or teaching, is probably also rising. As in adult psychoses, measurable biochemical and even biophysical differences can be detected between the brains of affected children and 'normal' children, which is hardly surprising. Since brain behaviour operates biochemically, so that anger or despair are each accompanied by measurable chemical shifts, different behaviours will inevitably generate at least transient biochemical differences. However, if some biochemical intervention can be found that improves behaviour more or less consistently, this creates an opportunity for diagnosis and medication. Doctors who want to help children and their parents may feel justified in exploring that opportunity, and companies in search of new markets will be only too eager to assist them. This begs another much more important question: why are these children unhappy, or why is their behaviour impossible for parents or teachers to cope with? If we knew the answers to that, we might address causes rather than modify effects by starting children on medication while their brains are still growing and their behaviours are still most easily modified.[64] But perhaps that question is too big, would take too long to answer, or the answer might lie beyond the power of doctors, parents or teachers to apply. The prudent, middle of the road course is just to carry on prescribing whatever pharmaceutical companies have developed to replace their old products, as each in turn becomes discredited, and so the long list of medically approved abuse continues through its eternal cycle of alternating credulity and disillusion.[65]

The perceived incidence of childhood depression, attention–deficit hyperactivity disorder (ADHD) and autism have all been rising steeply over the past two or three decades.[66] In Britain the incidence of first diagnosis of ADHD seems to have peaked in 1996, and changed little between 1996 and 2001, suggesting that whatever it is,[67] it seems now to have stabilised at a prevalence of about 5.3 per thousand boys age 5-14, compared with between 40 and 260 per thousand in different surveys in the US.[68] ADHD behaviour usually improves when these children are given methylphenidate (Ritalin), a drug closely related to amphetamine.[69] For a stimulant drug to help already overstimulated children seems paradoxical, but empirically it seems to be so, with benefit sufficiently obvious to impress even sceptical parents and clinicians. Diagnosis and treatment in Britain have lagged far behind the US, leading some doctors and many parents and media commentators to claim that the NHS and our schools are neglecting a remediable problem.[70] In the US, on the other hand, the new fashion prompted enough concern among educators that behavioural disorders were being over-diagnosed and over-treated, for the Federal Drugs Administration (FDA) to commission an inquiry by the United Nations Narcotics Control Board, through researchers at the University of California. Its report showed that in 1994, 50% of children diagnosed as needing methylphenidate treatment for ADHD by 380 paediatricians had not received any psychological or educational testing, but were diagnosed and treated without any formal assessment. Between 10% and 12% of all boys aged 6-14 were using the drug.[71] Most seriously of all, this study confirmed others that have shown that methylphenidate also improved concentration in 'normal' children not diagnosed with ADHD, again bringing into question whether ADHD can usefully be regarded as a disease, rather than an extreme normal behaviour.[72]

British child psychiatrists and psychologists seem still to be divided on this issue, between unrepentant advocates of more active diagnosis and treatment, and sceptics calling for caution.[73] A Working Party of the British Psychological Society has warned against the rush to label naughty inattentive children as needing treatment for a disease.[74] However, most special-needs teachers know children receiving treatment from GPs, where the children have never had any skilled formal assessment. This was bound to occur after so much public discussion in news media, with distraught parents appealing for prescriptions directly to their family doctors, often after a diagnosis made by parents themselves after trying out the 'miracle tablets' recommended by their neighbour next door.

These parents and neighbours may also be familiar with amphetamine, popularly known as 'speed'. This was originally used to keep commandos and bomber pilots awake and concentrating long after their bodies told them to sleep, and later by all-night dancers and people needing to lose weight, anorexia being one of its side effects. When I came to Glyncorrwg in 1961 I found addiction to and dependence on amphetamine (readily available from an alcohol-dependent local chemist) was a major local problem, though at that time the pharmaceutical companies denied any risk of addiction or dependence, and most expert psychiatrists agreed with them. By the mid-1960s addiction to amphetamine and dexamphetamine was recognised everywhere as a major problem, and by the 1970s most countries had legislation to limit its use. Why should methylphenidate, its close chemical relative and with a similar stimulant action, prove different? As with earlier experience with amphetamine, manufacturers now deny any risk of dependence or addiction, but there is already plenty of anecdotal evidence that this is a growing problem among teenagers prescribed this drug, and this has been accepted by the FDA as a real risk.

In reaching these extremely complex judgements, children, parents, family doctors and child psychologists and psychiatrists can be sure of simple and unequivocal advice from at least one source that entertains no doubts whatever. In 2001, these ADHD drugs became the first prescribed drugs to be advertised directly to the US public, over the heads of their doctors, to create consumer pressure for diagnosis and treatment.[75] In 2003 the companies launched a sales offensive on the UK and other European countries to promote prescription of methylphenidate and dexamphetamine for ADHD. Per capita sales in the UK were still ten times less than US sales, and 20 times less in France and Italy, but rates were rising and sales were good. Though both drugs had been listed by the FDA as having addictive potential, prescribing in the US still rose more than seven-fold between 1992 and 2000, so that between 4 and 5 million US children out of a total child population of 80 million under 18 were estimated to be taking stimulant drugs, a legal market worth about US$ 1 billion annually.[76] Something is happening to all market-driven societies, which its leaders seem unable to admit even to themselves.[77]

Pressures on consultation time lead to hasty, impulsive clinical decisions using inadequate evidence, either evidence from what patients say and think, or evidence from professional knowledge. Pressures from pharmaceutical companies, and any other agency where profits depend on clinical decisions, offer simplified and attractive but biased choices that distort those decisions. Consultations are a delicate construct, which should be treated with more care, respect and protection from commercial pressures than they now receive.

Stories

About 85% of the evidence used to reach any final medical diagnosis comes entirely from what patients say – from their own stories. Physical examination adds about 7% to this, and investigations like X-rays, blood tests and so on add another 7%.[78] Accurate diagnosis therefore depends overwhelmingly on careful, thoughtful, unhurried talking by patients and listening by professionals to patients' stories. Diagnostic weapons cannot be aimed accurately and economically without a diagnostic hypothesis, which only talking and listening (and sometimes some waiting and seeing) can establish.[79] This must include the 50% of usually minor symptoms that eventually turn out to be self-limiting disorders of small consequence. In otherwise healthy people, policies of delayed labelling, waiting-and-seeing for two weeks or so, rather than rushing straight to complex investigations or referral, are safe, effective and still acceptable to most UK patients, though advancing consumerism makes such cautious approaches increasingly difficult. Providing patients get intelligible and truthful explanations of what is going on, a balanced assessment of risks and assurance that their carers are always open to new evidence and revised opinions, few have persistent symptoms they cannot live with for two weeks.

Somatised mental illness

Minor and usually transient symptoms caused by emotional states, particularly by fear or minor depression, generally respond well to a combination of attentive listening (with particular attention to patients' own ideas about possible causes), careful examination and possibly some simple investigation and explanation in simple terms, together with a positive invitation to return for later review. This is a field in which inappropriate investigations and treatment are not just wasteful, but dangerous. In the words of Jerome Frank:

> with many patients the placebo may be as effective as psychotherapy because the placebo condition contains the necessary, and possibly the sufficient, ingredient for much of the beneficial effect of all forms of psychotherapy. This is a helping person who listens to

the patient's complaint and offers a procedure to relieve them, thereby inspiring the patient's hopes and combating demoralisation.[80]

A minority, around 5% of patients consulting in primary care, have a major problem of somatised mental illness.[81] Some of these originate from patients presenting initially with minor symptoms, whose anxieties have been reinforced by early resort to defensive measures designed to exclude problems they probably do not have in their bodies, with little or no effort to find what they probably do have in their minds. Patients with major somatised disorder tend to get disposed of by hasty and excessive disease labelling, investigation, referral, cross-referral and inappropriate surgery.[82] They become 'thick file' patients, dreaded by doctors and often off-loaded to a series of specialists (ending with a psychiatrist) incurring mounting costs as they go.

Somatisation disorder is therefore a big problem, with big effects on NHS costs, effectiveness, efficiency and morale of staff and patients. It seems to be much commoner in people who have suffered physical or sexual abuse in childhood, the results of which in adult life seem to be identical. Surveys in the UK, the US, Germany, Switzerland and Australia all show around 20% of women and 8% of men admitting to experience of sexual abuse as children.[83] Among patients who consult their doctors often, around 25% admit to experience of either sexual abuse or serious domestic violence in childhood.[84] Looking at it the other way round, about one-third of people who experienced such abuse have a reported psychological problem, compared with about half as many in people who deny such experience.[85] As for domestic violence between adults, that social iceberg only began to be revealed in the 1980s, but has always generated huge undeclared fears.[86] Most people are surprisingly tough, but as Katon, Kleinman and Rosen said, if the only way you can draw attention to sadness or fear is to have a headache or palpitation, that is how you learn to complain.[87]

All this is confusing, as complex and difficult as most other aspects of human biology. We are a complicated species. But our greatest problems arise not from the always doubtful, uncertain and ambiguous nature of human health and behaviour, but from cocksure refusal to admit this, and belief that putting human problems into a dehumanised black box with medication or surgery as its sole instruments can produce a useful output.[88] If doctors or patients can find any reason, however implausible, for a mechanistic explanation of symptoms or a somatic label, most will seize this with relief, rather than enter the bog of their innermost fears and anxieties. Doctors may share these as much as patients. If any trace of even the most doubtful evidence of somatic disease can be found, preferably with some apparently simple surgical solution, both doctor and patient can return to short consultations about body engineering and repairs, and keep away from the threatening ground where causes lie. On the other hand, to have any hope of rational care with measurable health outcome, we must pay the price in more staff, longer consultation times, and wider, more sceptical and more compassionate imagination:[89] a black box designed from experience of handling human problems, not management of assembly belts.

Discretional surgery

So far, we have considered the black box of primary care, and rightly so, because 95% of first consultations end at this point, and decisions at this level largely determine not only whether people are referred to hospital-based specialists (secondary care), but who they will see and what will be done when they get there.[90]

The simplest and most familiar examples of specialist care, which have almost monopolised media attention to the NHS since it began to be pushed back into the marketplace, come from planned, discretional surgery – coronary bypass grafts, hip replacements, cholecystectomies and so on. Surgeons necessarily work in a culture of decision and vigorous interventions of an engineering kind. However, rational surgical practice is as complex and replete with difficult choices as rational medical practice, and requires equally sceptical shared decisions, unbiased either by management pressures, or by economic rewards or penalties.

Common surgical procedures in this discretional (elective) category include tonsillectomy and adenoidectomy for recurrent sore throats, grommets for middle-ear disorders, hysterectomy for excessive menstrual bleeding, cholecystectomy for gallstones and otherwise unexplained abdominal pain, hip and knee joint replacements, and the different operations now available for grafting or stenting diseased coronary arteries, all with great latitude for decision even within evidence-based consensus guidelines. As surgical procedures are applied at ever-increasing ages, decisions to operate entail increasingly complex judgements balancing inevitably transient health gains against immediate losses, in which patients and their families need to participate, confident that professional judgements are unbiased either by economic incentives or clinical aggression.[91]

For example, for hysterectomy alone, there are huge differences between countries, even between those with advanced economies and supposed to share a common evidence base. US and Australian rates are twice as high as British, but British rates are half those in Norway, despite similar prevalence of rational indications for hysterectomy in all four countries.[92] It has been said that to study the indications for hysterectomy is to study the interface between medicine and society.[93] Hysterectomy removes more than a uterus. For some women it assures a welcome end to reproduction, for others this finality seems a disaster. For some it justifies withdrawal from an unhappy sexual role, for others it threatens a good sex life.[94] Surgery may have placebo effects at least as great as medical treatment.[95]

Evidence-based decisions

Evidence-based medicine (EBM) is a concept introduced in the 1980s, with David Sackett the best known of its many parents. He defined it as 'the conscientious, explicit, and judicious use of current best evidence in making decisions about the care of individual patients'.[96] This is a statement with which few doctors could ever have dared to disagree for the past several hundred years, but behind it lay three new developments that gave these platitudes new force:

1. After the Second World War clinical research shifted from intensive before-and-after studies of handfuls of interesting cases in a few teaching hospitals, to randomised controlled trials with hundreds, thousands and eventually hundreds of thousands of patients, either networked in many hospitals, or in people sampled from many communities. The content of medical journals shifted from anecdotal accounts of interesting cases and intuitive reasoning about their significance, to reports of randomised controlled trials with reasoning based on formal logic and statistical analysis.[97]
2. Beginning with mechanised information technology (IT) in the 1950s and electronic IT in the 1960s, data could be accumulated, stored and selectively accessed, at first centrally, later peripherally at points of clinical production, at vastly higher speed and lower cost in office labour than in the days of case-notes, marginal perforated cards or Hollerith machines. By 1995 almost 90% of

UK practices used computers, and 55% used them to access clinical data or other information during consultations.[98] Medical brains could be used less for remarkable feats of memory, releasing them for better informed and more sceptical thought.

3. By the 1990s worldwide evidence from human experimentation in trials and meta-analyses of trials became available in concise summary form to every clinician with access to IT. This is now centrally reviewed and edited by the International Cochrane Collaboration (ICC).

Worldwide health care reforms are intended to rationalise care by applying this evidence, and reducing use of procedures still unsupported by controlled evidence that they are effective. Selected and condensed into clinical guidelines,[99] systems of managed care try to make routine practice more consistent with evidence from clinical trials.[100]

Sackett estimated that just to keep up with new evidence in the field of internal medicine, clinicians needed to read 19 articles each day for 365 days a year. According to their own probably optimistic claims, NHS consultant physicians actually spent an average of less than one hour each week on this task. What at last made systematic application of evidence feasible 'at the bedside' was IT, and through this a central store of cumulative summarised knowledge, the ICC. This was initiated by Iain Chalmers, one of Archie Cochrane's apprentices, who had already pioneered evidence-based obstetric practice, delighting most midwives but infuriating many in the medical obstetric establishment. The ICC brought together a global network of expert committees able to produce meta-analyses merging data from numerous small trials to reach consensus conclusions, and from these to develop guidelines for everyday practice. All this cost money, readily forthcoming from governments convinced that if medical care could be made rational it would also be more cost-effective, more susceptible to management, and more compatible with conventional economic thought in the post-Keynesian era.

Guidelines can help to apply useful knowledge about human biology more effectively, but as soon as we try to use them in the real world, we meet two difficulties. First, few (often none) of the experts responsible for developing them have enough experience of the real conditions in which they will have to be applied to understand how they should be designed or propagated, or their limitations in practice, particularly their implications for staff workload outside their own centres of excellence. There seems to be an unstated but implicit assumption that quality of care must naturally deteriorate with increasing distance from these centres, and that the job of experts remains what it has always been in the past – to set a standard to which others should aim, even without proper resources, and regardless of the feasibility of attaining them.

Second, they reinforce the tunnel vision natural to specialists but wholly inappropriate to generalists, by formulating guidelines for single problems, ignoring the fact that primary care generalists must usually deal with multiple co-existing problems. In the real world of advanced economies, most patients are also old, usually needing a long learning period to accustom themselves to regular medication and follow-up, if they ever learn this at all. We still have insufficient research and therefore few guidelines derived from experience of caring for these real older people, but one thing we know: their progress depends on continuity of care, in the sense that the whole care team is known personally to the patients, and all the patients are known personally to the team. This does not sit easily with the often-fragmented tasks listed by guidelines, where the objective may soon become entirely one of ticking boxes to reach targets rather than achieve control over disease. Particularly is this so when staff become paid according to outputs measured in this way, as they are under contracts in the new health care market.

For example, guidelines produced by the US Preventive Services Task Force in 1993 required the average patient attending for outpatient care to have 15 different risk factors assessed, requiring decisions about 25 different possible interventions.[101] For guidelines to be followed intelligently rather than by rote, staff need to believe in them. The best way to achieve this is for staff to participate in the development of the guidelines. Guidelines prepared centrally by experts are at best only a starting point for staff expected to apply them in the field. Despite these caveats, guidelines are necessary and useful. A study of 24 East London practices in 1994, all of which had already established disease registers (and were therefore of above average quality), showed that only about one-third of all diabetics had ever had their weight recorded, and less than a quarter had smoking status recorded.[102] Just over one-third of all asthmatics had ever had any aspect of lung function recorded, and less than 20% had smoking status recorded. Of course these tasks needed urgently to be done, rational care was not possible without them, but consequent staff workload had either been ignored or grossly underestimated by NHS authorities.

All this has encouraged extremely sceptical if not cynical attitudes to guidelines from clinicians in the frontline. Because their earnings are increasingly tied to evidence that guidelines have been followed and that their targets have been met, this rejection may be superficially concealed, but for most medical and nursing staff it remains a chilling truth. EBM and its guidelines have often made their work more difficult, without making it obviously more effective.

General use of guidelines entails two inevitable risks. First, in practice, they easily become tramlines, not guiding judgement but replacing it by a checklist of ritual actions, performed whether or not the performer understands or believes in them. At worst, these checklist actions may be undertaken by different health workers who seldom if ever consult to interpret them, and thus gain some sense that their work has been useful for patients, rather than for attainment of targets. Such effects are easily visible in current medical and nursing practice, particularly where performance, funding and legal defence all depend on having every box ticked.[103] The new GP contract operating since 2004 adopted this pattern, with an apparently rapid effect on GP behaviour: ticked-box output rose rapidly. This raised practice income and resources, and it also raised the value of primary care as a business, for any corporate predators competing in this new market. GPs fear that attainment of ticked-box targets will be used to construct league tables to encourage competition between practices similar to those already being used to encourage competition between hospitals, with new health care companies bidding against them for customers. Outputs and productivity measured in this way by evidence of completed process are likely to relate little to outputs and productivity of health gain. They will promote responses to consumer demands, but not to health needs of communities. Consumers with already high expectations will demand and receive relatively more, communities with low expectations will have these confirmed. Government could mitigate this effect of any market by regulation, but this will be seen as intrusion on an otherwise natural and spontaneous process, always vulnerable to deregulation in the name of freedom and choice.

Second, if pharmaceutical companies, or any other sectional interest, can influence the content of nationally adopted guidelines, this may have economic implications too large for professional integrity to resist. Researchers in Toronto who studied 200 authors of 44 clinical guidelines used in North America found that 87%

were experts with undisclosed financial links to pharmaceutical companies.[104] We all hope that equivalent British agencies like the National Institute for Clinical Excellence (NICE) will manage to stay free from corruption of this kind, but it has already had to be warned by WHO about the company connections of some of its advisers.[105] The ICC probably will stay independent of commercial pressures if this is possible. It devoted a world conference with around 1,000 delegates to this subject in 2004, but increasing commercial penetration of university departments, encouraged by government, makes independence for any influential agency extremely difficult.

Evidence from patients

These problems will be much easier to solve when we all accept that EBM as generally understood still lacks a necessary dimension, namely evidence from patients. Substantial progress is probably impossible without it.[106] We have already seen that at least 85% of personal diagnoses derives from listening to patients' own stories, and that outside hospitals, patients or their informal carers become 100% responsible for actually carrying out whatever treatment has been agreed. Failure by patients to perform either of these tasks impedes production of health gain just as much as failure by professionals. Patients are just as able to benefit from guidelines, and they are equally confused by guidelines devised by experts ignorant or careless of the world in which they must operate.[107] Cumulative research evidence about patients' experience of illness and treatment is as necessary and feasible as cumulative research evidence about medical or nursing experience.

Thanks mainly to Andrew Herxheimer, this evidence is becoming available through the International DIPEx Library and website (www.dipex.org), from which I have already quoted an example earlier. This excellently designed user-friendly website at one stroke replaces all the books ever written as aids to lay understanding of illness and its treatment, at minimal cost and in far more accessible forms. It also provides essential learning material for all health professionals, which is now beginning to be used for undergraduate and postgraduate medical education. DIPEx provides a potential foundation for Chief Medical Officer Liam Donaldson's imaginative programme to facilitate development of expert patient networks throughout the UK, giving further education to volunteers with experience of particular chronic disorders to assist their own care.[108]

Though as I write government plans seem not to include developing some of these expert patients to help others with similar problems, it is hard to believe this will not eventually occur, and develop into an important new counselling occupation within the NHS.

Discussion about the Expert Patients Programme, now in its third year with over 2,000 patients having gone through a six-week educational course, has mainly concerned gains for these patients in managing their own care, as if they were consumers more than citizens, and mainly needed help in choosing alternative retailers. As yet, few doctors seem ready to welcome patients positively as co-producers, rather than embarrassingly well-informed critics. In 1999, only 21% of doctors in a random sample welcomed the Expert Patients idea, 58% predicted it would increase GP workload, 42% thought it would increase NHS costs, and only 12% thought it would improve doctor–patient relationships.[109] Another poll in 2003 found that 76% of pharmacists, 63% of doctors and 48% of nurses thought better-informed patients would take up more of their time, be more demanding, and be harder to deal with.[110] Objective studies of patients receiving more education about how to manage their disease show exactly the opposite, reducing medical consultation rates by at least 42%.[111] Typically, the response has been not more vigorous promotion of policies based on evidence, but retreat in the face of stubborn intuitive fears. A *BMJ* editorial on the subject welcomed suggestions that Expert Patients should be renamed as Involved Patients, Autonomous Patients, or Resourceful Patients;[112] anything, so long as health professionals did not in practice have to accept that patients have intelligence, information and expertise, which could assist care rather than obstruct it if they were encouraged to have a more active role.

Used as a foundation for the development of Expert Patients as an extension of teams both in primary and hospital care, and combined with evidence from controlled trials through the ICC, DIPEx could provide a complete patients' international database to complement the Cochrane Library, which now also accepts inputs from patients. From these two sources truly evidence-based practice could be developed at all levels, from international and national policies, to the most peripheral primary care units developing their own guidelines. Whether this possibility is actually realised will depend on whether professionals have enough maturity, self-knowledge and political realism to welcome more informed and assertive patients as their allies, or, as the evidence cited in the last paragraphs indicates, they continue to see them as just one more problem. As professional fears are already refuted by evidence, their perception could change, but this will depend on courage and imagination presently very scarce on the ground. It will depend also on whether enough patients retain their dignity as citizens, and refuse demotion to consumer status – in fact, for both parties, it is a political and social challenge rather than a technical problem.

Managed care: who for?

Accessible databases of professional *and* patients' evidence are preconditions for EBM, but do not of themselves ensure that decisions in practice will become evidence based.[113] This requires escape from a deeply rooted traditional culture of medical dominance and patient submission expressed at best through paternalism and at worst through trade, which systematically ignores, minimises or embezzles the always-necessary but customarily invisible contribution of patients to diagnosis and treatment.

As always, this escape can choose either of two directions. Patients' evidence can be used to encourage more discriminating selection by individual consumers in markets of competing providers. This eventually self-financing trade would be peripheral to core services still provided by the state as an ultimate human right for the indigent, preserving token loyalty to the NHS as conceived in 1948. New developments would occur at the new commercial periphery, not at the residual NHS core, so that the system could eventually become a self-financing commodity market, its proportion of all health care determined by what the market could bear. In this case providers and consumers would confront each other as in any other transaction – caveat emptor; let the buyer beware. This process would proceed at the same pace as gentrification of the population as a whole, which has no natural limit. People still unable to pay for necessary care would get it, in suitably spartan form, from what would remain of the NHS, but as more wealth spilled from the tables of the rich, everyone might eventually get included, state care could wither away, taxes could fall, the consumer would be king, and doctors would finally be put in their place – regulated by government, managed by their corporate employers and restrained by their own need to charm customers. Suitably regulated to restrain outright fraud, this consumerist scenario is the solution toward which global capitalism is now moving, led in Europe by New Labour.[114] Regardless of the declared intentions of policy makers, in this consumerist scenario evidence from providers and consumers would remain divided, because they would serve opposed interests. Each might learn from the other, but only as all providers and consumers must try to understand what the other is up to.

The alternative is that patients and professionals combine their two sets of evidence to form something new: a human biology including the full range of human experience and behaviour, its cultural and behavioural foundations as well as its material basis in anatomy, physiology and pathology. In this way medical practice could begin not just to use science, but itself become part of science, unique among sciences in that we would be both its subjects and its objects. Having made huge gains in effectiveness through respect for scientific thinking, health professionals continually seek new ways to bring their practice closer to scientific methods, recognising the essentially experimental (because not fully predictable) character of all interventions in health care. This has brought some of our most conservative professionals to recognise that without developing patients as equal partners, health care cannot advance beyond episodic repairs for end-stage pathology. Effective action to promote and preserve health depends on often very simple tasks undertaken jointly with all of the people, not just the minority already in obvious health breakdown. In this practical and material fashion, most health professionals are already entering a de facto alliance with their patients and the populations they serve. However uncertainly, their feet are already set on a path toward participative democracy and a broad alliance.

With socially informed imagination, virtually all consultations provide opportunities to develop new relationships between professionals and patients, in either of these two opposed directions. At first, their divergence may not be obvious, but if we look at populations as a whole, it quickly becomes so. As consumers, an already confident and well-informed minority of usually affluent and conventionally educated patients will become ever more confident and better informed as it picks its way through an NHS of diminishing scope, and avails itself of a widening variety of commercial alternatives. The NHS Expert Patients Programme could create a powerful collective force of citizens participating in a stronger NHS, but as matters now stand in England, with its published initial plans couched throughout in consumerist language, it seems more likely to accelerate disintegration into competing units, though this was probably not intended by its authors. With personal expectations already beyond the capacity of public service to meet them within presently conceivable resources, these Expert Patients could destroy the few barriers still left between public service and private trade, resulting in an even swifter inflow of commercial attitudes.

Most people with the most difficult and complex health problems, on the other hand, would be left to survive as best they could with core services, designed for crisis salvage rather than for continuing care, provided by staff they would no longer trust, who would in turn fear their patients. Finally, increasing numbers would bypass failing primary care to enter the revolving doors of A&E departments already familiar in the US, filled with people who need never have had accidents nor ever have become emergencies, had elementary continuing care been available from people they knew. Whether this will occur depends not on the intentions of government, but on what the first cohorts of Expert Patients decide to do with themselves. Despite all pressures from consumerism, their wish to help others in similar situations may prevail, and in this they would have support from most NHS staff.

For patients to develop their full potential as co-producers of health, trusting relationships have to be rebuilt on a new basis, not on faith or deference but on evidence. The old trust in professionals rested on myths of omniscience, supported by both sides. Doctors in competitive trade could not afford to admit either that science as yet had no answer, or even if it had answers, they did not know what they were. Doctors in competitive trade could not afford to say 'I don't know, but let's find out' and then reach for a book or search a website in front of their patients. They could not afford to reveal in practice that biological science rests on doubt, not engineering certainty, and that doctors' heads are not books. When their useful knowledge was small, medical pretensions of knowledge seemed almost infinite; the medical profession behaved as though it knew everything and patients knew nothing. Both parties colluded in this deception, because placebo effects were virtually the only means they had. Placebo effects depended on faith, a fragile asset best left undisturbed. Though now severed at its roots, much of this culture of mutual self-deception still persists; rubbish that must be actively swept away by patients together with professionals.

Reification of disease

Scientists look for questions that seem answerable. Searching the border between their expanding knowledge and the consequently expanding volume of perceived ignorance, to have any hope of success scientists must break this actually continuous boundary into manageable sections, simplifying and therefore to some extent falsifying reality so as to get a better look at it, analysing one bit at a time. In practice this reductionist approach has proved useful and effective for solving real health problems. An important consequence is that once any new field has been well developed, new advances tend to occur along its outer boundaries with other specialties, rather than at its obvious core.[115] This re-integrates fields that once were separated, in an endless cycle of initially useful but eventually counter-productive divisions, followed by rediscovered unities.

Applied to human health, such reductionism led to the extremely useful concept of diseases as entities distinct from their individual human hosts, though in fact these are inseparable: no disease can exist by itself, all are particular forms of the human condition, occurring in diverse individuals.[116] In recognisably modern form, this idea began in the 18th century, along with the Linnaean classification of animals and plants. It reached its zenith toward the end of the 19th century, when a period of extremely rapid advance in bacteriology provided a model for disease as a bestiary of predatory parasites, occupying their human hosts and thriving at their expense. This reification of disease was powerfully reinforced and vulgarised by medical practice and above all by the medical trade, which needed ways to simplify the otherwise unmanageably complex health problems of real patients, and simplified language in which to explain and think about them.

This had negative as well as positive consequences.[117] Medical students and nurses learned encyclopedias of disease, as if diseases were independent species, stalking life's jungle in search of human prey, in which patients as people could be treated with veterinary indifference, uninteresting vehicles of interesting diseases. Pharmacologists looked for magic bullets with which to shoot them, designed so far as possible to hit the diseases but not the patients. Both sets of ideas worked better than any previous philosophy: arsphenamine targeted syphilis in 1910, sulphonamides targeted streptococcal infections in 1935, penicillin targeted staphylococci and many other infections in 1943, and for the next couple of decades new breakthroughs in treatment of infectious disease became almost annual events.

However, reification of disease disintegrates whenever we move back from end-stage diseases to their origins. Late or post-mortem diagnosis – from which our entire classification of disease and system of clinical thought has grown – concerns converging probabilities in people sick enough to enter teaching hospitals, established as museums of gross, end-stage pathology.[118] On the other hand, early diagnosis, the chief concern of all health professionals in primary care, concerns diverging possibilities in people not yet sick, most of whom we hope to keep out of hospitals of any kind. We need a different system of thought, incorporating management of end-stage disease because this will not go away, but far wider in scope to include the earliest beginnings of disease, often much sooner in life, where the future is hugely less predictable; widening possibilities rather than narrowing probabilities.

This new way of thinking has already united hitherto separate end-diseases into more useful single categories of potential disease closer to their causal origins. For example, most central obesity, high blood pressure, type 2 diabetes and disease of coronary and other major arteries, can all be gathered into the single category of insulin resistance (the metabolic syndrome),[119] easier to understand and modify as a graded health problem than as a qualitatively distinct entity.[120] Most professionals working in primary care still assume that all scientific innovation comes from hospitals, but hospital-based specialists may find it more difficult to merge their specialties as this evidence suggests they should. Few in primary care have yet recognised this new category as more effective and efficient for organising anticipatory care than separate clinics, though this has long been obvious to researchers.[121] If primary care can escape from its present tight industrial management, this development will certainly occur.

Cascades of misfortune

By the 1960s, few people in developed economies were dying young from infectious diseases. As major causes of premature death, infections were replaced by injuries, cancers, auto-immune diseases and degenerative diseases of the brain and circulation. None of these resembled invasions by parasites, though this was still the way most people had learned to think about them. They were more like internal mutinies.[122] With an appropriate weapon aimed accurately by a correct diagnosis doctors could kill pneumonia or meningitis with a quick burst of fire over a few days, with little risk of injuring their patients, and little need or opportunity to get to know them before they returned to their anonymous lives. Internal mutinies were different; they were inseparable from patients' lives, often requiring lifelong supervision and follow-up, and substantial investment of staff time to help the patients understand their disorder so that they could participate intelligently in monitoring and modifying its course.[123] We have research evidence that investment in this shared understanding greatly improves productivity of health gain.[124]

We have already seen in Chapter Two that multiple problems are commoner than single problems. Misfortune provides its own multiplier. It's just one damned thing after another, a cascade of misfortunes, social as well as medical, each downward slide accelerating the next, drawing new problems into a rising and finally irresistible flood. There is no mystery about social class differences in morbidity or mortality, which increase at every stage of human development throughout life.[125] Every experienced worker in primary medical or social care knows families so beset with multiple and multiplying problems that their highest aim is simply to survive from one day to the next, a minority group of shifting composition that sets some of the sternest tests faced by any inclusive care system, but is so far as possible ignored by the care market.

This cascading process is hugely significant for the economy of health care. Early interventions, requiring little technical skill but much time and thoughtful social experience and judgement, can be far more cost-effective than late crisis interventions using high technology and expertise.[126] Yet over and over again, resource-starved acute services are compelled to steal from anticipatory care budgets, so as to sustain crisis care and thus hopefully avert public scandals, pillorying by journalists, and the ire of politicians whose careers depend on the next election. No one with their feet on the ground can justify withholding care in a crisis because anticipatory care for those not yet in crisis would be more cost-effective, but crisis care is our everyday reality in most public services, social as well as medical. When services are grossly underfunded overall, as they were in UK for at least the last three decades of the 20th century, anticipatory care of people not yet seriously ill is forced into grossly unequal competition with heroic end-stage salvage, and loses every time.

Medical and nursing records[127]

Clinical records provide most of the evidence we have from which to measure quality of the decisions initiating processes inside the black box. They provide the verifiable material links between clinical episodes, between different professionals in a single unit, between units in the generalist–specialist referral hierarchy, between the NHS and other social agencies, and between the NHS as a whole and the population it serves.[128] Most errors and inefficiencies arise at these linkage points, not in performance of the clinical tasks they connect.

By most professionals even today, records are tolerated rather than loved. They provide verifiable evidence about decisions often so blurred by doubt and uncertainty that some errors are inevitable, a fact which managers, lawyers and journalists often ignore. For many NHS staff much evidence actually used to make important decisions seems safer in their heads than when written or entered into a computer. They see records as evidence used for administration to apply either punishments or rewards, rather than their own indispensable aids to effective, self-critical work as independent creative workers.

For primary care of industrial workers and their families, medical records scarcely existed before the NHS, normally consisting only of lists of medicines prescribed and certificates of incapacity issued, with at most a cursory diagnostic label. They rarely contained any of the evidence on which such diagnoses were supposed to be based. Though most GPs knew their patients fairly well, they carried their life and health stories in their heads, inevitably with gross simplification and stereotyping – caricatures of real lives.[129] In almost all cases, the only elements in these records containing any usable evidence were hospital letters from specialists, usually stuffed into the record envelope without regard to date order, and then rarely consulted. These letters were often useful, because most consultants wrote them primarily as succinct case-summaries for their own use, with information to GPs as a byproduct. Somewhere in the patient's record it was important for hospital staff to have a summary making some sense of what seemed to be going on. If this could be found at all, it was in these letters.

When evaluating different international care systems, quality of primary care records is a good indicator of maturity in the system as a whole. Slowly and erratically, GP records worth reading began to appear in a few UK practices in the 1960s, became commonplace in the 1970s, and were almost universal by the 1980s. Today well over 90% of all NHS GPs use electronic computer-held records for at least some aspects of patient care, and since 2004 GPs' contracts have become virtually unworkable without them. In mid-2004 over half of all UK practices were either using a computer-based medical record as their sole clinical record, or were close to doing so, and 80% are expected to reach this stage by 2006.[130]

Plans are now in hand for all UK patients to have direct access to their online primary care records,[131] and there is evidence of substantial popular demand for a patient's right to enter their own data in them.[132] A small but growing proportion of practices with fully computer-held records have direct links to local hospital diagnostic and outpatient departments. The rate-limiting factor for development of a single unified NHS record, usable at any level, is the still generally primitive and uncoordinated state of hospital records compared with GP records. Much less hospital data is computer-held, and a single NHS record usable throughout all levels of the service remains a promise possibly ten years ahead if we are lucky, though we are still paying for similar promises made periodically at colossal cost since the 1970s and still unfulfilled.[133]

Several explanations have been offered for the backwardness of hospital IT compared with UK primary care, including the fact that patients referred to specialists tend to present more difficult clinical puzzles, poorly suited to the still primitive capacities of computer programmes depending on essentially obsolete systems of disease labelling.[134] A more fundamental problem is that in order to develop a viable system, programmers must understand the processes their programmes will serve, in biological, social and economic terms. These purposes are probably better agreed and more clearly defined in primary generalist care than in hospital specialist care. Primary medical care is not divided between rival specialty fiefdoms, and largely thanks to the Royal College of GPs (RCGP), has developed a unified postgraduate teaching programme with a coherent philosophy over the past 50 years. This still cannot be said of the hospital physicians, surgeons, obstetricians, anaesthetists and diagnostic specialists who together compose hospital medical staff, or of their various Royal Colleges. In the absence of clear leadership from clinicians, development of IT in hospitals has depended on managers, few of whom now have backgrounds in health care. Their main aims have naturally been to satisfy higher management and government demands to control waiting times, bed occupancy and staff deployment, rather than to help clinicians to work more effectively.[135] Of course, these process measures are important, but they should follow from clinical process, not lead it.

I have already referred in Chapter One to the 'Choose and book' function included in the new IT system (National Programme for Information Technology: NPfIT) now being developed for England at a presently estimated final cost of £30 billion, but rumoured among experts in this field to be more like £60 billion. It seems scarcely credible, but this system is being developed without regard to any of the existing IT systems already in use by virtually all primary care teams for many years, enough to have accumulated a great deal of experience of their possibilities, limitations and pitfalls. The plan seems to be that if and when this programme is completed, this product of theory without practice will then displace the IT systems now functioning in primary care.[136] Both hospital-based specialists and politicians still seem to assume that all worthwhile innovation has to come from hospital systems, even though government policies encouraging consumerism were originally presented as 'a general practice-led NHS'. To anyone familiar with how referral pathways upward and discharge pathways downward actually operate, it is obvious that the way to avoid another immensely costly IT disaster would be to build on what already exists in primary care, extend it upwards to hospital specialist care, and from this to create a truly integrated system. This would have no need to include trading functions that nobody except the private sector lobby wants or has asked for. Though there are still several different competing primary care IT systems, all of these are already able to exchange data between them, and there is already a single system used by about half of all teams. There is a real danger that in England, by the time these problems begin to be recognised by government, too much will already have been invested to allow dignified retreat. There is a real opportunity here for devolved governments in Wales and Scotland, which so far have stayed at arm's length from the English IT project, to take the lead and develop rational programmes from where they actually are, with the people they actually have.

Computers perform in milliseconds necessary drudgeries that once occupied years of human labour. They make locally, nationally and internationally coordinated networks for upward, sideways and downward communication readily feasible, which were formerly hard even to imagine. Paradoxically, some of their major advantages lie in their inhumanity. Soon after they were introduced, imaginative pioneers discovered their value for gathering human evidence without making judgements, so that patients could open their real lives without the embarrassment of a human listener. After an initial computer-led search for concealed problems like alcohol dependence or abusive relationships, evidence so gained could provide a basis for subsequent more realistic human assessment, jointly with health professionals, to reach fairer judgements.[137] The ruthless logic of IT and its assimilation of data to statistical form reveal truth and make deception readily detectable.

However, with these powerful virtues come dangerous new sources of error. Most obviously, it may produce doctors who spend more time interacting with their computers than listening to their patients, and who place computer screens so that patients can only guess what is going on. It may dehumanise consultations and confine them to even narrower and less imaginative agendas.[138] This issue is now generally tackled well in undergraduate teaching, and clear ground rules have emerged that could humanise the use of computers in consultations.[139] Use of check-lists as a framework both for care and for rewards and penalties required by management is a growing and dangerous trend, closely bound up with IT, which threatens yet again to replace judgement by ritual — a degradation of medicine that has occurred repeatedly throughout its history.

To write a viable computer programme dealing with human decisions it is essential to start from a valid model of how these are actually reached in best practice. Fundamental philosophical problems of the nature of clinical information are rarely addressed. Examples cited in this and earlier chapters show that present diagnostic practice is often closer to chaos than clarity, but at least chaos can provide flexibility, choice and a human face. Once locked into the logic of a computer programme, such qualities may disappear. Computers conscript users to theoretical models on which their programmes have been based. This presents exciting opportunities for rationally planned development, but also dangerous possibilities for the imposition of fundamental error, built into the foundations of entire health care systems and dictating their modes of thought.

Clearly, we need one single national, and eventually international, IT language in which the evidence used by medical science can be expressed. This single language must necessarily incorporate assumptions about the nature of the evidence it describes. In its widest sense, human biology must include sociology because we are social animals. The evidence used by medical science is not a growing and potentially limitless pile of independent facts, but the story of an extraordinarily complex species, told by itself to itself, for its own use to make its own future story more human than its past. It is conceivable, though probably unlikely, that our foreseeable future might still be constrained by the requirements of commodity trade, but medical science cannot in any circumstances accept that its universal language should incorporate this assumption and deny alternatives. If we did, we would close the door to real competition between the recent and — it is to be hoped — ephemeral philosophy of care as a business transaction, and our ancient but evolving philosophy of care as an expression of human solidarity.

Confidentiality

All four nations in Britain are now trying to develop regionally networked records interchangeable at all levels of the NHS. Costly past experience suggests we shall get viable systems later rather than sooner, but ten-year targets are probably feasible, given sustained political will to overcome sectional interests. Obviously these systems must be accessible to all staff using data from them and adding data to them, but with electronic records duplication is easy. Less obviously, their inputs and outputs should be accessible to patients. Present policy in Wales is committed to records designed around patients' life stories, and therefore readable and understandable by them and their families. Obviously these will include some data that are not readily intelligible to patients, or even to non-specialised staff, but these technical data will be peripheral to the life stories at their core. Consequences for present assumptions about confidentiality and ethics, often remote from real experience of necessary choices between evils rather than between bad and good, will be shattering.

Since invasion of the NHS by commercial providers, confidentiality has entered new dimensions, as yet virtually ignored in public discussion. In primary care, the NHS already holds computed lists of people itemised by their health problems, often inseparable from social problems, together with their names, addresses, telephone numbers and e-mail addresses. To invite commercial providers to share these with non-profit public services in a single universal NHS electronic record, constrained only by promises to ignore their huge potential for targeting accurately defined consumer groups, is simply not credible. A company specialising in continuing care of diabetes, for example, will naturally expect to have access to lists of people with that problem. From there it is a small and logical step to identify subsets with kidney failure, retinal damage or erectile failure. Where do we draw the line between informing potential consumers, and promoting a competing company or its products? Confidentiality would then be defended only by business ethics – which is to say, it would not be defended at all.

Apart from these threats to confidentiality from commerce, serious personal problems will in any case arise from a more open and honest approach to recorded stories: for example, past histories of interrupted pregnancies, domestic violence, sexually transmitted disease, or suspected but unconfirmed major disease, all need to be recorded, but will present major problems for sharing information within families, though such sharing will be inevitable.[140] These problems can be overcome providing innovative culture is allowed to follow innovative practice, each learning from the other as they have in the past. The most important point is that patients should begin to hold records themselves and gain access to their information, in stepwise fashion that recognises and respects such initial difficulties in moving toward a more open, tolerant and trusting society.

Only such records can provide material evidence that patients' participation in health creation has moved from rhetoric to reality. Fortunately these systems will take some years to evolve, giving us time to ensure that they are flexible, adapted to learning as we go. Providing that the NHS remains accessible to all citizens, that new electronic record systems are made accessible to direct patient inputs, and fragmentation of NHS care does not continue to the point where defined catchment populations no longer exist and audits of total performance against a population denominator become impossible, these records will provide opportunities to merge data in many different ways, longitudinally in time and laterally in populations. Such systems would provide powerful new tools for improving individual patient care, for monitoring performance of the system as a whole, for developing large-scale observational research and even some kinds of experimental research, for redefining both professional and public attitudes to science, and for raising professional–patient relationships to a qualitatively higher social level. Development of national systems on these lines could provide evidence of the relative effectiveness and efficiency of planned, socially inclusive national services, compared with services dis-integrated to become commodity markets.

Black boxes: dehumanising or humane?

This chapter has provided a few examples of what happens at some important points of decision within the NHS black box. They were chosen to illustrate ways in which they differ fundamentally from what happens at typical points of production in the black boxes of industrial commodity production, which are designed to eliminate human decisions, and have largely succeeded.

What about our NHS black box? This also uses machines, but it is difficult to find any that replace rather than augment and extend human labour and human decision. Even IT, which has raised productivity in its own field by several orders of magnitude, has not displaced any labour I can think of; all it has done is to create new and extremely useful (indeed, ultimately revolutionary) tasks that were previously unimaginable. Electrocardiograph (ECG)[141] machines now analyse their own results, and do so more accurately and reliably than most non-specialist doctors were previously able to do. No doctors have become unemployed as a result; they simply have more time for other tasks requiring more sensitivity and imagination. The same applies to surgical interventions, which since the advent of flexible endoscopy, closed-circuit television and minimally invasive procedures, is coming to depend entirely on advanced technologies. Far from displacing human labour, this surgery requires an ever-growing number of staff with extremely specialised skills, working to much higher standards of quality. For the sorts of shared decision exemplified in this chapter, IT can also make a huge new contribution, indeed without it shared production of health gain would probably be impossible, but it does nothing to reduce the human workforce required. On the contrary, to use IT intelligently and humanely we need many more people, with much higher skills, particularly the human skills of caring and communication.

Our NHS black box is qualitatively different from, and in important ways diametrically opposed to, the black box of Henry Ford and commodity production for the market. It has to deal with hugely complex biological and sociological uncertainties wholly unlike the world of engineering. Even in fields that seem most mechanical, for example hip replacement, apparently apt engineering metaphors are illusory. Demand for hip replacement cannot depend only on objective evidence from X-rays or scans: a large population study in Sweden found that fewer than half of older patients with substantial radiological evidence of joint damage had any complaints,[142] other studies have shown people with severe pain despite normal X-ray appearances. To target joint replacement accurately requires a wide range of carefully evaluated evidence from patients, including subjective assessments of pain, disability, co-existing illness, and social functioning, as well as assessment of joint rotation and X-rays.[143] These criteria can be quantified and standardised, but always depend on careful, shared assessments of patients' evidence as well as inhuman evidence from machines.

When such criteria are applied to whole populations they reveal total needs for replacement about 6% greater than NHS supply, an important difference, but not an infinite gap. With political will, it could be closed.[144] Those who deny this seem driven by their need to find impossibilities to justify their 'reforms'.

Post-modernists may discount the relevance of Henry Ford's black box to contemporary industrial production, but for those who still have jobs in commodity manufacture or marketed services, 'post-Fordist' black boxes differ from their predecessors only by dehumanising commodity production even faster than before. Management policies derived from industrial production, however indirectly and however modified to recognise at least some of the real clinical world, succeed mainly in demoralising staff and stifling all but commercial initiatives. The internal processes of our NHS black box depend on becoming more human, more labour-intensive, more imaginative, more trusting, with closer and more sustained relationships between staff and patients, disentangled from pursuit of profit so that mutual trust can grow. To develop this new model of shared creative production we have to do much more than reject the industrial model, but until this first step is taken, we can't even begin.

Summary and conclusions

At points of production most critical for its outputs and efficiency, the NHS care system operates in ways entirely different from commodity-producing industries. Progress in health care depends on developing professionals as sceptical producers of health gain rather than salesmen of process, and on developing patients as sceptical co-producers rather than either cynical or credulous consumers searching for bargains. Productivity in health care depends on complex decisions about complex problems, involving many unstable and unpredictable variables. These decisions require increasingly labour-intensive production methods, with deeper, more trusting and more continuing relationships between professionals and patients. Though machines may increasingly be used, they should be subordinated to human decisions free from either rewards or penalties. To apply either rewards or penalties to the judgements of professionals or patients can only impair trust and make appropriate decisions more difficult.

By contrast, industrial production of commodities depends on a diminishing number of human decisions, with increasingly exact duplication of standardised mechanical actions, eventually eliminating human decisions completely. It starts by reducing workers to machines, and ends by discarding them from production. Industrial commodity production moves toward elimination of human judgement and labour, other than at its design stage.

When applied to health care systems, management policies derived from industrial commodity production, and incentive systems of reward and punishment based on that model, are demoralising to staff and patients and thus reduce productivity. Health care requires an entirely different body of economic theory, only the outlines of which are beginning to become clear, to which health economists have so far contributed little. Progress and productivity in this field depend on new social relationships between public, patients and health professionals, based on levels of trust unattainable within commercial transactions. Beginnings of these already exist, but cannot develop rapidly without separating the NHS gift economy and culture from the dominant economy and culture of commerce.

Notes

[1] For example:

> ... the failure of the market to insure against uncertainties has created many social institutions in which the usual assumptions of the market are to some extent contradicted. The medical profession is only one example, though in many respects an extreme one. All professions share some of the same properties. The economic importance of personal and especially family relationships, though declining, is by no means trivial in most advanced economies; it is based on non-market relations that create guarantees of behavior which would otherwise be afflicted with excessive uncertainty. Many other examples can be given. The logic and limitations of ideal competitive behavior under uncertainty force us to recognize the incomplete description of reality supplied by the impersonal price system. (Arrow, 1963)

[2] The word 'free' has many contradictory meanings. Here I mean free for entrepreneurs to buy, sell and invest, not that patients do not have to buy care as a commodity.

[3] Trisha Greenhalgh (2005) has provided a beautifully simple example of this. Commenting on a worthy but orthodox paper on factors relating to obesity in childhood, she found that though the authors rightly remembered to control for differences in education in mothers, which – like other effects of social class – are closely and causally associated with obesity, they completely omitted this from their list of potential interventions to prevent or treat obesity. As she rightly remarks, 'interventions aimed at increasing the health literacy of the primary care giver have far greater potential [than clinical interventions] for achieving a slimmer cohort of primary school children'. The omission is typical.

[4] Spence, 1960.

[5] Hoffman et al, 1997.

[6] The shameful story of evaded state responsibility for care of the older chronic sick has already been told earlier. In the era preceding this turning point, care rose above the level of Poor Law warehousing in only a minority of pioneering geriatric units (Rodgers, 1982). Most remained little better than in Charles Dickens' time (Townsend, 1962 and 1981). A huge new investment was needed to meet the needs of an ageing society (Acheson, 1982). Without any public consultation or electoral mandate, the ruling consensus solved this problem first by declaring it insoluble (Jeffreys, 1983), then by turning its back on it, and handing responsibility to private nursing homes run for profit. Whereas healthy growth of geriatric medicine for all of the people in Britain was betrayed, in the US it never even existed (Carboni, 1982).

[7] Dowrick et al, 1996.

[8] Follow-up analysis of patients admitted to hospital in Australia found that 16.6% of admissions were prompted by acute events occurring within already established continuing disease. Roughly half of these events were judged readily preventable by continuing anticipatory care in the community – preventable, but not prevented (*Medical Journal of Australia* 1999, vol 170, pp 411-15).

[9] Oye and Bellamy, 1991.

[10] Cook et al, 2000.

[11] A characteristic example of what happens when care is fragmented between specialists, with no one person responsible for overall coordination of care and everyone minding only their own business, was reported recently. Care of an older woman with toxic effects from lithium treatment for depression was spread across three sites delivered by six teams. She died from treatable kidney failure (Gannon, 2005).

[12] About one-quarter of new entrants to British public health now have substantial prior experience in primary care as trainee GPs, many of them mature students who have shifted their careers. These form an entirely new and refreshing force in what had become a dangerously stagnant and complacent specialty.

[13] A contemporary local colleague always treated all acute childhood illness with broad-spectrum antibiotics, with or without any precise diagnosis. Such an indiscriminate policy might have prevented this death. On the other hand, community prevalence of antibiotic-resistant bacteria, including MRSA, is closely and causally related to rates of prescribing antibiotics in primary care. Prevalence in hospitals is much higher, mainly because antibiotics are far more heavily prescribed there. Blunderbuss clinical medicine is no solution.

[14] BC 41(3), from DIPEx website www.dipex.org, quoted by Herxheimer (2003).

[15] Department of Health, 1998.

[16] Freeman et al, 2002.

[17] Ridsdale et al, 1989.

[18] Verby et al, 1979.

[19] Mechanic, 2001.

[20] Beckman and Frankel, 1984. When a similar study was repeated in 1998, average time before interruption had risen to 22 seconds (Marvel et al, 1999).

[21] Hart, 1995b.

[22] Grol et al, 1999.

[23] Squires and Learmonth, 2003.

[24] Andersson and Mattsson, 1989.

[25] Švab and Katic, 1991. This study was so simple, and its evidence so counter-intuitive for most older health professionals, that it deserves to be used regularly as a learning experience for undergraduates, illustrating most of the main qualities needed for original research in unexpected settings.

[26] Cromarty, 1996; Pollock and Grime, 2002.

[27] Gottlieb, 1969.

[28] Speckens et al, 1995.

[29] Bridges and Goldberg, 1985; Weich et al, 1995.

[30] Slater, 1965.

[31] Crimlisk et al, 1998.

[32] Sims, 1973; Sims and Prior, 1978; Maricle et al, 1987; Lloyd et al, 1996; Moncrieff and Kirsch, 2005.

[33] Stewart-Brown and Layte, 1997.

[34] Schulz et al, 2000. Despite this convincing evidence of the lethal consequences of depression, meta-analyses of randomised controlled trials show little evidence of clinically (rather than statistically) significant net benefit from antidepressant drugs (Moncrieff and Kirsch, 2005). Despite this poor evidence, they remain a gigantic international pharmaceutical market.

[35] This should not be misinterpreted to mean that people can make all parts of their bodies do anything they want simply by thinking and wishing hard enough, any more than the world can be changed by thinking and wishing about it.

[36] Kroenke and Mangelsdorff, 1989.

[37] Katon and Walker, 1998.

[38] Bosanquet and Pollard, 1997, pp 98-103.

[39] Fijten et al, 1993.

[40] For a balanced assessment favourable to surgical intervention, see Crawford, 2005.

[41] Ciatto, 2003.

[42] Punglia et al, 2003.

[43] Lenzer, 2004.

[44] Creese, 1997.

[45] Evans and Barer, 1990, pp 80-5.

[46] Moses et al, 1992; *Lancet* Editorial, 1992.

[47] de Sardan, 2004.

[48] Williams et al, 1986.

[49] Corney, 1990.

[50] Goldberg and Williams, 1988.

[51] Barsky, 1992.

[52] Starfield et al, 1981. Though doctors like to imagine that they can predict their patients' decisions about their care, we have excellent evidence this is not so. Joel Ménard ran an excellent hypertension follow-up clinic at a Paris teaching hospital, where staff knew patients well and maintained continuity of care. Objective measures of how assiduously patients adhered to their treatment plans showed no correlation between predicted and actual behaviour, nor any association of behaviour with education or social class, though doctors thought these would be powerful predictors (de Goulet et

---

al, 1983). Similar results were found in the Netherlands when predicted and actual behaviour were compared for patients' capacity to change diet, smoking or exercise habits (Verheijden et al, 2005). In both cases, researchers reached a simple conclusion: nobody knows what patients can do until they are allowed to try, which means that they all have to be asked, and all their answers have to be listened to.

[53] Burack and Carpenter, 1983.

[54] In a classic experiment, eight sane researchers presented at 12 psychiatric hospitals in five states of the US, falsely claiming they had heard voices. They otherwise behaved normally. Persuading staff that they were sane, and could leave hospital, took from 7 to 19 days. All but one was diagnosed as schizophrenic on admission. Out of 118 real patients these researchers met on the admissions ward, 35 thought they were sane, and were probably doing an experiment, but none of the pseudopatients was detected by staff. The researchers then warned staff at a teaching and research hospital, which had denied that this could have happened there, that over the next three months one or more pseudopatients would present for admission in the same way. Though none were in fact offered for admission, 41 out of 193 patients presenting for admission were diagnosed confidently as pseudopatients by at least one member of staff (Rosenhan, 1973).

[55] Pringle, 1974.

[56] *Lancet* Editorial, 1989.

[57] Wing, 1987.

[58] The lifetime risk of schizophrenia is 1% for all social classes, with true prevalence unrelated to social class, but average age at first hospital admission for schizophrenia is 28 for most affluent patients, more than 8 years earlier than for poor patients, with others ranked appropriately between these two extremes. In other words, the inverse care law applies.

[59] Followed up 15 years after a first episode of schizophrenic disorder, about 25% have recovered completely and no longer need treatment (Wiersma et al, 1998). See also Turner, 2004.

[60] This was established by the important MRC studies at Northwick Park (Johnstone et al 1986; Crow et al, 1986; MacMillan et al, 1986a and 1986b).

[61] 'Psychosocial interventions for schizophrenia', *Effective Health Care*, August 2000.

[62] Rollin, 1979.

[63] Bagley, 2001.

[64] Timimi, 2002.

[65] Medawar, 1992.

[66] Taylor et al, 1991, pp 93–113.

[67] Consensus criteria for diagnosis of ADHD in the US are as follows: six or more out of nine frequently observed inattentive behaviours, and six or more out of nine frequently observed hyperactive or impulsive behaviours. Some of these must have been present before age seven, and some must cause impairment in two or more settings (for example, at home, at school or at work). They must provide clear evidence of clinically significantly impaired social, academic or occupational functioning, and they must not be more readily attributable to some other mental disorder (American Psychiatric Association, 1994). On these generous criteria even US prevalence rates seem surprisingly modest.

[68] Jick et al, 2004.

[69] 'Stimulant drugs for severe hyperactivity in childhood', *Drug & Therapeutics Bulletin*, (2001) vol 39, pp 52–4.

[70] Kewley, 1998.

[71] Roberts, 1996.

[72] Levine and Oberklaid, 1980.

[73] Guevara and Stein, 2001. Arguments for and against were presented by David Coghill and Harvey Marcovitch respectively in *British Medical Journal* (Coghill, 2004; Marcovitch, 2004).

[74] Mayor, 1996.

[75] Kovac, 2001.

[76] Marwick, 2003.

[77] Timimi, 2005.

[78] Hampton et al, 1975; Peterson et al, 1992.

[79] For practice to follow scientific method, diagnosis should follow a hypothetico-deductive pathway, forming successive hypotheses which further evidence is designed either to validate or refute. We have good evidence that this pattern is rarely followed in practice; most clinicians, most of the time, rely on recognising patterns familiar from experience. We also have good evidence that most serious errors occur in this pattern-recognition rather than hypothetico-deductive mode. Progress in part depends on a general shift to more scientific modes of thought, by both professionals and patients.

[80] Frank, 1983. Placebo is usually a misnomer, because it implies intention to deceive (Latin *placebo* = I please). A better term would be 'caring effects', because the main operator seems to be the patient's belief that at last she has found someone competent and willing to help (Hart and Dieppe, 1996). To assess their real effects, placebo or caring effects need to be measured not against active treatments, but also against an active drug, and against no treatment at all. This has been done, showing virtually no independent effect of placebo pills; the important ingredient is not the pill, but the person who gives it (Hrobjartsson and Gotzsche, 2001). More or less supportive environments in which treatments are given influence their effectiveness. For example, having a view of trees through a window seemed to speed recovery from surgery (Ulrich, 1984). Such environmental effects seem to be general (Di Blasi et al, 2001). This may not be surprising, but should be taken into account in design of NHS buildings. Most primary care health centres in Britain still look like our schools – cheap and rapidly dilapidated.

[81] De Gruy et al, 1987.

[82] Escobar et al, 1987; Fink, 1992.

[83] Davies, 1998.

[84] Portegijs et al, 1996.

[85] Hooper, 1990.

[86] Richardson and Feder, 1995.

[87] Katon et al, 1982.

[88] Dunea, 1991.

[89] Howe, 1996.

[90] Angela Coulter and colleagues tracked the full sequence from self-selection by patients through referral by GPs to final selection for hysterectomy for excessive menstrual bleeding (Coulter et al, 1995). They found that most critical decisions were made not by specialists, but at primary care level. Once people got referred into the hospital pipeline, few escaped surgery. Most significant choices were made by GPs, shared sometimes with patients, more often unshared, particularly with working-class women. The quality of primary care thus became the main determinant of surgical efficiency, chiefly depending on the extent to which patients' full health agendas were considered, without hasty resort to referral for surgery as a way both to save consultation time, and to ensure that patients were satisfied that something substantial was being done. Hysterectomy rates for this indication are now rapidly falling, to about two-thirds less than a decade ago (Reid and Mukri, 2005), and now show little variability between different NHS areas. This contrasts with cholecystectomy rates, which still show huge unexplained variation between areas, and have not been subjected to similar intelligent scrutiny (Aylin et al, 2005).

[91] Chris Gunstone (2005) gives a good account of five recent cases illustrating this point, with which most experienced clinicians or surviving relatives are likely to sympathise.

[92] Coulter et al, 1988.

[93] Lilford, 1997.

[94] It seems strange that nobody has yet developed a simple technique for measuring menstrual loss objectively, but perhaps there is not much demand for this. At the Oxford John Radcliffe Hospital, Margaret Rees (1991) used accurate research measurements of menstrual flow to see whether treatment could address patients' real concerns more accurately and rationally, with less resort to surgery. She studied 17 patients aged 30-45 referred for treatment of heavy menstruation, but with measured menstrual blood loss between 15 and 60 ml, way below the consensus threshold. She gave them a clear explanation of how they compared with other women, and then explored related problems constituting their own personal patterns of illness, rather than the standard disorder defined as menorrhagia. Three years after being told their blood loss was normal and did not need treatment, she found 14 had accepted this, a huge gain in efficiency. However, two were still taking medication for menorrhagia and one had managed to get herself a hysterectomy.

This suggests that more rational discussion and better communication has a more than 80% success rate, but there is other evidence that the other 20% may feel happier after a hysterectomy, and this includes a lot of people. Coulter and her colleagues found that of patients who had complained of mild to moderate menorrhagia, 83% who had had hysterectomies were satisfied with their treatment compared with only 45% of patients treated by medication, though objectively these treatments were equally successful in controlling bleeding (Coulter et al, 1994). Results were only marginally different for women complaining of severe bleeding. Her study of consultations about heavy menstrual bleeding between 483 patients and 129 GPs showed that when given an opportunity to choose between treatment options (medication, hysterectomy, or other operative techniques such as endometrial ablation) about one-third of patients wanted to participate in this decision and had a strong treatment preference. Strongest predictors for this wish were higher education and previous consultations for gynaecological disorders – patients who were more confident, knowledgeable and assertive. This must partly account for the astonishing fact that UK women who left school without any educational qualification are 15 times more likely to have a hysterectomy than women with a university degree. With much greater cost barriers, there are similar social differences in the US.

[95] Ligation of internal mammary arteries in hope of improving perfusion of heart muscle in coronary heart disease became popular in the US in the late 1940s, with convincingly high early success rates. By 1954 initial enthusiasm had waned sufficiently for a search for scientific evidence to be possible. Using random allocation to sham and real operations on internal mammary arteries for treatment of angina caused by coronary heart disease, Beecher showed that both were equally effective for about one-third of patients in terms of consumer satisfaction at short-term follow-up, though obviously sham operations had no objective effect on coronary bloodflow (Beecher, 1961; H. Benson and McCallie, 1979). Such experiments are no longer possible, but I see no reason why more recent procedures should not have similar positive transient subjective effects in the same proportion of patients.

[96] Sackett et al, 1996.

[97] For political and cultural reasons that deserve more study than they have received, this happened much earlier in Britain and the British Commonwealth, Ireland, the US, the Netherlands and Scandinavia – broadly, the English-reading medical sphere – than elsewhere in Europe. With the outstanding exception of Cuba, it was ignored or suppressed by states trying to build socialist economies.

[98] Sullivan and Mitchell, 1995. Ominously, this study found that doctor-initiated and medical content increased with computerisation of records, but patient-initiated social content fell.

[99] Spenser, 1993.

[100] Fairfield et al, 1997.

[101] Vogt, 1993. Stupidity on this scale is less common today, but from what I see by following the literature on population control of high blood pressure, not much. Guidelines issued by the National Heart, Lung and Blood Institute of the US National Institutes of Health now declare an official threshold for cardiovascular risk at an arterial pressure threshold of 115/75mmHg. They apply the disease label 'hypertension' from a threshold of 130/90mmHg, and designate the range 120-9/80-9mmHg as 'pre-hypertension' (7th report of the Joint National Committee on Prevention, Detection,

Evaluation and Treatment of High Blood Pressure). The British Hypertension Society has produced an almost equally absurd set of guidelines for the NHS (B. Williams et al, 2004). These provide excellent strategies for expanding medical and pharmaceutical trade, but either as human biology or as public health strategies they are grotesque. For anyone responsible for care of whole populations rather than a minority of profitable customers, they are logistically impossible to implement, and ignore the implications of applying disease labels to well over half of many populations.

[102] Feder et al, 1995.

[103] Ford and Walsh, 1994; Heath, 1995.

[104] Choudhry et al, 2002.

[105] Kuvietowicz, 2003.

[106] Hart, 1997.

[107] Williamson, 1995.

[108] Department of Health, 2001.

[109] Association of the British Pharmaceutical Industry, 1999.

[110] Market & Opinion Research International, 2003.

[111] Lorig et al, 1999; Barlow et al, 2000.

[112] J. Shaw and Baker, 2004.

[113] Greenhalgh, 1998.

[114] From cautious critic of a marketised NHS during Conservative administrations, Professor Julian Le Grand of the London School of Economics has become a zealous advocate, and adviser to Prime Minister Blair. At a recent conference he suggested that patients with chronic health problems be given their own NHS budgets to spend at whatever points of retail sale they might choose for their

health care. Our latest Health Minister, Patricia Hewitt, has promised to consider this proposal carefully (Harding, 2005).

[115] Marinker, 1973.

[116] Campbell et al, 1979.

[117] Positive consequences should not be underestimated, and have still not been fully understood or accepted by most historians. W.H. McNeill's wonderful book *Plagues and Peoples* (1979), introducing his original and liberating idea of human microparasites and macroparasites, reveals the immense continuing value of this paradigm.

[118] Foucault, 1973.

[119] Reaven, 1988; Eckel et al, 2005.

[120] MacMahon et al, 2005. For the arterial blood pressure component of this problem, George Pickering had reached the same conclusion four decades earlier, but the message is still unheard by most clinicians. Labelling is easier than physiological thought.

[121] Salomaa et al, 1991; B. Williams, 1994; Brunner et al, 1993.

[122] Hart, 1984.

[123] Riddle, 1980.

[124] Greenfield et al, 1988.

[125] G.D. Smith et al, 1998.

[126] Mold and Stein, 1986.

[127] In US terminology, charts.

[128] This function depends on continued existence of stable, registered populations in primary care, and defined population catchments for hospitals. Both of these are threatened by present policies promoting consumer choice, self-referral to a variety of competing

sources of primary care, and multiple competing pathways both for entry to care and for referral to specialist advice. Fortunately new patterns of staff and patient behaviour take time to get established, particularly when change is imposed from above, has little support from public opinion and still less from professional opinion. Despite more than 25 years of encouraging critical choice, first from Conservative and then from New Labour government, patients remain overwhelmingly loyal to their GPs and rarely move from one practice to another unless they move to a new home; competition between GPs is probably less now than it has ever been. What little competition exists between specialists or between hospitals still depends almost entirely on experience and opinions of primary care staff, hardly at all on the experience and opinions of patients as consumers. Any government decision to retreat from consumerism would almost certainly be greeted with relief by staff, and all but a small (though probably influential) class of patients.

[129] Interviewed about his recollections of practice when he started in the 1950s, soon after the NHS began, a Paisley GP described the then customary attitude to medical records in Scottish industrial practice:

> We had Lloyd George [records] and we kept them in cabinets … these were our receptionists's pride and joy and not taken out at any time. They were stored, everything was stored there, but we never used the files. The files were not brought out for us to use. So [as an incoming partner] I didn't have any knowledge of the patient coming to see me. The patients would come with all their bottles, with all the medication, and say: 'Doctor, that's what I'm getting', and I would just write out what the medication was. But we never got the files out. The partners' attitude at that time was 'Well, we know the patients, we don't need files – I've known them all their life … why would I want to write anything down? We kept the letters from the hospital in a pile, which just got bigger and bigger.' (Michell and Smith, 2003)

As a locum in the 1950s and 1960s, that was exactly my experience.

[130] Professor Mike Pringle, personal communication July 2004.

[131] Ward and Innes, 2003.

[132] Pyper et al, 2004.

[133] My nearest city, Swansea, is served by two large NHS hospitals, Morriston and Singleton, both now quasi-independent Trusts. In the pre-'reform' NHS they had similar paper records, and exchanged information freely, though inefficiently; about 12% of records were missing at any particular time. 'Reform' introduced competition between these hospitals, so each Trust developed its own IT system, each incompatible with the other. Fortunately competition did not develop very far, the Trusts agreed to specialise in different, complementary fields, so outpatients still moved frequently from one to the other. Whereas paper records could follow them on loan, there was, and still is, no way to transmit computer-held data between them.

[134] T. Benson, 2002a and 2002b.

[135] Langton, 2003.

[136] J. Williams, 2005.

[137] Dove, Wigg et al, 1977.

[138] Brownbridge et al, 1985; Ridsdale and Hudd, 1994; Sullivan and Mitchell, 1995. On average, consultations using a computer-held rather than written record add almost one minute to consultation time. In the British NHS situation where average time available is eight minutes or less, seldom more than ten minutes, though doctor-initiated clinical content tends to increase, patient-initiated social content tends to fall.

[139] Progressive teaching of this sort depends on having sufficient staff for teaching in small groups, close to real patients. According to a recent report the number of UK clinical academics has declined from 4,000 in 2001 to 3,500 by 2005, with the number of clinical lecturers falling by 30% over the same period, while medical schools are trying to double their intake of medical students and double output of doctors because of serious staff shortages at all levels. The decline in teaching staff was attributed to lack of career structure, inflexible patterns of clinical and academic training, shortage of

supported posts, and income differentials favouring clinical rather than academic work. The government has now pledged an initial £2.5m for 2005/06 to establish a new integrated training programme for clinical academics – a drop in the ocean.

[140] Spokespersons for the Ministry of Health have assured the press that data of these sorts will be excluded from the future shared NHS patient records now being developed in its National Programme for Information Technology (NPfIT: www.connectingforhealth.nhs.uk). This assurance is a typically glib conclusion from people whose model of NHS activity is episodic surgery, as though illness could ever be wholly separated from the people that have it. Data will certainly have to be partitioned in various subsets, with different levels of access, an extremely difficult task which can succeed only if patients are supported by professional carers with sustained and intimate experience of their family circumstances.

[141] In US usage, EKG.

[142] Bagge et al, 1991.

[143] Naylor and Williams, 1996.

[144] Frankel et al, 1999.

FOUR

Ownership

The argument of this book is organised around the NHS as a production system. How does the idea of ownership play out in these terms? Production systems may or may not have shareholders, but all have managers, operatives and material resources – land, buildings, equipment and so on – that, combined with labour, enable them to create their product. For each of these players, ownership is always an important question, and for each of them ownership is conceived and defined differently. As we saw in the last chapter, patients must increasingly be recognised as co-producers of health gain, and so their views on ownership are as important as those of professional staff.

Origins of property in health care

Together with specific treatments made possible by knowledge gained almost entirely in the past hundred years, recovery from illness assumes the same factors as those required to maintain normal health, knowledge we have had for thousands of years: nutrition, hydration, hygiene, shelter and security. Social conditions providing access to these for all well people should be the primary aim of rational public health policy, and their active provision for sick people is a precondition for rational care. For an overwhelming majority of people in the eras preceding industrial capitalism, the tasks required to care for people too sick to care for themselves were provided within families, almost entirely by mothers, daughters and grandmothers.

Shift from the common, unspecialised (but gender-divided) labour of subsistence agriculture to the divided, specialised labour of industrial capitalism made it impossible either for well people to maintain their own health, or for sick people to restore it, without aid from their employers or from the state. Most of this was designed to support nursing aid still provided by families, chiefly by cash benefits so that families with a sick breadwinner could survive until he recovered. Doctors for the common people had to find ways to introduce medicine and surgery into this family support system.

The first person in Britain to think quantitatively about the nation's health as a whole and in economic terms was Sir William Petty in 1690.[1] Most remarkably, he recognised the population as a measurable economic asset rather than a liability. Two centuries later the foundations of our state health service were laid by Sir John Simon in the 1860s,[2] but this was strictly confined to Public Health, sanitary laws and their local enforcement. It excluded personal care except for epidemic infectious disease and warehousing of the insane or indigent. The reason for this strict separation of Public Health from personal care arose from the medical profession's determination to keep ownership and control of clinical trade in its own hands. Doctors as entrepreneurs kept everyone else out of any activity that might be done profitably, but so far as possible avoided responsibility for anything patients could not pay for. By the mid-19th century public health began to be understood as indivisible; poor sick people fortunately created enough risk for rich well people to ensure some action by the state, both through safe water and effluent systems and sanitary laws, and by barracking the indigent poor where they could not infect the rich.

In Manchester, Britain's first centre of mass industrialisation, by the middle of the 19th century roughly two-thirds of all deaths had received prior medical attention of some kind, a rough indicator of the extent to which this had become regarded as important either for survival, or at least for a dignified death.[3] Doctors who could afford it lived entirely from fees from those who could afford to pay, but this certainly did not reach anything like two-thirds of the population. Doctors scaled their fees roughly in proportion to their estimates of the value of their patients' homes. The richest areas were therefore most attractive to medical trade, generally getting those able to spend longer as unpaid junior staff in hospitals to get wider clinical experience. Richer patients paying larger fees allowed doctors to give patients as much time as full application of contemporary medical knowledge required. These areas provided opportunities to develop state-of-the-art personal clinical medicine and surgery.[4] To doctors they therefore appeared the natural growing points for any eventual public service (the eternal argument for 'levelling up, not levelling down'). In fact they never became so. The origins of NHS primary care lie in prepaid systems developed for the care of industrial workers, not in genteel fee-earning practice in market towns or white-collar suburbs.

Care without fees

Wherever income from rich patients was insufficient to maintain a medical family,[5] doctors looked for other work, either for the state, through extremely ill-paid salaried service for the Poor Law Boards of Guardians, or to groups of workers able to organise subscription schemes for prepaid care, generally known as clubs. To distinguish them from trade unions (which were by the 1799 and 1800 Combination Acts made illegal until 1825) they were called 'friendly societies'. These were compelled to register after 1793, so their subsequent progress can be measured. By 1891, almost half the adult male UK population, and a majority of employed industrial workers, were members of such societies.

Some societies became huge national institutions. By 1855 the Odd Fellows had 200,000 members and the Ancient Order of Foresters 100,000, and by 1872 both of these had more than doubled. Despite their size, these were still largely organised and controlled by their members through local lodges, where everybody knew everyone else and could watch how their pennies were spent. They provided burial expenses, subsistence during unemployment, illness or injury, and a usually narrow range of prepaid medical and nursing care, often for dependants as well as subscribers. Costs were low because almost all administration was by elected committees of volunteers, and all profits were accumulated as reserves for future benefits. They paid doctors better than the Poor Law, but not much.

In 1896 the *Lancet* sent a correspondent around Britain to report on the terms and conditions of service of doctors serving industrial workers and their families, resulting in publication of a classic work, *The Battle of the Clubs*.[6] In Southampton the *Lancet* correspondent found about a quarter of the population registered in club schemes, from which doctors earned 4 shillings a head annually for unlimited access to medical advice and medicines. The Southampton Board of Guardians contracted medical care for its 2,000 indigent poor for an annual fee of £5 a head. In 1893 these 2,000 had 500 medical visits at 2½ pence per visit. In Portsmouth, the Medical Benefit Society contracted for unlimited access to advice and medicine for dockyard workers and their families for a weekly fee of ½ pence a head. One GP contracted to this scheme kept a ledger showing 1,958 home visits and 4,650 office consultations for fees totalling £38 11 shillings and 11 pence, an average 1.4 pence per consultation. For larger specific items of service there were higher scales.[7]

To understand these sums one needs to know something of contemporary prices and earnings. From 1883 to 1913 the value of money stayed almost unchanged. The purchasing power of £1 in 1883 fell over the next 100 years to 3½ pence by 1983, 3.5% of its original value. It may be more meaningful to look at a few prices around 1905. A new brick-built terrace house cost about £150, or £100 if built in stone; an iron and brass double bedstead cost £2.5 (£2 10 shillings). Adult miners' earnings by 1914 averaged around £145 a year, with large differences between younger, fitter men able to hew high tonnage from the coalface, and less fit or older men working on transport, timbering, repairing and the many other skills needed to keep a mine in production. Hewers worked underground for an eight-hour day, six days a week, cutting and loading coal entirely by hand. Boys of 14 started at £0.6 a week, £31 a year. All this compared well with £15 a year for a 6½-day week for girls forced by absence of local paid work into exile in London as living-in housemaids.[8] It compared badly with economist Alfred Marshall's estimate of £500 a year as a reasonable income for a university professor, or the £1,000 a year inherited by Beatrice Webb on her marriage to Sidney, to support their lifelong enterprise as theorists for mainstream English social democracy.[9] Coal miners were never rich, but they were not too poor to afford subscriptions of around 6 pence (£0.025) a week for their medical aid schemes.

Miners' medical aid schemes

Pit villages had to make their own social institutions for themselves, drawing from egalitarian social theory implicit in dissenting interpretations of the Christian bible dating from the Puritan movements of the English civil war, from ideas about temperance born from bitter family experience, and finally (from about 1898) from socialist ideas.[10] All three sets of ideas frequently fused. Marxism had little impact until around 1910, but then rapidly became a powerful force in the South Wales coalfield, at least in simplified form. Valleys socialism had strong elements of syndicalism, derived from the fact that engagements between lodges of the South Wales Miners' Federation, and boardrooms of the Coal Mining Employers' Federation, were the battles from which all the most important social and political decisions derived. These often led government policy. Local government was incomparably stronger than it is today, and every local election was a struggle between miners and coal owners for supremacy.

The miners' medical aid schemes were the most developed of the club systems. The clubs employed doctors either on contract or salary, paying the going rate for labour in a then over-manned and extremely competitive professional market, in which medical poverty was still a reality. Whereas schemes in England depended on fixed rates of subscription, all the miners' medical aid schemes in South Wales eventually adopted poundage schemes (usually around 3 or 4 pence for each £1 earned), in which subscriptions proportional to earnings were deducted from wages at the colliery office – in effect, a local income tax.[11] Employers generally favoured these schemes as a stabilising factor in their otherwise precarious industrial relations, and as a means of attracting doctors to the often remote communities in which they needed doctors for their own families. The poundage system became a critically important feature, creating possibilities for development of comprehensive services impossible elsewhere.

In all these schemes the doctors' duties were: to adjudicate fitness for work and entitlement to benefit, and exclude from benefit categories of illness attributed to 'immoral behaviour' (mainly alcohol and venereal disease); to treat frequent industrial injuries; and to provide medicines and diagnostic labels for all illness presented to them, with unlimited free access. Major injuries and surgical emergencies like fractures or strangulated hernias were managed by GPs, all of whom were expected to have elementary surgical skills as soon as they qualified.[12]

The friendly societies and miners' medical aid societies were strongholds of probity, sobriety, dissenting religion, and a balance between servility and solidarity depending on the conflicting influences of religion, self-help and militant traditions descended from the Chartists of the 1840s, according to the relative strength of these traditions in different communities. Socialist and Marxist ideas had little impact in Wales until the Cambrian Combine colliery dispute in 1910, after which they grew rapidly. Advocates for self-help turned readily to local employers and gentry for whatever they might give, either as cash or influence. In most of the earlier schemes, employers hired and fired the doctors, expecting and often getting loyal support from them in their many disputes with their workmen. After the 1897 Workmen's Compensation Act made employers liable for some of the more flagrant consequences of industrial injury, employers' influence over doctors became a major issue, and eventually most schemes came under full workers' control. This was not generally regarded by employers as a fundamentally important issue; where workmen were militant enough to press their case, employers gave way and operated poundage schemes through their pay-offices, even if this upset the organised medical profession, and loosened the employers' influence on doctors' 'expert' evidence in court for compensation disputes.[13]

As miners' doctors had to deal with frequent fractures and other injuries, they encouraged their various sponsors – mainly local government and the aid societies but also local employers and charitable donors – to build small cottage hospitals, usually with only ten to 15 beds, with a small theatre in which to operate. Moral ownership of these hospitals, and control over access to them for surgical practice, were frequent matters for contention. Local bigwigs were often more generous with their names than their money. The coal-mining valleys of South Wales and the slate-mining valleys of North Wales filled with cottage hospitals variously built and maintained by rates from local government and by local public subscription, their public face and administration often virtually monopolised by gentry whose cash contributions were often much less than the funds raised collectively by mining communities and through subscriptions from poundage. Speaking of cottage hospitals in the mining valleys in the run-up to the NHS, Bevan claimed that, though government described them as voluntary hospitals, many got 97.5% of their revenue from miners' subscriptions.[14]

Unsupported by the state until 1911, the friendly societies excluded the very poor, but in all areas of heavy industry they included most employed workers. In Welsh coal-mining communities, the medical aid societies included all dependants, and by annual or weekly personal subscription, all council workers, small business people, shopkeepers, teachers and other minority occupations surrounding the coal industry.[15]

The most comprehensive miners' medical aid schemes developed in the South Wales coalfield, because of its unique character concentrating whole valley communities around production of coal, iron, steel and tinplate.[16] The small valleys towns became culturally self-sufficient, with their own highly developed representative and participative democracy.[17] The poundage system provided funding and administration sufficient not just to maintain primary health care, but also to allow some investment in staff and buildings. The communities did their best to provide for all their own social needs out of their own human resources. The doctors they employed had common interests with the communities they served to establish better facilities for care, chiefly through building small cottage hospitals as surgical units and for the isolation of infectious fevers.[18] The doctors also had property interests of their own, wherein lay seeds of conflict. Development, control, staffing and ownership of these GP hospitals soon became central to contention between three well-defined local forces: doctors, miners and gentry.[19]

Miners' medical aid schemes as models for socially inclusive care

Though most South Wales doctors saw their ownership and control of local hospitals as inseparable from ownership and control of the leading edge of their work, there were important exceptions. Social service ultimately implies social funding, social funding implies social accountability, and this in turn implies either social regulation, or social ownership. If you really serve the people, you must also be answerable to them, which means salaried service (so that value added by doctors' work can be used to expand the range of health care, beyond the scope of GPs), not entrepreneurial ownership (whereby GPs could mainly expand their own work and incomes, with lower priority for investment in care). Though almost forgotten today, there were powerful advocates for salaried medical service in the valleys within the profession, most notably Dr Henry Norton Davies in Rhondda. He believed that poundage efficiently administered could support better-than-average salaries for doctors, who would then not need further income from private practice. He believed it could expand health care to include a range of specialties far more imaginative than contemporary general practice – the beginnings of modern integrated referral.

Several of the miners' aid schemes demonstrated this. In Tredegar, by the 1920s the medical aid society included 95% of the town's population, and employed five GPs, a specialist surgeon, two pharmacists, a physiotherapist, a dentist and one domiciliary nurse, as well as free rail transport for access to larger hospitals in Newport. In Rhymney, Dr Redwood was employed by the miners' aid scheme at an annual salary of £700, together with a free house, a dispenser, a cottage hospital and nurses – a better living than most of his 'independent' local colleagues.[20]

These examples show that salaried service, with locally representative lay control, was a viable option, and could be more innovative both socially and clinically than medical shop keeping.[21] These schemes survived even through the period of mass unemployment that devastated the South Wales coalfield from 1926 to 1941, by reducing subscriptions for the unemployed to 3 pence a week, by employing unemployed men as collectors, and by reducing the cost of its contracted doctors (because, through the poundage system, their earnings fell at the same rate as those of their subscribing patients; the salaried doctors escaped this penalty). With imaginative leadership from a state serving all of the people, salaried service could have lifted all British medical practice to become a source of national pride rather than the squalid disgrace it actually was in most UK industrial areas when the NHS began,[22] and mostly so remained until the 1980s.[23] By then well over 80% of investment in buildings, equipment and non-medical staff was being met by the state. With rare exceptions, GPs in industrial areas invested huge amounts of their work, but little of their money in even the minimum of staff, equipment and buildings expected of any other business.[24]

Most GPs held stubbornly to what seemed to them self-evident. It was, they thought, their job to know what was best for their patients, and this included definition of professional tasks, the scope of services, the nature of staff, planning and ownership of land, buildings and equipment, and how access to these might be divided between routine patients prepaid by insurance or medical aid schemes, and more profitable private patients. In this they were powerfully supported by the British Medical Association (BMA), whose central principle was total rejection of any kind of lay control; all regulation of doctors must be by other doctors.

The central issue of dispute between the miners and the doctors lay in control of poundage funds.[25] The miners presented their case in these simple terms, but the BMA claimed higher motives, saying the elected committees of the miners' medical schemes would try to control the doctors' clinical decisions. As public funding inevitably meant public accountability in some form, this became an argument against any kind of state funding for health care. Though from time to time the BMA made progressive proposals in theory, every attempt to make direct state investment in staff, equipment or buildings for primary care was resisted by the BMA until 1966 – and was conceded then only because most NHS general practice in industrial areas had become so squalid that it faced collapse of recruitment.[26]

As most of the documentation about the many disputes between miners' medical aid schemes and their doctors comes from the *BMJ* we have little evidence about how the miners presented their case, but I have never been able to find any example, either written or anecdotal, where miners, or any other group of workers, actually did challenge the opinions of doctors in their own field of clinical expertise. On the contrary, miners seem generally to have taken a more deferential view than was justified by the real state of contemporary medical knowledge, though such was the authority of doctors that it was probably prudent not to challenge their opinions head-on, even if their claims to expertise were obviously being used to disguise economic self-interest.[27] Though letters to the *BMJ* at critical times often show miners' doctors more sympathetic to their patients than to coal owners, these sympathisers were not linked with the minority of radical top doctors advocating a state service, and there was then no political party able to make such connections.

To coal-owning employers, their relations with organised workers were more important than their relations with unorganised doctors, easily replaced from an over-filled profession, so they generally agreed to cooperate with the medical aid schemes, even though the men now controlled them and they powerfully reinforced emerging trade union and socialist political culture. Recognising that optimal work from the doctors required their undivided attention, in 1905 the Ebbw Vale Workmen's Medical Aid Society instructed their salaried doctors to cease private practice in the area. Supported by the BMA, which they had now joined, the doctors ignored this instruction. The *BMJ* refused to advertise any salaried post, and the BMA threatened to expel any member who accepted a salary from the Miners' Aid Society on terms it had not approved. The BMA maintained the incomes of doctors sacked by the society, and in these ways turned the tables. The society retreated to a 10% limit on private practice, but the BMA was now on the offensive, fearing extension of salaried schemes first to the whole Welsh coalfield, then to the rest of industrial Britain.

The BMA demanded that virtually all poundage be paid directly to the contracted doctors, thus eliminating the main advantage of salaried service by putting investment back into the hands of the doctors. The society retaliated by recruiting non-members of the BMA to replace its existing medical workforce. This raised new issues of principle. What was the difference between the solidarity of self-employed GP entrepreneurs, and the solidarity of employed industrial workers? That there was indeed a real difference is not in doubt, but it was a question of greater complexity than has generally been recognised.

From 1905 to 1913 the doctors and the aid societies fought for the loyalties of mining communities in Ebbw Vale, pulled one way by collective ties to their union and the other way by personal ties to their doctors – both substantial forces, because these doctors lived within the communities they served, and often played major roles at critically important moments in their patients' lives. The doctors continued to practise in the area and publicly appealed to their patients to claim repayment of poundage so they could give this to their own doctor. This succeeded in detaching about 10% of the Ebbw Vale society's members. Closely followed by the *BMJ* and by all the other miners' schemes, the dispute grumbled on without a clear victory for either side until 1911, when Lloyd George's National Insurance Act took the ground from beneath their feet.[28] With similar smaller disputes erupting elsewhere in many parts of the coalfield, it became a major item for public discussion in South Wales, then the most dynamic part of the British economy, and Lloyd George's own political base. In designing his Act, he must certainly have had its resolution in mind.

In historical retrospect, the most important issue of this dispute was whether investment in health care for the people would be socially controlled serving social aims, with doctors' incomes a subordinate charge on this social fund, or be privately controlled by doctors as their own personal incomes, with any further investment for wider aims coming from their own pockets. All experience confirms that however it may have been obtained in the first place, once money enters the pockets of professionals, spending for any social purpose has to compete with personal acquisition of carriages, cars, holidays and privileged education for their children, and rarely emerges as the winner. Capitation-paid independent contractor status proved to be an effective way of limiting the costs of primary care while leaving responsibility for consequently squalid services firmly with doctors rather than government.

Lloyd George and the 1911 Insurance Act

In Wales in the 1870s, 60% of all land was owned by about 570 people, nobility and gentry. The landed aristocracy was still fattening from royalties on coal found by chance beneath their estates, to whose production they contributed not one penny, nor any drop of sweat or blood. Popular hostility to this injustice provided foundations for a Liberal ascendancy throughout Wales as complete as the Labour ascendancy that began to replace it in the 1920s, and finished it off by 1935.[29]

An alliance of miners, steelworkers, industrial employers, tenant farmers and slate quarrymen confronted idle landed aristocracy. They were led by David Lloyd George, a small-town lawyer, in the last battle of a revolution started by the English civil war of 1642. After the election of 1906 a newly transformed industrial and imperial Conservative Party began to supersede the dominance of landed nobility, drawing big industrialists away from the Liberal Party as their workers began shifting to the Labour Party. Since the socialist revival of the 1880s, socialist ideas had begun to compete successfully with Liberalism, from Fabians close to the top to militant trade unionists close to the bottom of society.[30] Recognising that the social foundations of Liberal ascendancy were crumbling, Lloyd George embarked on social reforms that gave the Liberal government a few more years of power before its permanent extinction, provided his Labour successors with their eventual agenda for the rest of the 20th century and finished landed aristocracy as an independent political force. As Chancellor of the Exchequer, Lloyd George attacked the aristocracy's economic power through inheritance taxes in 1909, and their political power in the House of Lords through the 1911 Parliament Act. Finally he set foundations for state pensions, unemployment and health insurance through his 1911 National Insurance Act, all these providing a new basis for popular consent to Liberal rule, with minimal disturbance to industrial power and property.

For an answer to nascent socialism, Lloyd George turned to Germany. Bismarck had simultaneously made the Social Democratic Party illegal, and stolen its most popular social policies for mutual aid on lines similar to the UK friendly societies and miners' medical schemes, but endorsed by the state. This policy had some success. The German Social Democrats became the world's largest and leading socialist party, developing an internally inclusive independent culture that before 1914 seemed on course eventually to provide the world's first socialist state, but Bismarck's insurance schemes shifted the Social Democratic agenda from revolution to reform, and helped to ensure that by the end of the 19th century the revolutionary legacy of Karl Marx seemed safely emasculated.

Lloyd George intended a similar system for the UK, chiefly to support wage earners during short periods of sickness, and provide retirement pensions for the usually brief lives of men following retirement at 65.[31] Ever since 1840, the Poor Law had been punitive in intention, deliberately stripping its supplicants of their homes and possessions as a precondition for minimal relief, designed to drive rural labour into the mines, mills and factories.[32] Knowing from his own experience as a lawyer that illness was a major cause of irreversible pauperism, Lloyd George designed his Insurance Act mainly to prevent this, by assuring a subsistence income of 10 shillings (£0.5) a week for wage earners during periods of incapacity up to three months, falling to 5 shillings (£0.25) a week for 13 weeks thereafter. Beyond this period, they again fell into pauperism and the grip of the Poor Law. These benefits would be paid for by compulsory weekly contributions: 4 pence from workers, 3 pence from their employers and 2 pence from the state (promoted to voters as 'ninepence for fourpence').[33] Though elementary medical care was included in the Act, the main function of its doctors was, even more than in the miners' medical schemes, to justify selection for benefit by certifying incapacity for work. Again this became the central feature of medical work in primary care, around which anything and everything else had to be built.

Though Lloyd George took his strategy from Bismarck's Germany, the social customs needed to root it in British soil had already been developed by organised industrial workers, above all by miners. He simply nationalised the social machinery already in existence, and extended it to virtually all workers on a weekly wage. This solved some problems, but created others. It largely eliminated nascent trade union control either of benefit systems or local investment in medical care, and put an end to all experiments in local participative democracy that might otherwise have limited the authority either of doctors, or of the state. On the other hand, it also destroyed the local social control that had previously limited abuse of benefits. State insurance came to resemble state taxation – too large, too remote and too unshared a property to retain the universal respect once given to locally owned and organised mutual aid. Those playing the system had little respect from their communities, but were no longer regarded as thieves.

Opposition to the 1911 Insurance Act in 1912, and to the NHS in 1948

Through the BMA, the organised medical profession mounted furious opposition to both these historic steps to shift medical practice from trade to public service. In 1911 opposition was led by the top of the profession, the teaching hospital consultants in London, Edinburgh and a few other large cities, who then dominated the BMA. They were backed up by established senior GPs who dominated and exploited their many young unestablished assistants.[34] In 1948 similar resistance was led by the bottom of the profession, by established GPs, mainly with large industrial practices, who took over the BMA. Consultant specialists concentrated on their own interests in the Royal Colleges of Physicians, Surgeons, Obstetricians and Gynaecologists. They saw no alternative to grudging acceptance, on the generous terms offered by Bevan, and in the eyes of most contemporary GPs, betrayed their colleagues by agreeing to work in NHS hospitals.

A great mystery surrounds these two similar events. On both occasions, well over 80% of GPs rejected new legislation already overwhelmingly endorsed by Parliament and by the electorate. On both occasions, similar majorities of doctors declared that their work would be impossible under the new Acts, that they would therefore refuse to work under the Acts, and that the Acts would therefore collapse as unworkable in practice. On both occasions, virtually all doctors were working within the Acts within a few days or weeks of their starting dates; threatened doctors' strikes never materialised. On both occasions, a large majority of doctors stood to gain both more money and greater security under the Acts, and following both Acts they actually did so. On both occasions, by the time medical opposition had peaked, no political party, and only the most reactionary sections of the press, dared any longer to support the BMA's obviously impossible position.[35] So why did they do it?[36]

On both occasions, the basic answer to this lay with the GPs' contemporary sense of ownership. Both times they believed that without ownership and control of medicine as a trade, they would lose ownership and control over their lives, their work and their future as a profession moving reluctantly but inexorably toward a scientific basis for all of its work. Sir Clifford Albutt, a leading and innovative teaching hospital consultant with a strong though patrician sense of social responsibility, wrote about this in the following letter to *The Times*. He accused Lloyd George:

> ... of some vague notion of village clubs ... 'take the mixture, drink it regularly, and get well if nature will let you ...' ... the treatment of disease is first and last a matter of searching diagnosis ... the man who leaves us for

practice is schooled in all these methods; he can examine
the blood, counting and comparing its corpuscles; he
can perform the ordinary bacterial examinations; he can
estimate the chemical values of secretions and excretions;
he is skilled in the use of instruments of precision, of
blood pressure machines, of endoscopes for the eye, the
larynx and other internal parts.... Now if we are to say
that the general practitioner is to be but a stop-gap and
that every malady of importance is to be sent to some
central institution, is not this to take the heart out of our
very efficient students, and to degrade the career of
medicine? Gloss it as we may, contract practice will stand
lower in public esteem, and will be of lower efficiency
and much less humane ... push them back to old-
fashioned routine and to ill-remunerated and therefore
undervalued service.... It must be admitted that, *where
clubs made the bulk of a practice, it was very perfunctory work,
and fell in the hands of perfunctory men.* ... The solution is
no contract, but payment for work done on a standard
tariff.[37] (my emphasis)

Albutt assumed that clinical innovation and investment depended
on medical ownership, medical trade and access by GPs to hospital
practice, because this seemed to be the sole growing point for new
medical knowledge, which was conceived almost entirely in terms
of personal clinical interventions and body repairs. In that critically
important era, when medical education all over the world was
acquiring its modern form, the two most important figures in
English-speaking medicine were Sir Clifford Albutt and Sir William
Osler. Though they were regarded as the greatest physicians in the
contemporary English-speaking world, both repeatedly insisted on
the pre-eminence of public health as having a far greater impact on
health than personal clinical interventions, but this was not what
their most influential audiences wanted to hear, nor what they
themselves felt able to bring about. Public health was social action,
and therefore lay self-evidently outside their responsibility, whereas
clinical interventions gave professionals something obviously useful
to do in a more or less recognisable commodity form and therefore
attracting payment, even if evidence showed it to be far less effective.

In the last years before the Second World War, British GPs
performed an average of three surgical operations each week, nearly
all privately and mostly in cottage hospitals.[38] As a large majority

did no surgery at all, those who did operate did so much more than three times a week. These GP surgeons were expelled from all but a few NHS hospitals after 1948, and replaced by fully trained professional surgeons. In a letter to the *Lancet* ten years after the NHS was born, headed 'The decapitation of general practice', Erich Geiringer restated Albutt's argument almost exactly, this time reinforced by experience between the two world wars:

> Bad practice ... originated at the turn of the century, partly from genuine attempts to provide some kind of general practitioner service for the poor, partly as a result of the panel system.... Under the *per capita* method of payment this type of pauper medicine is still profitable, and is no longer, as formerly, confined to the poorest section of the community ... a fee-for-service system ... would eliminate them in a few years. The real tragedy of the present situation lies in the relentless process of passive hospitalisation which forces even the best practitioners into doing bad general medicine.... The attraction of a fee-for-service system is that it would automatically rehabilitate general practice, simply by the working of economic laws ... [it would be] a hotbed of abuses, but at least it would allow good medicine to survive.[39]

Generalists, a threatened species

In France, Germany, Holland and above all in the US, Albutt and Geiringer got the fees-for-service they wanted, with the predictable result that by the mid-20th century, specialoids (specialists without a significant hospital base) became commonplace and rich, and GPs were becoming an endangered species.[40] Any doctor claiming clinical expertise wanted at least a toe in the door of a local hospital, without which their claims to specialist status (and fees) were scarcely credible. Until the 1960s, imminent extinction of GPs seemed to many a logical consequence of their obsolescence and redundancy to any serious medical task. If you wanted a real doctor, you looked in a hospital.

Then as now, politicians in search of ideas about the future travelled to the US to see what was going to happen everywhere else. The proportion of GPs had fallen from 76% in 1940 to 36% by 1965, mostly old men, and 40% of US citizens no longer had a family doctor.[41] Every component part of the body had its own host of competing specialists, their number depending on the fees pool that fed them,[42] but ever-fewer people had any generalist doctor to bring these parts back together to make a comprehensible story and take responsibility for it. This had frightening economic consequences. Costs of state medicine in Europe, and of state-subsidised medicine in the US, were escalating each year much faster than the general rate of inflation. Britain alone seemed to have discovered how to control costs, delivering much the same clinical service but spending less than 6% of its GNP to do so, compared with around 9% in other West European countries, and over 12% in the US.[43] The main differences seemed to be that Britain still had family doctors acting as generalists, and as gatekeepers to ensure rational referral to hospital-based specialists, that none of these had an economic interest in promoting their wares to consumers, and that funding through general taxation avoided the administrative costs of often extremely fragmented national insurance systems.[44] Albutt and Geiringer notwithstanding, general practice under the NHS had thrived as none other, though GPs seemed to have lost everything they had believed essential to independent clinical work.

Rebirth of general practice

Shut out of their hospitals and cut off from those specialties that depended on the organisation, staff and technology that hospitals alone seemed able to provide, NHS GPs had been forced to look for new tasks. Liberated from having to seek fees rather than problems needing solution, the most innovative GPs found plenty of serious problems not being addressed by any trained staff. These 'new' problems were mainly those emphasised in earlier chapters of this book – early symptoms of illness before the end-stages recognised in medical schools, complex interactions between the brain and other systems and organs, complex interactions between social and biological problems, complex interactions between different diseases in the same patient, and all the problems considered either too trivial to command attention from specialists, or too difficult for them, and therefore best passed on to somebody else. The pioneers of NHS general practice who defined this new agenda, mostly between 1960 and 1980, set world standards for what became recognised as a new speciality – the community-based generalist, based mainly on communication skills and knowledge of physiology and social behaviour rather than mastery of technology.[45]

Evidently it was not necessary to own a public service in order for it to work well. GPs actually worked more imaginatively as contractors for a state franchise than they had as struggling entrepreneurs. Perhaps they would work better still if they could be relieved entirely from the running a business, and were allowed to concentrate on the work they want to do and have been trained to do. Doctors in Tredegar and Rhymney were already able to do this in 1912, and their salaried successors are now beginning to do so in the small pockets of salaried practice now established by the Welsh Assembly at almost exactly the same sites.

Ownership concerns dignity as much as property

Writing in 1993, Andrew Wall had the following to say about ownership not of property, but of work, in the new conditions introduced by imposition of the purchaser–provider split on the NHS (a first step in the still-continuing transition of the NHS from being a provider of services and employer of NHS staff, to becoming a purchaser of services from a wide range of competing contractors, including corporate providers working for profit):

> The benefits of the Purchaser–Provider Split, now seemingly the gospel of the public services of the western world, are by no means self-evident. Organisations need to have the capacity to learn if they are to be flexible and adapt to circumstances. At a very fundamental level of work, anyone at any level of the hierarchy will have ideas about how their job could be done differently and better. *The purchaser–provider split introduces something inherently unnatural because there is a forced division between those who do the job and those who plan the job.... People and organisations are motivated by the prospect of being able to have a significant say in their futures. Rob them of that, and they become lacklustre, unimaginative, and in the end obstructive, if only to attempt to recover some sense of power.* (my emphasis)[46]

Wall was writing about the NHS, but his conclusion applies to all work in any field. For anyone who cares about the future of society, the last three sentences of this quotation should be engraved in memory. They reach the heart of Marx's most important and fundamental perception, the division of mind entailed in all production for market demands rather than human needs. This division, which he called alienation, had raised productivity for commodities to unprecedented heights, but stripped of the social frame that once preserved at least a condescending humanity, it is dragging down creativity and self-respect to unprecedented depths, filling our prisons with alienated youth and poisoning people's minds with fear of their neighbours. In this sense – and *only* in this sense – all who operate any production process want and need to retain or recover ownership and control of their work, and thus regain community status, self-respect and dignity.

Nobody has ever willingly forsaken control over their own work. When English, Scottish, Welsh and Irish peasants lost access to land and streamed into mines, mills and factories in the 18th and 19th centuries, they did so for the same reasons as Chinese, Indian and Vietnamese do today; they could no longer make even a subsistence living on land of their own, or land shared with others in their community. Factory work was their only means of escape from a collapsing rural economy. Nobody wants a boss. Providing they know and understand the product they are supposed to produce, how they produce it should be their own affair, because people at points of production have the most effective ideas about how their work could be done differently and better. This alone gives them dignity and status in their own eyes and within their community. Doctors feared loss of control over their work in the same way as did the silk loom weavers of the 18th century, when machines suddenly transformed them from skilled craftsmen to unskilled labourers.

Albutt's 'perfunctory care by perfunctory men' was an accurate description of most GP care in most British industrial areas well into the 1980s.[47] Most of the innovative general practice born in the 1960s was concentrated where it was easiest to do: in prosperous market or university towns and leafy suburbs. Where occasionally innovation occurred in industrial or inner-city ghettos, it relied on socially committed evangelists willing to defeat the perfunctory tradition by lifetimes of often unsustainably selfless work to create something better.

However, Albutt, Geiringer, the large majority of their contemporaries who agreed with them, and GPs still clinging to independent contractor status have been fundamentally mistaken in four ways:

1. They assumed that ownership of their work process as a personal responsibility was equivalent to ownership of health care as commercial (or, as they always prefer to call it, professional) property. There was and still is little evidence that *as property*, professional ownership of any level of care assures quality. There is plenty of evidence from our own experience that *as responsibility*, professional ownership of work processes is essential to motivation, and to effective and efficient clinical judgement. These two kinds of ownership – of property, or of responsibility for work process – need to be understood as wholly distinct, and ultimately opposed to each other, if our aim is to serve whole communities. *As property*, ownership is at best irrelevant to progress, at worst its most serious obstacle.

2. They ignored the effect of fees-for-service in consolidating a transactional, provider–consumer model for care, inhibiting development of public health responsibilities, and inhibiting development of a cooperative model for care through which patients could develop as co-producers. Though capitation methods of payment created stable registered populations, and therefore created the possibility of planned and audited anticipatory care for whole populations, barely a handful of NHS GPs actually did this until government constructed new contracts to reward them for doing so, and penalise them for failing to do so. Progress is not spontaneous.

3. They ignored the positive consequences on professional motivation and public understanding of any system, however primitive, that included either more of the people through National Insurance, or all of the people through an NHS.

4. Finally, they were wrong about lay control. They ignored the possibility that when it came to health care policies rather than individual clinical decisions, lay people often saw further and wider than doctors, that with substantial lay input, health care might be more imaginative and wider in scope than in any medical monopoly, and that public respect for medical and nursing science was far more robust than they feared.

By 2005 these issues are losing their meaning, either for doctors, who have been forced by circumstances to recognise a truth that has long been obvious to everyone else, or for governments, for whom professional monopoly now represents a pre-capitalist survival, obstructing free play of the market, wherein lay control is expressed through consumer demands. For citizens and for NHS professionals, development of new, democratic forms of lay control remains by far the most important issue, and must eventually fight its way to the top of the political agenda.

Ownership of hospitals

The central strategic decision of Nye Bevan's 1948 revolution was the nationalisation of hospitals. This initiative was entirely his own, unexpected and contrary to the views and expectations of virtually everyone else in the postwar labour movement.[48] This was understood by Charles Webster, official and pre-eminent historian of the NHS, and by George Godber, its principal architect in the medical civil service, as the central feature of the NHS that ensured its success. Its deletion has been understood by New Labour as essential for return of the service to the market. A centrally planned NHS could not be privatised.

Bevan was far more confident than either his cabinet colleagues or the press, that in his confrontation with the BMA, he would win. He understood that the centre of gravity of the profession now lay with the hospital-based specialists, not the GPs. The specialists could work effectively only in hospitals, with their large teams and technical and logistic backup that individual medical entrepreneurs could not provide. The hospitals were all either close to bankruptcy or beyond it, kept going during the war (like much other ramshackle British industry) by government subsidies and regulation. Nationalisation entailed not confiscation, but transfer to the state of mortgaged assets for which nothing had been paid for many years. Consultants and specialists knew where they stood. Without government help, solvent hospitals could not exist. They had no choice but to cooperate, and this they did, albeit usually through gritted teeth, publicly bared. Their leader, Lord Moran, exulted in the excellent deal he had made, through which consultants were handsomely compensated for anticipated loss of private practice (which for most of them never materialised), and given indefinite rights to do private work in NHS hospitals, on top of their already handsome NHS salaries. They obtained effective dominance over hospital governors and investment in competing specialities, guaranteeing that essential but unromantic specialities like geriatrics and psychiatry stayed safely at the bottom of the staff ladder and the end of the resource queue.[49]

The NHS transformed British hospitals, not by building new ones (none were built until the 1960s) but by redistributing medical labour away from their previous concentration in university cities, to wherever they were needed to provide all major speciality functions everywhere in Britain; a task no market could ever have achieved, or would ever have attempted, as US experience has confirmed.

In primary care, little changed after 1948 except that there was a much higher workload, because care was now free for the whole population, and there were now facilities for specialist referral outside London and other cities with teaching hospitals. Bevan seems to have shared the general contemporary belief that all significant clinical decisions depended on specialists in hospitals, not GPs. This probably reflected his personal experience, both in Ebbw Vale and Tredegar, and later in London. He seems to have been impressed by the specialists he met, perhaps because they had some connection with then rapidly advancing medical science. Few GPs seemed to have any such connection. In 1948 the GPs had demanded to be left alone, so he left them alone. Though his civil servants had prepared plans for a nationwide network of health centres more or less following the Soviet polyclinic model, and these had raised high hopes for the future among many of the younger doctors in its plebiscite of 1944, the BMA poured scorn on them: 'Platinum blondes in chromium-plated offices,' ranted Charles Hill, the BMA secretary and radio doctor who led the doctors against the NHS. So most of NHS primary care was left to GPs as a shop-keeping function, to stagnate for another 18 years of maximal earning and minimal spending, with local government public health departments providing whatever socially necessary functions the GPs found too unprofitable to perform. Community paediatricians, midwives, home nurses and public health nurses therefore worked in isolation from GPs, and it was an uphill task even to get the idea of primary care understood. All serious new investment and expansion went into hospital equipment and staffing, and all clinical innovation was expected to come from this source.

Nationalisation meant that the state became the legal owner of all but a handful of hospitals, but power – de facto ownership of hospitals as perceived by themselves and at least tolerated by politicians and the public – remained with the consultants until the neoliberal era after 1979.[50]

Ownership of the NHS

Industrialisation and commercialisation of the NHS since Thatcher's accession in 1979 implies that ownership of medical care, for which doctors contended first with locally organised workers and then with the state over the past hundred years, could end in the hands of neither doctors nor workers nor the state, but with large multinational companies operating to maximise profit for their shareholders, with any contribution to health as their byproduct. All established main political parties are converging toward agreement that, as consumers, patients might no longer care who owns the NHS.

Commercialisation of public services is a worldwide process, reaching every nation accessible to global investment and disinvestment through the World Bank, International Monetary Fund (IMF), and the World Trade Organisation (WTO), their policies applied through the General Agreement on Trade in Services (GATS) legislation. Though created in 1946 as agencies of the United Nations, all three institutions are effectively controlled by the US, representing the interests of its wealthiest investors, extending their markets to occupy fields traditionally reserved for collective ownership through the state and thus answerable to electors. Though different arguments have been presented to voters in different countries, the motivation everywhere is the same: to expand the scope for profitable investment by multinational corporations (based mainly in the US) and transform national care systems from their traditional role as public service planners and providers, into bulk procurers in a health care market.[51] The US government, which denies accountability of itself or its citizens before any international court and has unilaterally withdrawn from all international treaties limiting its weapons or how they are used, uses its command of these international economic institutions to replace traditions of public service by its own commercial ethics.

Before much of the lay public understood what was happening, British doctors, led by the BMA, the Royal Colleges (mainly the London Royal College of Physicians), the NHS Support Federation and the NHS Consultants' Association, embarked on a big public campaign to defend the NHS. The BMA drew public opinion to its side under the slogan 'Who do you trust, the government or your doctors?' Knowing the limitations of his enemy, Kenneth Clarke stood firm. The Labour Party, even in opposition, evaded joint action with doctors,[52] but public opinion overwhelmingly supported the BMA and so did many influential journalists.

Faced with the imminent possibility of victory, the BMA and medical Royal Colleges seemed to have no idea what to do next. Though the medical profession had wonderfully changed from opposition to the NHS in 1948 to its vigorous defence in the 1980s, to work with mass support in a popular alliance with patients and other NHS unions was (and still remains) unthinkable for this generation of leaders. In November 1994 the BMA and Royal Colleges convened a summit meeting on core values, at which it announced its terms of truce. The keynote speech was delivered by Sir Maurice Shock, former rector of Lincoln College Oxford, a pillar of the establishment (but interestingly, not a medical doctor). He was reported as follows in the *BMJ*:

> British doctors were unprepared for the *Blitzkrieg* from the Right which overwhelmed them at the end of the 1980s.... They seemed to imagine that they were still living in Gladstone's world of minimal government, benign self-regulation, and a self-effacing state ... [but now] instead of the rights of man we have the rights of the consumer, the social contract has given way to the sales contract, and, above all, the electorate has been fed with political promises ... about rising standards of living and levels of public service.... Doctors cannot swim against the tide and must recognise that this is an age of regulated capitalism in which the consumer is courted and protected, encouraged to be autocratic, and persuaded of his or her power.... Doctors must be willing to get their hands dirty with making decisions on allocation of resources, must speak authoritatively and sensibly to the consumer.... If [doctors] organised themselves in these ways the government would have to work with doctors, because a *Blitzkrieg* can conquer, but cannot occupy.[53]

Such moments of frankness are rare. Sir Maurice's choice of historical parallel reveals an amazing ignorance of its meaning to anyone aware of 20th-century European history as it appeared to those who actually experienced its consequences.[54] In Sir Maurice's view, the profession had somehow to regain its role as faithful servant to the few who rule, even after being discarded as redundant to an economy no longer challenged by any credible alternative.[55]

An alternative strategy was obvious and, up to a point, had already worked. Had the doctors stood firm and made it clear that they were prepared to act jointly with the Royal College of Nursing (RCN), UNISON and other NHS unions, they could have retained overwhelming public support. Even the Labour Party would probably then have recognised a force it could no longer afford to ignore. In fact, faced by a strong government determined to lead rather than follow public opinion, retreat by an even stronger army – as the BMA, RCN, NHS unions plus majority public opinion plus the Labour opposition certainly were – became a rout. Sir Maurice Shock's proposal for abject capitulation and alliance with a commercialising government against the public as demanding consumers signified exactly that. The *Blitzkrieg* has continued its advance ever since, and consolidated its grip over Britain's intellectual and media establishment. Apart from a few activists in the NHS Consultants' Association and the NHS Support Federation, medical resistance has so far consisted of hand-wringing, though today (in November 2005) we may well be on the brink of change. A new campaigning alliance has been formed called 'Keep Our NHS Public', supported by the NHS Consultants' Association, the NHS Support Federation, UNISON and a large and impressive list of leading doctors, nurses and lay celebrities, most notably Mrs Clare Rayner. If this keeps going, and can ultimately bring the BMA and RCN on board, this pessimistic judgement will have to be revised.

Why public ownership of the NHS will continue to grow

Sir Maurice Shock's offer to collaborate was the end of an era whose fate was already sealed by the final and complete defeat of Britain's miners in 1985, and the collapse of 20th-century experiments in socialism in 1990. However, an embryonic alternative economy still exists within the NHS. It will probably continue to grow even in the worsening conditions of state-promoted corruption and consumerism. If it grows even in the US, where the social organisation of health care is more primitive and there is no mass experience of any alternative, then surely it will grow in Britain.

This embryonic new economy at the heart of the NHS depends on the growth of an element it always contained, which has only recently, and slowly, been recognised: the power and necessity of patients as co-producers. The idea of an NHS owned by the people needs to be taken more seriously, and to be considered in more material terms. Once released from deference, public expectations become an irresistible force, providing initial elements of democratic accountability can be retained and rapidly extended. If voting remains confined to agendas introduced from above, this force will be deflected to consumerism, but this strategy, shared by leaders of both New Labour and Conservative Parties, will probably fail, at least in the residual public service always necessary to serve unprofitable purposes in unprofitable parts of society. The private sector of health care cannot prosper without a residual NHS to do the work that its investors do not want to, including not only mass care for the poor, but also super-specialised care for rare conditions even for the super-rich. Despite an average 4% swing to Conservatives in the general election of May 2005, enough voters who rejected neoliberal policies in 1997 still reject the Conservative Party, even though New Labour has developed all its policies on the NHS from the Conservative agenda rather than its own annual conferences, or the policy forums offered to the membership as token alternatives to conference voting. We still have the NHS economy as a potentially independent force, terribly damaged and much of it mortgaged to private contractors, but with huge social reserves as yet unused, and a parliament still empowered to do anything it really wants, when it reaches a generation that rediscovers confidence in active, participative democracy.[56]

Despite its relentless advance, the drive toward industrialisation and commercialisation of care carries within it internal weaknesses and contradictions. It is simply not delivering the savings in cost or improvements in quality confidently predicted by its designers. The much higher cost and lower bed capacity of PFI-funded hospital projects compared with traditional government funding is slowly becoming apparent to MPs and local government councillors who went with the flow in the high tide of privatisations forced through by New Labour. Effects on access of substituting health care markets for public service in the world beyond Europe and North America have shaken even its authors at the World Bank.[57] Henry Ford's capitalism was convincing because its products were real, incontrovertible material evidence that for production of cars, it worked. Did it work as production of a useful social function, as sustainable mobility? Of course not. On the contrary, in these terms of social function it can now be seen as a growing disaster; but it worked at the primitive level of making cars for customers to buy, in individual struggle to keep moving within collapsing public transport systems. Can the same be said for health care produced as a commodity? Certainly not. The now rapidly growing UK private health care sector had 40-50% unused capacity until government shifted 15% of NHS referrals to it by administrative order, not market choice, and guaranteed this for the first five years of the new health care market.[58] A few (very few) research papers have by hook and crook contrived to present bits and pieces of the world's least efficient and most extravagant care system as though its production of routine body repairs provided a model for the less inefficient, less extravagant quasi-socialist systems developed in Europe, but they can refer to no popular experience comparable with the products of Henry Ford. Except to people with a career interest in believing them, they are simply not credible.[59]

Though far too slowly and timidly, patients and health professionals in primary care are moving toward functional alliance at personal levels of care on a mass scale, and (much less frequently) on a local community scale. This could develop a new culture based on citizen needs rather than customer demands. As yet such development is incoherent and spontaneous, but it includes a large and possibly growing minority of UK practices, and of NHS hospital specialists. When, in November 2005, NHS staff in primary care woke up to the fact that Primary Care Trusts had been instructed to end their role as providers of care, and become only administrative commissioners of care by the end of 2008, there was a wave of anger never before seen. All district nurses, health visitors, physiotherapists, speech therapists, podiatrists – all primary care staff except those directly employed by GPs – were to cease employment by Primary Care Trusts or local government, and were expected to accept employment by whichever provider agency got the contract in a competitive market. Health Minister Patricia Hewitt forthwith climbed down and promised to rethink this policy.

What this movement still lacks is what we had in Britain and the rest of Europe from 1942 to 1948, of which flashes briefly reappeared from 1968 to 1974: a mass forward movement of opinion toward social solidarity, dominating all thought about the nature of society for an entire generation. Without that movement we would never have got the NHS, but its foundations were laid half a century earlier, where this chapter began, in struggles to build the original social institutions of mass health care. Without a rediscovery of human solidarity, in action not rhetoric, our planet will, within the next generation or two, cease to provide a basis for civilised life. Such a rediscovery is already beginning, and will continue to grow. We still are many, they are few.

Summary and conclusions

Before responsibility for health care was accepted by the state, ownership of health care systems in industrial societies was a matter for contention between doctors as entrepreneurs, and representatives of the communities they served. This was most obvious in areas of heavy industry like South Wales. Developments in coal-mining areas before the 1911 Insurance Act created models for local accountability and democratic control, which the Act brought to an end by enlisting doctors as independent contractors to the state.

Contemporary senses of ownership played a major role in the disputes between doctors and the state at the birth of both National Insurance in 1911, and the NHS in 1948. In both cases, doctors serving affluent populations, and therefore able to practise clinical medicine as they had learned it in their medical schools, feared degradation of their work if it escaped their ownership and control. Though some of these fears were justified, state funding opened free access to care for all of the people, with virtually no loss of independence in taking clinical decisions between 1948 and the onset of NHS 'reforms' after 1983. This actually expanded professional ownership as social responsibility, even though professional ownership as property diminished, to be haltingly replaced by public ownership (though this process is still incomplete).

Remodelling of the NHS on industrial lines is conscripting health professionals to essentially the same loss of control over their work as that experienced by hand loom weavers in the late 18th century, and other commodity producers ever since. Health professionals are becoming industrial employees, valued according to their productivity not of health gain, but of profit or economic viability to corporate employers in competitive markets.

Optimal creativity and productivity require a sense of ownership, in the sense of social responsibility, for those who do the work, with scope to modify it according to their own experience. These cannot be provided by the industrial model. Health care professionals cannot and should not own the parts of socially organised health care systems they operate, but they can and must aspire to regain responsibility for and control of their work within those systems. They will fail unless they learn how to ally themselves with their own patients, and with the communities they serve, to re-establish the NHS as a gift economy for all of the people, outside and beyond the world of business.

Notes

[1] Petty was the founding father of modern economics and public health, a genius who deserves to be better known. There is an adequate account of his work by Rosen (1958/1993), but the best of all short accounts is by Anikin (1975).

[2] Lambert, 1963.

[3] Evidence of Dr John Leigh, physician to the Manchester Union and Registrar of Births and Deaths, Parliamentary papers; Select Committee on Medical Relief, 1854, quoted in Bloor, 1980.

[4] Doctors with least training were glad to serve poor areas in any paid capacity, but had virtually no time or other resources to apply medical science as it was beginning to be understood in the most progressive teaching hospitals. George Bernard Shaw, who knew better than most the realities of care for the poor from experience as an elected member of the St Pancras Board of Guardians, provided a classic description in his preface to *The Doctor's Dilemma* (1907, pp 26–7):

> The only way [the GP serving the poor] can preserve his self respect is by forgetting all he ever learnt of science, and clinging to such help as he can give without cost merely by being less ignorant and more accustomed to sick beds than his patients. Finally he acquires a certain skill at nursing cases under poverty-stricken domestic conditions, just as women who have been trained as domestic servants in some huge institution with lifts, vacuum cleaners, electric lighting, steam heating and machinery that turns the kitchen into a laboratory and engine-house combined, manage, when they are sent out into the world to drudge as general servants, to pick up their business in a new way, learning the slatternly habits and wretched makeshifts of homes where even bundles of kindling wood are luxuries to be anxiously economised.

[5] In late 19th- and early 20th-century society, this implied enough to wear a suit, collar and tie, keep a bicycle or horse and trap (or after the First World War, a car), a wife, one or possibly two living-in servants, a varying but usually large number of children, and private education for them, usually with priority for boys. Doctors had relatively low social status until science began to give them some credibility. For example, Queen Victoria excluded army doctors from a royal ball for winners of the Victoria Cross in 1859, because they were not considered to be gentlemen (Cantlie, 1974). When a colleague who worked in the poshest practice in Port Talbot was called in the 1930s to the local mansion, he could enter only through the tradesman's entrance, though when royal physician Lord Horder arrived from London to confirm the diagnosis, he got in through the front door. The NHS virtually eliminated poor doctors, but this did not stop many of them looking back to imagined better days, when they were really appreciated.

[6] *The Battle of the Clubs* was a reprint of the reports of the special commissioner for the *Lancet* appointed to enquire into the medical aid societies. London: *Lancet*, 1896.

[7] Doctors were called only to difficult births beyond the capacity of midwives. In Portsmouth these calls earned a fee of 15 shillings. Bexhill Provident Medical Association served mainly farm workers. Its special fees included leg amputations, compound fractures and strangulated hernias, all at £5 each; £3 for closed fractures of the femur; and £1 each for fractured collar bones or dislocated shoulders.

[8] Data on prices and earnings from Egan, 1987; and M. Davies, 1992.

[9] Hobsbawm, 1987, pp 184-5.

[10] C. Williams, 1996. The best way I know to understand these ideas in contemporary terms is to read Robert Blatchford's *Merrie England* ([1893] 1976). The first edition sold 25,000 copies, leading to a reprint which sold over 700,000 copies within a few months, later reaching nearly a million. The Independent Labour Party, precursor of the Labour Party and the first British socialist party with a mass base, was formed in the same year. Before publication of *Merrie England*, there were fewer than 500 socialists in the whole county of Lancashire, an area of concentrated industry; 12 months later there

were 50,000. It was translated into Welsh, Dutch, German, Swedish, Italian and Spanish, and a US edition is said to have sold roughly as many copies as the original in Britain. Blatchford knew how to write for people only beginning to read newspapers. He was inspired mainly by William Morris, the first Englishman to develop Marxism imaginatively and to try to apply it to his own field of work. Blatchford was a vulgariser, whose popularity partly depended on trimming socialist ideas to fit existing common sense; whatever didn't fit, he amputated. Like others with such an eclectic approach, as soon as the 1914 war broke out, he became an equally successful propagandist for the slaughter of man by man.

[11] In 1911, the total annual income of all 32,000 British doctors was estimated by the *BMJ* at £8m, resulting in an average annual income of £250, and a median income somewhat less than £200. Compared with care for the rest of Britain's labouring poor in the early 20th century, the Welsh miners' medical schemes were well funded and their doctors well paid. This depended on the poundage system, unique to South Wales. Everywhere else, friendly societies took fixed subscriptions unrelated to income, but in Wales the schemes took 3 or 4 pence for every £1 earned, deducted at the colliery office, so that funding for health care rose and fell with earnings, which were linked in turn to the pithead price of coal and the prosperity of the entire industry. Coal prices fluctuated, often wildly, but tended to move upwards throughout the first two decades of the 20th century, when coal was the main source of energy and provided an apparently unlimited domestic and export market. In some schemes poundage was paid straight to the contracted doctors, in which case any investment in care was a deduction from their personal income. This guaranteed that little investment was made even in premises, equipment or clerical staff, let alone specialist doctors or nurses. But in the larger, more politically and socially conscious schemes, which are of much greater interest, poundage was paid not to the doctors, but to a miners' medical aid fund from which doctors' salaries were paid, leaving the rest for investment in better buildings, equipment, staff, training and whatever other measures the scheme committees thought conducive to the health of subscribers and their families.

[12] Until well into the 20th century, most operations were done in patients' homes on the kitchen table. In my own practice in

Glyncorrwg, my GP predecessors held a minor operating session every Sunday morning until 1948, when patients first gained access to free care at Neath and Swansea hospitals by fully trained surgeons.

[13] Dr Alastair Wilson of Aberdare told me how his father, a GP sympathetic to workmen and a rare medical supporter of the Lloyd George Insurance Act, would attend operations for hernia at the cottage hospital, alongside a GP colleague equally notorious for his unswerving support for Guest, Keen & Baldwin (GKB), the local coal and steel employers. Each would stoutly assert that the cause of the hernia – from exceptional work strain (for the Miners' Federation) or from a congenital weakness (for GKB) – was plain to see. There was in fact no visible evidence either way.

[14] Aneurin Bevan, in *Hansard*, 30 April 1946, vol 422, col 47. Quoted in M. Powell, 2000.

[15] Falk, 1966; Earwicker, 1981.

[16] Coal was mined where it was to be found, resulting in many relatively isolated settlements where every aspect of life became organised around this single industry. In South Wales isolation was reinforced by mountains dividing each valley from its neighbours, resulting in a characteristically mixed, often contradictory culture, common to all mining communities: independent self-reliance but also divisive parochialism, combined with disciplined solidarity against external enemies. Compared with England's ancient North-Eastern and Midland coalfields, deep mining was a late development in Wales except around the iron and steel industries in Merthyr Tydfil. Welsh coal mining became a major economic and social force only from about 1860, but from then onwards development was extremely rapid, leading to an international in-migration to the South Wales valleys at roughly the same rate as to the Klondike in the US over the same period.

[17] Day-to-day decisions about the schemes were taken by elected committees, initially dominated by colliery officials but from around 1900 by the South Wales section of the Miners' Federation of Great Britain, locally known as the Fed (Francis and Smith, 1980). Meetings of the kind where major decisions were taken concerning the medical aid societies and their disputes with the BMA have been well described by Steve Thompson (2005):

In any mass meeting of colliers or other workmen in south Wales, the usual practice was for anybody who had something to say to stand up and make their comment. Debate was open to anyone with anything to express on a particular matter regardless of position or status. Furthermore, oratory at these public meetings involved an interactive relationship between speaker and audience that ensured that the opinions and feelings of society members were clearly expressed. Newspaper reports of meetings show that speakers were constantly being interrupted with cries of approval or objection from those present, so that even usually inarticulate groups and individuals could make their feelings felt in a very direct way and play some part in determining actions and policies.

Such scenes are sometimes described as 'Athenian democracy', forgetting that two-thirds of the population of Attica were then slaves, with no rights whatever. Miners are among the founders of true participative democracy. The nature of coal mining is entirely different from factory production, leading to few national disputes but many local disputes with employers. At least until the 1930s, production of coal depended almost entirely on men working in extremely variable and often unpredictable conditions, assisted very little by machines. Miners were paid according to the amount of large coal they produced, and the workforce rose or fell according to world market demand, leading alternately to mass overwork and mass unemployment. This gave every trade unionist personal experience of wage negotiations at the point of production, a keen interest in the work of the union and a deep appreciation of the value of solidarity in all its aspects. Whenever local lodges of the Fed had to take important decisions affecting a whole colliery, or a whole village dependent upon it, mass meetings were held, well attended by everyone affected. For the concept of democracy to have any real meaning, it must in some way be measurable. Its most suitable yardstick could be the extent to which decisions are taken by people who will themselves suffer their consequences. Using this measure, the rise and eventual decline of the miners' medical aid societies was a rise and eventual decline of participative democracy. Even as late as the 1970s, long after every trace of local democratic control of the NHS had vanished, meetings of this kind were still possible where Welsh mining communities needed to discuss any major issue of common concern. A.L. Cochrane, the pioneer of epidemiology after the Second World War, got the miners' union to organise such meetings for him in the Rhondda Fach in South Wales, through which he gained informed cooperation from around 90% of his target population for a demanding programme of research into tuberculosis and pneumoconiosis, setting a new world standard for population response. Our research studies in Glyncorrwg for the Medical Research Council all began with whole-community meetings of this kind, with exactly the sort of informal participation Thompson describes.

[18] The first hospital in the Rhondda valleys opened in 1896 with only four beds serving almost 100,000 people. Even by 1914 provision had risen only to 88 hospital beds serving 180,000 people (Egan, 1987, p 90).

[19] Hospitals began to concentrate on effective care for the sick at the beginning of the 20th century. By its end they were close to monopolising it. To most people today, ownership and control of hospitals seems equivalent to ownership and control of the entire care system. In the first decade of the 20th century the British medical profession divided into what has remained its essential form ever since: community-based generalists and hospital-based specialists. These were connected by a referral system generally respected by both; that is, patients saw specialists only with a letter from their GPs, and specialists wrote back to GPs when they returned patients to their continuing care (a situation still not reached either in France or Germany, nor fully established elsewhere in southern Europe). This resulted from a trade war between doctors in the late 19th century, in which specialisation of any kind was initially regarded as unethical – that is, in restraint of free trade. To do their work well rather than merely pretend to do it, specialists needed staff and equipment, which could only be used economically in the shared, centralised facilities of hospital wards, surgical theatres, laboratories and clinics. In cities, medical ethics were redefined to limit specialists to episodic consultancy based in hospitals, and limit city GPs to continuing generalist care in the community, without this augmented staff and technical base. Rosemary Stevens (1966) was the pioneer historian of this important process. Her aphorism cannot be bettered: roughly from 1912 onwards, British GPs owned the patients, and specialists owned the hospitals. This division of patients' problems as traded property

(mainly in custom rather than law) was simpler and more complete in the UK than any other country, essentially because the UK was more completely urbanised and industrialised, providing a market for mass care. This division between generalists and specialists was never so simple or complete either in rural Britain, or in rural-industrial areas typical of coal mining, but it certainly dominated the medical profession as a whole, and provided the rational basis for our referral system and division between primary and hospital (secondary) care.

[20] Thompson, 2005.

[21] At a national level this opportunity was first recognised by Beatrice Webb in her Minority Report to the Royal Commission on Poor Law reform in 1909, though her proposals were ignored in the Majority Report. Far less known are proposals for a nationalised public medical care system oriented to public health aims made in 1911 by Dr Benjamin Moore (1867-1922), founder of British medical biochemistry and a pioneer of 20th-century health economics. He estimated that about 250,000 UK deaths annually could have been prevented by a medical care system organised to apply current knowledge fully to the whole population. His ideas were presented in his book *Dawn of the Health Age*, and through the State Medical Service Association (SMSA) formed by him and a small but authoritative group of like-minded medical intellectuals in 1912. This attracted much attention in the medical press for two years, until all progressive thought was submerged by war hysteria. It never seems to have reached doctors in the front line of care in industrial areas. Though discussion revived briefly in 1918, the SMSA lapsed into passivity after Moore's premature death in the postwar pandemic of influenza. The SMSA wound up in 1929, but some of its remaining members resurfaced in 1931 with the birth of the Socialist Medical Association (SMA, renamed Socialist Health Association (SHA) in the 1970s). The SMA was affiliated to the Labour Party, and introduced plans for a free, universal and comprehensive state medical service into Labour's national policy in 1934.

[22] Collings, 1950.

[23] Irvine and Jeffreys, 1971.

[24] Bosanquet and Leese (1986) studied GP investment strategies from 1966 to the early 1980s, when government began to support such investment with large subsidies. On five indicators of improvement (employment of practice nurse, improved or purpose-built premises, participation in training, possession of ECG, follow-up clinics) 32% of practices (high investors) accounted for 71% of positive scores. Nearly all the high-investing practices were in affluent areas. Even with large subsidies, investment in areas of continued industrial decline with falling populations made clinical sense, but no business sense.

[25] In the words of coalfield historian Ray Earwicker (1981) it was:

> ... the system of pay-as-you-earn deductions that gave the miners' medical clubs their strength. But it was the acquisition of financial control of the clubs through a Workmen's Fund and initiation of a salaried medical service that gave the South Wales clubs their distinctive character. Dispute over the issue of control was settled between the employers and workmen. Employer resistance was minimal.... The colliery doctors petitioned the employers against this change but it was promptly rejected. The doctors, poorly organised, were forced to acquiesce ...

This soon changed once the big disputes between miners and their doctors began in the early 20th century, when the BMA became as fierce a union as any other.

[26] I have dealt with this in greater detail elsewhere, see Hart, 1988.

[27] Though the miners had potential allies in Benjamin Moore and his eminent medical colleagues, these medical intellectuals were socially and geographically too distant from both miners and miners' doctors to form any effective political alliance. British doctors at the bottom of the professional pile rarely saw themselves as intelligentsia in the European and Latin American traditions exemplified by Chekhov, Semashko, Štampar, Evang, Guevara and Barghouti.

[28] The Ebbw Vale dispute was almost exactly repeated in 1934, when my father, Dr Alex Tudor Hart, together with several other doctors, was recruited by the South Wales Miners' Federation to work for the Llanelli Workmen's Medical Aid Scheme after the local doctors, supported by the BMA, withdrew from their previous contracts. The miners, tinplate and foundry workers of Llanelli were trying to develop a larger scheme similar to that in Tredegar, with major surgery performed by specialists rather than their GPs. They proposed to pay for these by reducing the proportion of poundage paid to their contracted GPs, who would also have lost fees previously paid to them for surgery. After a bitter and divisive dispute lasting 18 months, the old doctors still retained most of the patients, though the new scheme was generally recognised as a more rational system. The BMA's chief negotiator was Dr Charles Hill, who later led BMA resistance to the NHS. The dispute was finally settled by arbitration, giving the BMA most of what it wanted, but allowing recruitment of enough salaried specialist staff for the influential Political and Economic Planning Report of 1936 to propose it as a model for the future NHS (R. Davies, 1995).

[29] As Rhodri Morgan (who became leader of the Labour Party in Wales against sustained opposition from Blair) is fond of recalling, the Conservative Party in Wales has never succeeded in winning an elected majority, in the whole time since common people began to get a vote. This is in profound contrast to Scotland, where Conservatives still dominate rural areas.

[30] The imperialist wings of the Liberals, Conservatives, Fabians and reforming civil servants like Sir Robert Morant led a vigorous pre-emptive reform movement on the eve of the First World War, which laid the foundations for 20th-century education and welfare services, completed after the Second World War. This was a conscious effort to assimilate vulgarised socialist ideas to an imperialist programme, assuring British citizens a privileged status as servants of a dominant imperial power. In this way the perceptions of Charles Darwin, which had destroyed the hold of the Anglican Church over the minds of industrial workers, were easily adapted to social Darwinism and the ranking of races. Social Darwinism provided the seeds for Fascism. The close association between eugenic concepts of racial purity and the birth of modern state welfare is a necessary and useful embarrassment for socialists, deserving more thought than it has so far received. The depth and extent of change needed in state

services to make them into services of, by and for the people, rather than means for social control, has always been underestimated.

[31] Lloyd George knew from his actuaries that male life expectancy in 1911 averaged only about 12 months of life after retirement at 65. Proposals today to raise retirement age to 70 would mean that in many unhealthy inner-city areas, pensions might again become 'affordable' to the top of society, in much the same way. At present death rates, if retirement age were raised to 70, 30.6% of men would never collect their pension because they had already died. Biggest losers would be in the poorest London boroughs, of which Hackney is the worst, where 48.3% never reach their 70th birthday (Trades Union Congress, 2004).

[32] Even the Poor Law, however, was intended to strengthen existing social hierarchy by heading off revolution, not just repressing it. William Farr, one of Britain's foremost 19th-century pioneers of public health wrote in the 1870s that 'without abuse' the new Poor Law was 'an insurance of life against death by starvation, and of property against communistic agitations' (quoted by Terris, 2002).

[33] Grigg, 1978, p 325.

[34] These divisions were well described by Francis Maylett Smith in his little-known but excellent autobiography (1981).

> When our local branch of the BMA met, those present were mostly owners of practices.... The assistants, who did most of the work ... greatly outnumbered their seniors, but they were seldom heard because they were hardly ever present. The establishment therefore had little idea of what was going on in the minds of the rank and file. Now that the state was to take over the medical care of wage-earners, through doctors enrolled on the panel, the owners of the profitable medical monopolies became alarmed lest the assistants should go on the panel and set up practice on their own, detaching for themselves most of the wage-earning patients. It looked as if the lucrative system of running large practices through low-paid assistants was about to receive its death-blow ...

No such death-blow was ever delivered. Lloyd George understood this professional division, and adapted his strategy accordingly. 'A deputation of doctors', he said, 'is always a deputation of swell doctors. It is impossible to get a deputation of poor doctors or slum doctors' (quoted in Cox, 1966).

[35] Like Bevan, Lloyd George had a shrewd understanding that because his proposals would make most doctors richer and more secure, and because he had no intention whatever of imposing lay control over clinical decisions, most of this hostility would evaporate if he held to his course. Three weeks before the National Insurance Act came into operation in December 1912, BMA delegates voted by an 80% majority to boycott the panel. Three weeks after it started over half the GPs had signed on (Cox, 1966). Virtually the same humiliating scenario was repeated in 1948: six months before the NHS Act came into operation and with an 84% turnout, 90% of all doctors, and 95% of all GPs, swore in a BMA plebiscite that they would never accept contracts under the Act; two months after the NHS began, 90% of GPs had joined and 93% of the population was registered (Foot, 1973).

[36] A solution favoured by BMA loyalists is to claim that the BMA never did oppose the NHS (so far as I know they have never tried this on the events around 1911). In vain attempts to avoid total isolation, the BMA did offer counter-proposals to Bevan's plan, but they were never presented seriously, and this was not the issue as seen by any contemporary observer. Anyone inclined to believe this myth need only read a few copies of the *BMJ* for 1947-48 to see the hysteria then prevailing in the profession, initially stirred up by Charles Hill and Guy Dane, then getting out of their control, as ridden tigers do. Both in 1911 and 1948, doctors who supported state service publicly were ostracised by most of their colleagues. It is also worth recalling that the Conservative Party voted against the NHS Act in 1946 at all three stages of its progress through Parliament.

[37] Albutt, 1912.

[38] Hill, 1951.

[39] Geiringer, 1959.

[40] Rational primary care cannot compete with the irrational and counterproductive patterns of reward created by either professional or corporate trade. In 1981, at the height of the international fashion for talking about primary care, US primary care physicians could earn three times as much from common in-house laboratory investigations as through listening to their patients, examining or advising them. US surgeons could earn three to seven times, gynaecologists five times, and urologists ten times more per hour for operating as for talking or listening to their patients, and gastroenterologists could earn six times more per hour for endoscopy than for consulting with their patients (Eisenberg, 1988). Such income gradients fail to reflect the skills required for effective talking, listening, and making clinical judgements, and they discourage development of simpler, earlier, more effective and economic interventions. They encourage superfluous, later and more costly but less effective interventions. Above all they encourage technical interventions, by highly trained staff inappropriately deployed.

Governments from time to time rediscover their interest in primary care, always for the same reason: it seems cheaper than hospital care. When this rediscovered interest moves from rhetoric to reality, we find these income gradients are modified, so that the earnings of medical and nursing generalists, whose main tools are their ears and tongues, begin to approach those of medical and nursing specialists. This happened in the 1970s, when half of all UK doctors were GPs. For the first time, most of these actually *wanted* to be GPs. They were no longer just failed specialists, and occasionally broke the hearts of their sometimes eminent parents who feared their talents would be wasted. However, good primary care is probably not in fact cheaper than hospital care. The advantages of primary care lie not in its cost but its humanity, effectiveness and efficiency compared with trying to do everything in hospitals, and its greater accessibility to patients, not just geographically, but culturally. Primary care is less intimidating, and closer to patients' real lives, at home and at work. When governments understand this their interest in primary care wanes. The income gap between community generalists and hospital specialists then resumes its normal growth through operation of the professional labour market. As I write, we are still in such a time of retreat, and medical career preferences have shifted accordingly.

[41] Fulton, 1961.

[42] In the 1960s there were eight times as many specialists per head of population in the US as there were in Britain, but unprofitable areas still had no adequate specialist cover. In New York, 196 neurologists served 6.5 million people, while in West Virginia two neurologists served 2 million people (Battistella and Southby, 1968). By contrast, planned distribution of specialists in the NHS ensured that by the 1960s, no part of Britain lacked real specialist cover.

[43] Schieber and Poullier, 1990; Evans and Barer, 1990.

[44] Even in 2005, after consolidation of many small local insurance funds, there are still 280 different sickness funds in Germany, all independently accounting for each item of service, a major reason for costs running at 10.7% of GDP in 2001 and still rising, compared with 7.6% in the UK. Despite such evidence, there is still much pressure for NHS funding through insurance rather than taxation from so-called expert opinion in market-oriented think tanks. Derek Wanless estimated the per person annual cost of such a move at £700 (Needham and Murray, 2005).

[45] Almost all this work was achieved through the Royal College of General Practitioners founded in 1951, partly because its aims coincided with those of the medical civil service when it was led by Sir George Godber, a man who devoted his life to the birth, infancy and early youth of the NHS. Godber gave the college responsibility for developing a training scheme for young GPs throughout Britain, and made sure this was properly funded. This provided a material foundation for what might otherwise have been little more than a talking shop.

[46] Wall, 1993.

[47] Though industrial general practice was indeed a low form of clinical medicine, young doctors in training at London teaching hospital casualty departments were prepared through embarrassingly similar experience, of which Albutt may have been ignorant. As casualty officer at St Bartholomew's Hospital in 1879, Dr Robert Bridges saw 30,000 new patients a year personally, with an average consulting time of less than one minute (P. Benson, 1979). Contemporary students' ledgers show that in these conditions they

dealt with many common but serious disorders, for example leg ulcers, rodent ulcers of the face and scalp, tuberculosis affecting skin, lungs, kidneys and testicles, fungating cancers of the breast, and every kind of open or closed fracture and dislocation. Medical care as taught in the early 20th century was still brief, brutal and almost veterinary in culture, except for tiny minorities of patients either paying large fees, or allowing themselves to be taught or experimented upon in teaching hospitals.

[48] Rivett, 1998. This confirms the view strongly held by George Godber and expressed by him many times.

[49] Nationalisation of all hospitals was a huge leap forward, and Bevan evidently judged he could not, at that time and in those circumstances, go any further. Through Lord Moran, president of the Royal College of Physicians, he negotiated a compromise with the hospital specialists. He allowed them to work part time in the NHS while continuing in private practice, using NHS resources. He feared that otherwise they would work in their dangerous private nursing homes and neglect their NHS duties (as some still do today). Anticipating that free NHS care would rapidly erode demand for private care, he gave a secret committee of senior consultants full control of substantial additional pensionable income (Distinction Awards, also known as Merit Awards) for them to give to those who might otherwise have earned most from private practice, using secret criteria to establish their 'outstanding merit' ('Our regular correspondent' (1949), 'Foreign letters: London. National Health Service', *JAMA*, vol 141, p 1236; Lee-Potter, 1993). Bevan famously said that he had choked the consultants' mouths with gold; more importantly, he stuffed their hands with power, giving them access to staff, buildings and equipment they could never have provided themselves, letting them use these resources more or less as they pleased, with only one important exception: they must give care free to everyone who needed it.

Thus he divided the professional opposition and reassured his cabinet colleagues, most of whom were appalled by his temerity (which several hoped would cause his downfall, predicted imminently by most of the press). He won, but paid a huge price for what some now see as a small victory. Their argument is consistent with the facts, but if I found it convincing, I would not have written this book. For those who believe that transfer of material ownership and transformation of any major commodity into a social gift is the most necessary but also the hardest step to take toward a sharing society, the case is made.

[50] Why did Bevan, a more principled socialist than any other Labour leader before or since, agree to this? He had few alternatives, having no confidence in local government to rise above parochial concerns at that time, though he later said that he hoped NHS hospitals would become locally accountable to elected local authorities. He liked most of the practising clinicians he met. He was impressed with their genuine enthusiasm for their work, and seems to have believed they were at least no greedier than those of their schoolmates who had chosen to go into business as capitalists, rather than to become extremely skilled (and well-paid) health workers. He seems to have had faith that once their feet were set on his new path, where health care would escape entirely from the world of business, they would steadily move away from medical trade, toward medical science serving the whole of society. I think he was right. In his excellent book Jonathan Neale (1983, pp 14-15) gave a vivid account of the complex relations of power within NHS staff hierarchies as they appeared in the early 1980s, little different from those in 1948 and still recognisable even today. After describing a crisis-ridden surgical operation, with its absurd but effective combination of unbridled consultant vanity, nursing deference and a ghastly downward cascade of condescension, servility and bullying through ranks of diminishing status, he reached an unexpectedly positive conclusion:

> Like a well-drilled army, everybody has done the right thing at the right time, with no orders given. Each works as a member of a team, and each trusts the others. They are united by their various skills and the importance of the work they do. This is a part of what makes hospital workers different from factory workers. The theatre has a more rigid hierarchy than any factory. But the hierarchy seems more justifiable to the workers. The surgeon isn't just using his class power when he behaves like a pig to a technician. He's also nervous. The team isn't just a pyramid of privilege, it's a group of dedicated people too. The nurses aren't spectators in their own lives. They're part of a great drama.

[51] For example, the main argument used to initiate 'reform' of the NHS in Britain was rising costs. This ignored the fact that the NHS

actually cost less than equivalent service in any other developed economy. The NHS was later officially admitted to be grossly underfunded (Beecham, 1991). In Sweden, which soon followed Britain with a similar programme (Walker, 1991; Nilsson, 1993), costs as a proportion of GDP had actually fallen from 9% in 1982 to 7.8% by 1992 (Gilson, 1993). In Sweden the argument was first, that every other country was already doing it, and second, that out-sourcing and internal competition were bound to give better value for money. In practice, these savings have not materialised, so some rethinking is going on (Whitehead, Gustafsson and Diderichsen, 1997).

[52] The most active organised professional force at that time was the NHS Support Federation, led by Dr Harry Keen, professor of Medicine at Guy's Hospital, selected as pilot site for the Hospital Trusts first conceived by Thatcher's government and now imposed everywhere by Blair's New Labour government. Harry's repeated attempts to organise a public meeting with Robin Cook, then Labour shadow Minister for Health, all failed, so he finally gave up trying to organise any joint action with the Labour Party, of which he had been a lifelong member. That experience was typical. Even then, Labour leaders were wary of any close alliance with the medical profession. Though they like to attribute this to enduring memories of medical resistance to the NHS in 1948, opposition to doctors (or any other affluent professional group) still provides an easy and popular alternative to tackling serious concentrations of wealth and power.

[53] Shock, 1994.

[54] Like the Munich agreement it so closely resembles, this capitulation seems to have captivated enough of Sir Maurice's audience to suspend critical thought, at least for long enough to disarm collective resistance. A liberal friend distinguished enough to be invited to this great occasion was elated. 'I do wish you could have been there, Julian, you would have been so relieved to hear him. I think we really do have a resolution now to this dreadful situation.' Peace in our time?

[55] From the 1980s onward, the received wisdom became that doctors primarily served themselves rather than the public interest. Though obviously there was some truth in this, did it contain any more

truth in the 1980s than in the 1970s, or come to that, in the 1870s? Typical of this new establishment view was health economist Alan Maynard (1994): '... unless we tackle the doctors, health reforms will fail to deliver ... processes of health care are dominated by clinicians, who merely represent their own vested interests ... [we must] strengthen the role of health managers and economists, who would speak for society at large'. There is no evidence that this shift in trust, from doctors to NHS managers or to health economists, ever took place among the general public.

[56] In her excellent book *NHS plc: The Privatisation of Our Health Care* (2004), Allyson Pollock provides a wealth of irrefutable evidence that the NHS has already been sliced up, ready for serving to shareholders, in an already-irreversible privatisation by stealth promoted by the leaders of New Labour and Conservative parties, with apparent acquiescence from the Liberal Democrats. Even if the NHS has already been reduced to much the same objective state as our privatised railways, the fact that, unlike British Rail privatisation, this has had to be done secretly or by deceiving or confusing the public, puts it in a different case. Like railways, the NHS will eventually have to be renationalised simply in order to function efficiently and at affordable cost, as an essential social service for the whole of society. There is a huge force of public anger awaiting release when people generally come to understand the scale of this betrayal. This will certainly find some political outlet, either through some process of renewal within the Labour Party, or new developments in the wider Labour movement. In July 2005, the BBC invited listeners to nominate their choice for the greatest philosopher in world history. They expected about 6,000 people to vote, but in the event, 34,000 voted. Karl Marx led the field with 28% of the total, twice as many votes as the next runner-up, David Hume, despite desperate appeals from Lord Melvyn Bragg, hapless initiator of this game, from *The Economist*, and from other establishment figures alarmed by this unexpected tidal flow. We probably have a new generation ready for change.

[57] Abbasi, 1999. Though there were some indications of disquiet during the Clinton administration, President George W. Bush's appointment of Paul Wolfowitz, principal architect of the war on Iraq, as president of the World Bank in 2005, suggests no risk of any such humility.

[58] By 2005, the Department of Health had contracts with for-profit independent treatment centres (ITCs) for 250,000 operations a year in England, at a cost of £500m. Contracts assume 90% bed occupancy, though before NHS 'reforms', private-sector bed occupancy was generally below 50%. The Department of Health guarantees this rate of use for the first five years, whether or not patients can be induced to accept these referrals (*Health Service Journal* (2005), 'Government to pay ITC tab regardless of use', 19 May, p 7).

[59] After statistical contortions that would normally preclude publication in any authoritative peer-reviewed journal, a paper by Feachem et al (2002) claimed that the Kaiser Permanente scheme in California provided a better service than the NHS at a roughly equivalent price. Of many scathing refutations, one of the most restrained was from Smee, a health economist who had worked with Feachem at the London School of Hygiene (Smee, 2002). Smee was consulted about Feachem's first draft, and found its arguments poorly supported by evidence. He went on to conclude:

> Kaiser is indisputably much more expensive than the NHS per capita. At the currency conversion rate used by the authors and after their adjustments for differences in service and population coverage the per capita cost of the NHS is barely 60% of Kaiser – $1161 compared with $1951. If we are looking at the total costs or macro-efficiency of two systems it is simply wrong to adjust for differences in healthcare prices, over and above adjusting for general differences in prices. But to suggest that NHS per capita costs are 60% of those in Kaiser is to give the comparison a spurious accuracy that is not warranted by the data presented.... Alternative (and arguably more defensible) assumptions – e.g. about treatment of Kaiser's profits, their 'considerable' administrative costs, and the currency conversion rate – would reduce NHS costs per capita to barely half those of Kaiser.... The NHS has equity and universal coverage objectives that are irrelevant to Kaiser. The NHS also aspires to provide a range of health services that is significantly more comprehensive than is available under Kaiser ... from the data in this paper there can be no doubt at all that in terms of total

costs per capita or macro-efficiency, Kaiser is far more expensive than the NHS.

Feachem never provided a convincing answer to these criticisms, but this paper continues to be quoted by apologists for commercialisation of the NHS, as they have virtually no other.

FIVE

Solidarity

Human biology and the practice of medicine are based on a belief that people are sufficiently alike, that the secrets of disease in a king may be found by cutting up a pauper. Though doctors have often behaved as though patients had no brains, even they had to admit, if pressed, that this could never be true. Solidarity, a belief that humans are all of one species, that we are social animals who stand or fall together, whose survival depends on helping one another, has a sound foundation in the full science of human biology, which has to include scientific, evidence-based approaches to psychology, sociology, history and politics.

Medical fascism

Despite this humane tradition, doctors were in the front ranks of the imperial and eugenic movements in Europe and North America before the First World War, which laid foundations for Fascism, drawing initially on social Darwinism developed mainly in Britain and the US.[1] In 1933 Germany had the world's most advanced research teams and most innovative physicians and surgeons, just as the US has today, but they did nothing effective to save their country from regression to medieval levels of thought and behaviour. On the contrary, German doctors and nurses were foremost among the zealots heading over the abyss. Doctors formed a higher proportion of Nazi Party membership than any other professional group. In Germany, already by 1932, sterilisation legislation was prepared, and accepted by a wide range of Catholic, Jewish and socialist eugenicists. Most of the scientists involved in German eugenic policies remained in key posts related to human genetics after 1945. The Nazi euthanasia programme met no serious resistance either from public opinion or the various churches.[2] In the US, following the same vulgarised quasi-scientific theories, at least 60,000 people were forcibly sterilised in the first half of the 20th century;[3] similar measures were taken in Sweden in the 1930s.[4] They were certainly contemplated by government in Britain, with similar widespread acceptance of reductionist assumptions about the nature of inheritance, but fortunately were never implemented.

Obviously neither medical science nor clinical practice then provided inherent guarantees against even the most extreme forms of inhumane thought and behaviour. Wherever the full power of the state authorises violence by its uniformed servants or by criminal sections of its population against groups said to be enemies of society – as in the USSR, South Africa and most of Latin America since the Second World War and at present throughout the Middle East – only recently have medical professional organisations begun to organise serious resistance among their own members.

Fascist ideas depend on the solidarities of our prehistory, when tribal survival seemed the only consideration, and human survival was never in question. The answer must lie in refusing ever to accept exclusions from a single human species. For health professionals this is a much easier rule to apply than for most other occupations, because we have established institutional frames and customs that reinforce socially inclusive thought and practice. In all wars there have been exceptional, and occasionally not so exceptional, health workers who cared for their sick and wounded enemies as much as for their friends. The Geneva Conventions may not have counted for much, but they did count for something.

When I qualified in 1952, all NHS services were available free to anyone in Britain who needed them. To include people who were not British citizens may not at first sight have seemed logical, but if a Greek seaman or a French cook or an American visiting her sick grandmother happened to break a leg or get pneumonia, our first consideration was to help them, with no questions asked about who was to pay. Though foreign visitors could have been made to fill in a lot of forms and pay for their care, in an already cash-free economy the costs of collection were close enough to potential revenues to make this a gratuitous act of meanness, useful only to prove that nothing must ever be given without payment. The definitive experiment was finally made by Margaret Thatcher's government in 1983, when Sheffield Health Authority staff were compelled to quiz 50,000 patients in the first three months of the operation of the government's new procedure for charging overseas visitors. Among these they found a total of eight who were liable to pay. Their total charges amounted to £4,066, but almost half this amount was incurred by patients who evaded payment. The authority decided to resort to the courts only if this made economic sense, which of course it never did.[5] Like unpaid doctors' fees in the era of pre-NHS trade, bad debts to the NHS generally cost more to pursue through the courts than they were worth. In 1949, a year after the NHS began, tabloid newspapers floated alarming stories of waste in the new free NHS, including a tale that foreign seamen were streaming into Liverpool to get free NHS dentures, which then turned up for sale in a Baghdad bazaar. Attlee's cabinet feared this was true, so they set up an inquiry. This revealed a grand total of ten foreign seamen who had ever seen an NHS dentist in the first year of the service, with no evidence whatever of abuse by any of them, or of any NHS dentures in Baghdad.[6]

Solidarity is simple, and broadly speaking, true. The simpler we can make it, the truer it can be. Health care is a field in which generosity is a natural behaviour tending to create generosity in return. Despite many similar nasty stories, the common experience of both staff and patients in the NHS has confirmed this optimism. The stories turn out to be either tabloid rumours, like the seamen's trade in false teeth, or based on exceptional incidents remembered precisely because they were exceptional.

Solidarity has its origins in the survival advantages of pooled risk. If I help weak people when I am strong, then when I become weak I can expect to find other stronger people to help me: the principle of reciprocity.[7] All human societies have had this characteristic, which is even more obvious in the subsistence economies of hunter–gatherers and nomads than in more advanced economies with an agricultural or industrial surplus and an evolved care system. Systems based on wholly inclusive pooled risk are immensely more efficient than contributory insurance systems of any kind, above all more efficient than the individually calculated risks of privately marketed insurance.[8] If everyone is entitled to care according to their need, a huge bureaucracy of risk assessors, premium collectors, fraud detectors and millionaire or billionaire directors leading an army of investors are all made redundant. All we need to do is to pay our taxes on a single assessment of income. These taxes then fund the cash-free internal economy of the NHS (or any other service we decide to transform from a commodity to a shared human right), and there is the end of it. The pre-'reform' NHS worked because few people wanted to be ill, and most were intelligent and civilised enough to understand that it made sense to pay throughout their lives for a service they hoped to use as little as possible, or ideally, not at all. Even though our press and approved experts constantly tell us otherwise, this was and still is how most people think, because this view is reinforced by common experience of the NHS, even in its present mutilated state. The great weakness of the US is that neither its people nor its health professionals have ever had that experience.[9]

Solidarity is not altruism

Solidarity should not be confused with altruism. This is an area of thought that requires rigorous clarity and realism, not sentimentality. Adam Smith's opinion expressed in *The Wealth of Nations*, that most people most of the time act in their own interest, was correct. Sustainable economics deals not with exceptional people in exceptional states of moral fervour, but with ordinary people in their everyday thought and behaviour. The concept of altruism – motivation to act not for oneself but for others against one's own personal interest – is natural and appropriate for liberal academics, whose own experience continually reinforces their belief that a large social conscience is an economic burden, and that to act generously is usually against their own material interest. For generations of organised industrial workers this was simply not true; they thought in terms not of altruism, but of solidarity. Experience taught them that their personal interests, or those of their families, were almost always best served by acting in the interests of their whole work-based community. Institutions outside the market, like the NHS and public education were created by that solidarity, and by the response of rulers to the threat it posed to their privileges, not by the altruism of either party.[10]

The concept of solidarity as a fundamental guiding principle for health care has its diametrical opposite in the view that health care can be most effectively and efficiently provided as a commodity traded for profit. In 1999, after damning evidence against profit motivation in health care appeared in the *New England Journal of Medicine*, battle raged in its correspondence columns. None of the angry defenders of profit motivation presented any countervailing evidence. Where beliefs reach religious intensity, evidence becomes irrelevant, because even the possibility of doubt is excluded. The following passage comes from one of these letters:

> To claim ... that free market principles do not apply to health care is akin to believing that the law of gravity does not apply to certain objects on this planet. Upholding this myth can only be compared to clinging

to a pre-Copernican view of the universe.... When
money is the mission, everyone wins.[11]

The physician who wrote this is, like most of his generation, an
orthodox disciple of Friedrich Hayek, Milton Friedman and the
Chicago school of economists. Like many others doing well out of
the global market,[12] he had blind confidence in his own rectitude,
wherever this might lead him. The leaders of society say hard choices
have to be made. To make economic progress they must harden
their hearts without regard to immediate results such as mass
unemployment or destruction of skills, because in the long run this
will create more wealth. Some of this, they assure us, will eventually
spill down to the rest of society, and the higher the pile on the rich
man's table, the more crumbs will fall to the poor. There can be no
other way.

Such religious faith in a profit-motivated universe, where
economic theory is not tested against empirical experience, not
tested for its predictive power, and not asked to explain or solve
rapidly expanding social problems in the real world, is itself our
main problem. The pre-Copernican universe failed when it was
compelled to explain and predict real events in the real world. In
health care it is obvious that when money becomes the mission,
everyone ultimately loses. Fully developed free-market society
compels everyone to become either a winner or a loser. Both of
these states distort or destroy human creativity, our greatest source
of health and happiness. Even if some losers somehow obtain more
crumbs from the winners than they could produce from their own
subsistence production, eventually even the winners will lose –
first their integrity and self-respect, then our planet as a shared
habitat for our species. There is no ultimate escape from human
solidarity.

Does any informed person really believe that advances in medical
science or innovations in care have to be driven by greed rather
than ambition to serve well in our present and for our future society?
Does anyone really believe that the great pioneers of medical and
nursing science would have worked harder for profit, than for the
dignity and honour of having achieved something real to make the
world a happier place?[13] In a public service frankly committed to
meeting human needs rather than making a profit or promoting
top people's careers, motivation is rarely a problem.
Overwhelmingly, NHS staff love their work, and ask only to be
allowed to do it to the standards they have learned. If they come to

hate or fear their work, serious questions need to be asked, usually about wages, workload or bullying in the still-persistent staff hierarchy, but above all, whether the service is in fact devoted to meeting human needs rather than business-oriented management demands, and whether staff really control their own creative process.[14]

Solidarity works both ways. The NHS also depends on patients and communities helping NHS staff. When society itself begins to fall apart into a war of every man against every man, a lifelong battle between consumers where disciplined queuing has become a lost social skill, and personal demands become an all-consuming force (as they do, for example, in drug dependence) solidarity may seem almost impossible to regain: but it remains the only possible foundation for an evolving but sustainable society. To accept that we have lost solidarity is unconditional surrender to the past and betrayal of the future.

Internal inequalities in health and health care

My mother qualified in medicine just after the First World War and was in the first cohort of specialist endocrinologists. When she was 12 years old she had acute rheumatic fever, then a common disease among the poor, but often seen also in affluent professional families like hers. At 52 she had a dense embolic stroke from mitral stenosis, a late consequence of that childhood event. Five years later she had another embolic stroke and died.

Today, acute rheumatic fever has virtually disappeared in Britain. Working as a GP in relatively poor communities, I saw three new cases between 1953 and 1963, the last I ever saw. Students seeking experience of this now rare but formerly common disease will still find plenty in West Africa, Rio de Janeiro or India, and occasionally in Chicago, Washington DC and Harlem.[15] Acute rheumatic heart disease, and other disorders related to streptococcal infection like acute nephritis, are causally related to poverty, chiefly because of overcrowding. Material poverty of that degree is now rare in Britain, except in recent immigrant neighbourhoods. The lesson is that where affluent people live close to poor people, some of their children will share the diseases of the poor. The reflex *Daily Mail* answer is social segregation. Those who can afford it retreat to suburbanised countryside or gated urban communities, those who can be imprisoned or expelled from the country are thrown out, and those too poor and too British to do either of these are expected to shut up and behave themselves. Experience of drug addiction and AIDS shows that all gates fail and all frontiers are porous. Fortunately, so long as the poor exist, their diseases will threaten the offspring of the rich.

> The belief that subpopulations in one country are separate and do not operate as a single ecosystem affecting each other has propelled the US into a crisis of social and economic structure and of public health and public order which is so severe that even such crude measures as life expectancy show deterioration. It reflects a profound error: concentration is mistaken for containment.... Public policies or economic practices which marginalise vulnerable communities within Europe may be expected to create a crisis similar to that now raging in the United States.[16]

That was written in 1997, when Britain voted by a landslide for an end to the Thatcher era, and its retreat to the deregulated and detaxed capitalism in the US, itself regressing to the era of the robber barons before the First World War. We never got what we voted for. The gap in both income and health between rich and poor has continued to grow under New Labour as it did under Conservative governments, because, just as before, satisfaction of the immediate wants of big multinational companies still have priority over every other consideration.[17] Denial that everyone shares the same human ecosystem has made little headway among medical professionals, but this is already how affluent, educated and liberal people act in relation to their own choices of where to live and educate their children, because both alternately ruling parties have abdicated from collective choices that individuals cannot make, even if that is how they would prefer to live. This is the philosophy underlying the xenophobic attitudes now propagated by the Conservative Party and its press in Britain, and accepted by New Labour, as their own agenda.

Large mortality differences between social groups, and the even larger morbidity differences they approximately represent, are a danger to everyone. Though technical repairs later created personal clinical solutions to my mother's problem (mitral valvotomy, valve replacements, atrial embolectomy and lifelong anticoagulants) these remain inefficient and costly compared with preventive actions easily available for at least the past two centuries – rehousing poor people in the conditions we all want for our own families,[18] for which no serious national programme existed until after the Second World War, and even then was not sustained.[19] The parallel between rheumatic heart disease and coronary heart disease is almost exact – both are social epidemics for which there were two sets of answers: either extremely clever but costly and socially inefficient surgical repairs, or mass changes in planned social housing, education and food economy to develop people as intelligent citizens rather than passive consumers, and to provide conditions in which intelligent collective choices could be made.[20] That is no more impossible now, than was decent housing for everyone in the first half of the 20th century.

We also have consistent evidence over long periods of time, mainly from studies in California and Sweden, that people who live within larger, more integrated, sustained and participative personal networks of family, friends, neighbours and workmates live longer than those who are isolated. Real community matters to health. This is probably not linked to specific disease pathways, but to more general factors related to rates of senescence and resistance to disease.[21] Close, mutually supportive relationships are for most people a necessary part of healthy life. The grossly unequal, destabilised acquisitive society created by unregulated operation of market forces is therefore inherently unhealthy. Market forces propagate ill health, just as they propagate crime and every kind of selfish behaviour. Within established modes of thought that perceive health only as the absence of specific disease this is easier to understand than to prove, but it remains a stubbornly held popular belief because it confirms popular experience, as well as being the consensus view of most sociologists.

Global inequalities in health and health care

The dangers presented to national health by socio-economic ghettos have their obvious counterpart in dangers to world health presented by pools of uncontrolled disease in virtually all countries outside Europe, North America, Australia and New Zealand. This used to be the main agenda of the World Health Organisation (WHO) when it was a truly independent agency of the United Nations, not a poor relation of the World Bank (WB).

The World Bank began to take an interest in global health policy in the late 1970s, when this subject began to interest investors. From 1984 to 1989 WB loans related to health care trundled along at a steady US$ 0.25 billion a year, about half as much as the WHO budget. Between 1989 and 1990 WB loans for health care leapt five-fold to US $1.25 billion, well over the US $0.7 billion spent by the WHO. In 1996 WB loans for health care began an escalating rise still continuing today, taking WB investments in health care to more than double the entire WHO budget by 2000.[22]

This reflected changing patterns of US investment. In the US, more than one-third of economic growth between 1994 and 1999 was in service exports. The World Bank calculated that in less-developed countries alone, infrastructure development with some private backing rose from US $15.6 billion in 1990 to US $120 billion in 1997. About 15% was direct foreign investment in public schemes, with loans or aid conditional on new policies of privatisation and direct patient charges.[23] Effective socialised care services that once served as splendid examples of successful best practice, for instance in Kerala and Sri Lanka, were broken up and privatised under WB pressure, with predictably dire consequences for public health.[24] A struggle has been going on since November 2004 in the European Union between its Competitiveness Council led by Fritz Bolkestein, which wants a single market for all service industries, and defenders of EU Treaty Article 52 insisting that member states must each retain responsibility for their health services.[25] This struggle included politicians concerned to get re-elected, and 60,000 trade unionists who demonstrated in Brussels in March 2005 to remind them of that fact (unreported by mainstream British news media).[26] Effectively, bankers have replaced health professionals as directors of global health policy, where together with the World Trade Organisation, they opposed the consistent general direction of WHO policy from 1946 to 1990 favouring socialisation of health care, not because the WHO was wedded to an ideology, but because this policy manifestly worked.[27]

Despite weak leadership since the days of Hafdan Mahler, the WHO still exists. Like the NHS, it represents an immensely popular idea that is almost impossible to destroy by frontal attack. It is now surrounded by many non-governmental agencies, for example Médecins Sans Frontières, with even greater appeal to generations not yet worn down by cynicism and complacent despair. Except in a few almost entirely technical specialities, medical and nursing skills are much less internationally mobile than many people think. Clinically effective and efficient practice depends almost always on close relationships between carers and patients, requiring familiarity with customs, cultures and languages. However, there are also centuries-old traditions of caring across national, ethnic, religious and political borders, and of professional opposition to military and judicial murder and torture, which will increasingly make life difficult for politicians now inclined to discard international institutions like the United Nations, the World Court and now even the Geneva Convention, as obstructions to global trade, free movement of capital and free exertion of military power. Future combinations of real respect for local diversities, together with real internationalism, could support a rebirth of truly accountable global authorities, without which we shall have no future at all. The immediate threat of mutant avian influenza reveals the political consequences of abandoning WHO and other UN agencies through which rational policies can be developed and applied.

A new economics of shared risk

Public health depends on recognition that to maximise health, public health cannot be hoarded by those with most power, but has to be shared by everyone. Likewise, the advances in science required to support health gain beyond the point secured simply by ensuring that everyone eats, has shelter and has access to education, require investments so huge, so uncertainly profitable, and where the returns on investment may be so long delayed, that investment risks must be shared by the whole of society and across more than one generation.

If essential services become funded even in large part by for-profit investors, then market failure becomes intolerable not just to disappointed gamblers on the stock exchange, but also to society as a whole. The original reason that the state took responsibility for essential infrastructure such as education, health services, roads, bridges, docks and harbours, postal services, policing, prisons, armed forces, housing for the industrial working class and support for a multitude of creative arts and sports, was that none of these looked profitable enough for capitalists to undertake or sustain them on the scale needed by a developed economy. In virtually all countries, national railway systems ultimately proved unprofitable, and had either to be sustained by colossal subsidies from taxation, or nationalised as another responsibility for the state. In most European countries, the same thing happened to coal mines and other sources of power for the same reasons.

None of these state-owned industries was socialised, in the sense that the nature of work itself became less dehumanising. Henry

Ford's principles were applied in nationalised industries through the same management techniques as in private sector industry. However, workers in state-owned industries did make huge gains in security, because essential industries could not be allowed to fail, and their survival no longer depended on their profitability. For them, it was enough to break even.

This changed with the neoliberal era, though less so than its apologists suggested. They claimed that industries must learn either to stand unaided on their own feet, or fall into bankruptcy. The world, they said, must return to the disciplines of the marketplace, and both success and failure must be allowed to find their own natural limits. The 50% top rate of income tax prevailing when Thatcher was first elected became unthinkable for any political party in serious contention for government, while mass unemployment became thinkable for the first time since 1945 – not, of course, for people who might themselves become unemployed, but for people with power to determine the lives of others.[28]

The only aspect of this rhetoric applied in reality was mass unemployment and declining real wages in manufacture and basic heavy industries. Workers rooted in the now obsolete era of manual work were indeed left to sink or swim. But the biggest employers and investors, whose opinion makers had ensured Thatcher's and Reagan's elections, could be confident that their own transition to the new global economy would be as painless as government could make it. Governments that claim to have shifted the burdens of necessary social investment from taxpayers to private investors have not shifted the risks. If railways, schools, prisons or hospitals fail in market competition, they are, almost without exception, still kept in business through subsidies, still funded by taxation. The big change is that public undertakings that were once answerable to elected representatives of the people have become private business, wrapped in commercial secrecy, with rational central planning replaced by consumer demand, carrying added costs of profit for investors and astronomical salaries for top executives.

Mature capitalism can develop only as a closely regulated bureaucratic machine, so entangled with government that conflicts of interest have become the norm, and every successful politician can anticipate a great personal future in business, like his 18th-century predecessors in the heyday of graft and corruption. Colin Leys estimates that about half of all tax revenues now go eventually to profit-making companies, compared with just over a quarter in the mid-1970s.[29] Return to small government and the simplicities of a small-business economy remain central to the Conservative Party platform, but have no real place in the practice of any party close to power, and are now losing credibility with voters. To move from this new understanding that the risks of modern investment have to be shared by the whole of society, to understanding that this must apply also to its benefits, is a short step, though it crosses the deepest possible division in ideology.

Pooled risks in the pharmaceutical industry

Two industries typify this new relationship between government and corporate power more than any others: the arms industry, producing commodities to destroy life, and the pharmaceutical industry, producing commodities claiming to make life longer and happier – in the words of its trade association, a goal 'not only necessary but noble'. Both are motivated by profit. Is this motivation a necessity, or simply the way they have evolved so far?

There is no convincing evidence that motivation to innovate in health sciences has to depend on anticipated profit. What may be mistaken for such evidence is the fact that research, development and pioneering innovation have to be paid for. They entail work, their workers must have something to live on, so they can't be done for nothing. If government policy precludes public funding, innovators have no alternative to funding from the market, in return for expected profits to investors. Steady withdrawal of the state from ownership and direct funding has led to increasing commercialisation of fundamental research, with ever-closer links to pharmaceutical companies, though state subsidies through selective tax relief, price fixing and cost-plus contracts have continued to expand.

The contribution of states to progress in these industries has not in fact diminished, only their control over how this money is spent. Even in the US, most basic research from which new medications originate is still funded directly by the state and conducted in university departments. Even in 1990, the US Federal government still provided about 45% of all funding for pharmaceutical research and development, matched by another 45% from companies, and supplemented by 10% from charities.[30]

Though pharmaceutical industries in developed economies yield huge profits, normal market competition has virtually disappeared. All pharmaceutical product development, production and marketing is highly regulated by governments – to protect patients against unhealthy side-effects, to protect care systems against bankruptcy and to preserve profitability for investors so that their business can continue to expand, they can continue to pay taxes and to provide employment. Pharmaceutical companies invest a higher proportion of their revenue in research and development than any other industry except armaments and computing, about 16% of their total revenues in the US. In 1993, of all the compounds synthesised between 1961 and 1983, only about one in 60,000 made a global profit over $100m a year (the conventional threshold for commercial success), with an average lag of ten years between the original research idea and its marketing.[31] Though production costs tend to fall, research and development costs continue to rise. Risks of market failure are increasing rapidly as sales come to depend on millions of patients at diminishing personal risk from disease, but with constant risks from harmful side effects, many of which are not known before marketing.[32]

In Britain, profits of pharmaceutical companies are determined not by market competition, but through secret agreements whereby government, still an almost monopoly consumer through the NHS, guarantees a high rate of profit, in return for much lower prices than those paid for the same medications in the US or most of the global market.[33] As Alan Maynard wrote in 1991:

> Although often regarded as the epitome of capitalism, the pharmaceutical industry is the product of government regulation which ensures an absence of price competition … the Pharmaceutical Price Regulation Scheme (PPRS) requires firms to reveal trading details to the Department of Health; in exchange, Government permits the industry to adjust its prices to achieve a high target return (rumoured to be around 18-20% at present) on historical capital. This protection is administered by one part of the Department of Health; another branch increases development costs by overseeing the process of taking a drug from the laboratory to the patient … the UK has little tradition of independent business regulation compared with the USA, and the new mechanisms, instruments and techniques of regulation in the wake of the processes of privatisation and competition introduced in the 1980s have been designed in an intellectual vacuum unconfused by facts or precedent. These changes are not confined to the pharmaceutical industry, but only this industry has the additional complications of universal

patents, high barriers to new entrants (eg, costly safety and efficacy legislation), a sole buyer of its products (the NHS is a monopsonist) and product (not price) competition created and sustained by government. The secret complexities of the regulation of the pharmaceutical industry are changing, but their precise nature, and their efficacy, remain secret. Capitalists are the enemies of capitalism, seeking to achieve monopoly power and to corrupt the market to their own advantage by undermining the powers of the customer.[34]

Pharmaceutical manufacturing with a laboratory base began in the late 19th century, first in Germany, then in Switzerland and France. Largely because of demands for effective control of tropical diseases in its empire, Britain began to develop some independent research-based industry in 1894, with the Wellcome Laboratories. Research and development remained concentrated in Germany, where development of sulphonamides in 1935 made the first breakthrough into effective medication on a mass scale, with a really substantial impact on mortality. The Second World War and the Nazi occupation of Europe then revealed the weakness of this industry in both Britain and the US. Starting in 1941, both countries then made huge investments that effectively created new modern industries in both countries. Penicillin was its prime product, an immense advance over sulphonamides in both effectiveness and safety. Most of the fundamental research was done in Britain, while product development and manufacture were undertaken in the US, giving US industry a lead it has never subsequently lost, first in antibiotics, later in psychoactive drugs. By 1965 the global pharmaceutical market was valued at US $10 billion, rising to US $80 billion by the early 1980s, with about 25% in the hands of European countries and the rest divided between the US and Japan.[35] Many important medications are relatively cheap and simple to manufacture as generic (unbranded) products, so that countries like Sri Lanka, Brazil, India, Poland and Hungary all developed highly competitive industries of their own, without any substantial research base, but requiring great political commitment against huge pressures of every kind from the large multinational companies trying to protect and extend their copyrights, and states and international agencies acting on their behalf. This opportunity still exists for any even small country with sufficient imagination and courage to create such an industry both to supply its own care system with generic drugs, and to export them at low prices to other countries that need them.[36]

Pharmaceutical companies now penetrate government, the university medical schools concentrating clinical research, and university departments of basic science where fundamentally new ideas, followed by 30 or 40 years of profitless gestation, precede new explosions of profitability.[37] Pharmaceutical company support for medical research in the US almost doubled between 1980 and 2000, and now accounts for 62% of all medical research funding. About a quarter of US academic researchers now have links with industry that can and do influence their research and publications. Industry-sponsored research tends to reach conclusions favourable to the sponsor. For example, in 61 sponsored trials comparing non-steroidal anti-inflammatory agents, none found the comparison drug superior to the sponsor's drug.[38] Results of unfavourable trials were simply not published.

The industry in Britain was recently reviewed by the House of Commons Health Select Committee.[39] Its report confirmed that the UK pharmaceutical industry generates net exports valued at over £3 billion a year, with a research budget of £3.3 billion including about 90% of all clinical drug trials. It also has a marketing budget of £1.65 billion, compared with 0.3% of this sum spent by the NHS on independent information to prescribers. The industry funds over half of all UK postgraduate medical education, and pays its selected key opinion leaders up to £5,000 to give a one-hour lecture.

Though even the richest multinational pharmaceutical companies can operate only through state-organised and state-subsidised care systems, and have to accept tight state regulation to maintain public confidence and keep out smaller and often more unscrupulous competitors, they insist that innovation and efficiency depend on their continued functioning as companies operating to maximise profit for shareholders rather than health gain for everyone. Evidence that this is so, that researchers would work less tirelessly for public benefit than to make profits for investors and astronomical salaries for their top executives, does not exist. Following the thalidomide disaster in 1961,[40] first the Kefauver Committee in the US, then the Sainsbury Committee in Britain, reviewed the performance of their respective pharmaceutical industries, for the first and last time implying at least the possibility that they might work better as nationalised industries for the common good than to make money for private investors.[41] The companies' answer was to invest more in public relations and lobbying of Parliament and Congress, with the result that this question is no longer even discussed in polite conversation. However, there seems to be no cogent reason why the NHS, or any other care system should not research, develop, produce and market its own medications in competition with commercial companies, other than new EU and WTO laws designed to make such competition illegal. Experience of access for poor countries to life-saving treatment for HIV infection and AIDS shows that given sufficient political will, this issue can be got onto the agenda.[42]

Taking into account the entire global economy, efficiency in all sectors of production increasingly depends on an acceptance of shared risk, as more production becomes research based. Health services are in the best position to set the example, from which all other sectors might learn.

Are we approaching the end of solidarity?

Since the Second World War, virtually all mainstream experts on social change have agreed that the social base for solidarity has diminished. Employment in heavy industry and manufacture has declined, consumer choice is replacing trade union and political organisation as a means for people to improve their lives, and most of what was the working class is now said to have become middle class. Two years after he became Prime Minister, Tony Blair said he had: 'a 10 year programme to tackle poverty and social exclusion. At the end of it I believe we will have an expanding middle class ... which will include millions of people who traditionally saw themselves as working class, but whose ambitions are far broader than their parents and grandparents.'[43] With all those who have built careers on his patronage, he believes that the natural ideology of the aspirant middle class is consumerism. He is trying to reconstruct traditional one-nation conservatism on a broader mass base, the large but now almost spiritless carcass of the Labour Party.

Social class may be defined objectively by observed status, wealth or income, or subjectively, by the groups with which people themselves choose to identify. Considered as agents for social change, these subjective self-definitions are important; if people do not think of themselves as members of a class, they will no act as members of that class. Marx used social class as a means for analysis of the power structure of societies, assuming that in every society production of means for existence was the centre and source of all power. He defined classes in terms of the nature and extent of their control over the processes of production. In advanced economies with little or no peasant class, significant independent subsistence production has become virtually impossible, and even self-employed people have virtually no control over their work outside the requirements of those owning and controlling large enterprises. His perception of two great social classes, a small class of powerful owners and a large class of powerless and property-less operatives, is therefore more obviously valid now than it was when he wrote.[44]

Though this is a powerful device for social and historical analysis, there is no evidence that Marx ever intended it as a precise statistical tool. He set out not a detailed anatomy of the form of society, but an analysis of its function, its physiology, how society worked. So, starting from where most people are, and from available data, we have categories useful to business, government and social policy, rather for planning the transformation of society.

The following subjective data came from the Centre for Elections and Social Trends in 1999:

	1966	1979	1987	1997
People describing themselves as:				
Middle class	30%	32%	34%	36%
Working class	65%	63%	62%	61%
Don't know	5%	5%	4%	3%

We can compare this with the objective UK census rankings in 1951, based on occupation. If, as was once customary, we accept that the registrar general's social classes I, II, and III non-manual were the middle class, together these formed 27.8% of the population; and social classes III manual, IV and V, then described as working class, together formed 72% of the population. By 1995, the middle class thus defined had grown to 51.2% of the population, and the working class had declined to 48.9%.

This confirms that as a cultural group, the working class is in slow decline, with corresponding recruitment to the middle class. However, it does not support widespread adoption by UK media of US terminology, which describes virtually everyone in employment as middle class (the 'middle America' wooed by presidential candidates, corresponding to the 'middle Britain' which has become the pivot of all the gossip now passing for political discussion in UK media). In fact this terminology seems doubtful even in the US, where a high proportion of industrial workers still describe themselves as working class, whatever media discussants may think.

Market research targets various social groups as consumers with different capacities and inclinations to spend. As usual, they allocate most white-collar workers above the lowest grades to the middle class, and all manual workers, however skilled and well paid, to the working class, together with people without work, but competing for lowest-paid employment. Using their definitions, they confirm a rapid fall in the proportion of working-class people, from about 64% of the UK population in 1975 to about 52% in 1997, and a corresponding rise in the middle class from about 36% in 1975 to about 48% in 1997. This corresponds with the rapid decline in UK manufacture, which continues today.[45]

This conventionally defined working class has provided bedrock voters for the Labour Party ever since it overtook the Liberals as a popular mass party after the First World War, though there has always been a substantial minority working-class vote for the Conservative Party, rarely falling much below 20% even in Labour strongholds of heavy industry. Though there has been a catastrophic fall in the number of workers employed in mining, fisheries, agriculture, manufacturing and heavy industry, the British industrial working class still remains a huge potential force. Allied with the new kinds of worker generated by new kinds of commodity in a knowledge-based economy, it is potentially bigger than ever before. The actual composition of the 'middle class' seems extremely suspect, certainly containing many white-collar workers with no more power or property than blue-collar manual workers. Though white-collar workers generally lack the traditions of militant solidarity typical of workers in mining and manufacturing, they have in fact provided most new entrants to trade unionism over the past 30 years.

A middle with a bottom but no top?

The term 'middle class' implies that it has some higher class above it, and another lower class beneath it: or, if we prefer the North American myth of classlessness in a fluid society without significant inherited wealth, on either side of it. Either way it's a sandwich. The people beneath are the working class, the size of which depends on how many white-collar workers are allocated, or allocate themselves, to middle-class status, but there can be no doubt that a working class exists, comprising anything from one-third to four-fifths of the whole population. The great mystery is the hypothetical class above the middle class, presupposed by this terminology but undetectable by population censuses or surveys. According to market research, both in 1975 and in 1997, the middle class and working class together formed 100% of the population: a middle with a bottom but no top. Even the registrar general has no category for the super-rich, who are subsumed into social class I, along with all the other higher managers and professionals. Apparently no upper class actually exists.

Unlike any previous era, few wish to admit they belong to a class whose wealth and power is by orders of magnitude greater than anyone else's. It is now hard to find anyone too rich or too powerful to find refuge in the ubiquitous middle class, at least when the nature of society is being discussed. The English queen, with one of the world's largest personal fortunes, was recently described on the BBC as the embodiment of English middle-class values, though middle-class life is completely outside her experience. No candidate for high office, either in Britain or the US, can afford to be anything other than middle class, even if massive funding from billionaires is already a precondition for election to the presidency in the US, and is becoming so for increasingly presidential prime ministers in Britain. In fact, the super-rich are extremely few compared with the rest of the population, so few that no census bothers to categorise them, but this does not mean either that they do not exist, or that they are not important or that the mass of the people are unaware of their existence.

Transition of workers from manual to intellectual work does not necessarily imply a parallel transition from defining themselves as producers to allowing others to define them as consumers. The solidarity of coal miners, steel and tinplate workers, and their families, who stood together with their breadwinners to compel capitalism to construct an enduring social frame, outside and beyond their world of business, did not appear spontaneously, painlessly or inevitably. Though South Wales eventually became an area of industrial militancy matched only by the Clyde, and eventually employed a higher proportion of people in nationalised industry and public services than any other part of Britain, it took more than a century of bitter struggle to get there. The social base for solidarity has indeed changed, the need for it is greater than ever, so the real problem is how to reconstruct something like it, but from new social ingredients in the fundamentally different conditions of a knowledge-based economy.[46]

The spontaneous nature of consumerism makes it an extremely powerful force, but central to it lies a self-limiting contradiction. Market capitalism promotes people as avid consumers but degrades them as socially responsible creators of value. In exchange for fantasy worlds we can buy as commodities, it creates a real world of greed, selfishness and the death of fellowship. Self-respect is essential to health. How can we respect ourselves if we allow such a world to become our children's inheritance? Creation of a new social base for solidarity is the theme of the next and final chapter.

Summary and conclusions

Humane development of science depends on including the entire population within its scope, on the same footing – all for each and each for all. Internal equivalence of our species provides the foundation for medical science; social inclusiveness is the foundation for effective care systems. Solidarity created state care systems, and their shortcomings are largely attributable to a lack of it. Consumerism stands in opposition to this, posing every man for himself as a philosophy for our own times of predominant material affluence; solidarity is relegated to the past. Consumerism tells us we are now so rich we can no longer afford the generosity of the poor. Though this set of ideas now dominates people at the centre of affairs, they have failed to carry the rest of society with them. Public belief in solidarity, at least for health care, seems virtually undiminished, despite almost three decades of consumerist brainwashing.

The philosophy of consumerism ignores the real world even more than the most romantic myths of solidarity. It assumes we still live in an economy of small entrepreneurs, so self-reliant that they have little need of the state. No such economy in fact exists. Small entrepreneurs sink below the waves as fast as new ones set sail, and the state continues to expand under both New Labour and Conservative administrations, whatever their rhetoric. Before 'reform' of welfare economies, the state-funded and organised ventures were too large, and entailed risks too great, for any prudent investor to bear. The wave of privatisations of state industries, services and utilities has not reduced state funding. It has generally increased it, but diverted the money from direct investment in state property, with at least some public accountability through Parliament, into colossal subsidies to giant corporations now operating for profit where once the state operated only to break even. The new pattern for state enterprise is partnership with big business, where business takes the profits and the public, through the state, takes the risks.

Assumptions that solidarity is natural to the declining industrial working class but repellent to the rising middle class are illusory. Solidarity was not natural, it had to be built through experience and struggle. The so-called middle class is the working class in new conditions. It also will have to struggle to build and maintain solidarity, in new ways. Class analyses proclaiming a new era of peace based on a middle class to which almost everyone belongs, with the working class marginalised to vanishing industries or permanent unemployment, are based on superficial assumptions. The reality continues to be nations divided between a minority who live from what they own, and a majority who live from what they do. The future of the NHS depends on this majority.

Notes

[1] For a wonderfully ripe example of this see Sir James Barr (1912), president of the BMA on the eve of the First World War. Barr also led the BMA's cavalry against Lloyd George's Insurance Act, in similar eugenic terms (1911).

[2] Burleigh, 2002.

[3] Weindling, 1989.

[4] Armstrong, 1997.

[5] 'Gnat survives sledgehammer', *Times Health Supplement*, 11 March 1983.

[6] Webster, 1988, p 131.

[7] 'Wherefore putting away lying, speak every man truth unto his neighbour: for we are members one of another' Ephesians 4:25. Solidarity does indeed depend upon truthfulness, and recognition that if we want community, we can't choose our neighbours.

[8] At a Chicago Institute of Medicine panel discussion in 1995, *New England Journal of Medicine* editor Arnold Relman reported that for-profit insurance groups were taking 20-30% of premiums as profits, before paying out for care (Wolinsky, 1995).

[9] In 1988, 56% of US doctors said they would support a national health insurance programme but 74% thought most of their colleagues opposed it. By 2002, the number of US citizens without health insurance had reached an all-time high at 45 million (*Harper's Index*, 28 August 2003). In the US, paid lobbyists still have more power than voters.

[10] Though Adam Smith's belief that people individually and social classes collectively act most efficiently in their own interest remains true of any social system, this interest is defined by how it is perceived, and this is the real issue. There has been much usually futile and poorly informed discussion about how those who live from what they do rather than what they own perceive their own interest as either independent, opposed or consistent with the interests of those who live from what they own. There seems to be much less discussion about the capacity of some of the larger owners to see a bit further than their own immediate interests, and consider the long-term survival of themselves and our planet; never a majority, but always a significant minority. The position of the present British government is almost unique in Western Europe in its apparently inflexible resolve to open every corner of society to penetration by the market, exempt so far as possible from legal restraint in the interests of social justice or even global survival.

[11] Menendez, 1999. He was commenting on two key papers: Silverman et al, 1999; and Woolhandler and Himmelstein, 1999.

[12] Richard D. North (2005) has written a whole book in this vein, given prime space for discussion by the BBC.

[13] Röntgen refused to patent or copyright his discovery of X-rays. So did Fleming, Chain and Florey who developed penicillin, Waksman who developed streptomycin, Salk who developed poliomyelitis vaccine, Scribner who invented venous shunts for kidney dialysis, and innumerable other pioneers of medical science. The race to patent sections of the human genome, and then even some clinical procedures, is a recent development still generally regarded as disgraceful and illegal, even by the US Congress (Gene-Macdaniel, 1996). Though between 1981 and 1994, 1,175 patents were granted for human DNA sequences, three-quarters of them to private US or Japanese companies (Thomas et al, 1996), European centres working on the human genome oppose the entire concept

of intellectual property in this field, supported by some sponsoring multinational pharmaceutical companies who understand the fearful implications of this step for the continued advance of science (Berger, 1998). Intellectual property is a concept that is intoxicating some parts of the global market while it terrifies others, a struggle, the outcome of which is unresolved and has implications that are only beginning to be understood (Frow, 1996).

[14] Undeniably, profit provides powerful motivation, and competition soon drives idlers out of the market, even if it distorts the social objectives of production. Undeniably, many units in public service become stagnant, their staff content to meet the letter of their contracts, without imaginative commitment to proclaimed goals. The most effective treatment for this common disease is neither profit for employers nor tight management for employees, but inclusion of research and teaching as essential functions for all service units without exception. Research and teaching at some level ensure that staff continue to learn, that they participate in and contribute to the forward march of their profession, of its knowledge base and of public understanding.

[15] This has nothing to do with race, however defined, but everything to do with poverty. The US presents almost all of its public health data in terms of 'race' – black/white/latino – rather than social class. Evidence consistently confirms that income is a better predictor of almost all health-related variables than 'race' (the haemoglobinopathies – sickle cell disease and the like – are rare exceptions).

[16] Wallace and Wallace, 1997.

[17] M. Shaw et al, 2005. In 2002 the New Labour government promised to reduce the gaps between the poorest 20% of local government areas and the UK average for life expectancy and infant mortality by 10% between 1997 and 2010. In fact, between 1997 and 2003 (the most recent data available), the gap in life expectancy for men rose from 2.00 years to 2.07 (a 2% rise) and for women from 1.54 years to 1.63 (a 5% rise). Over the same period, the gap in infant mortality (deaths in the first year of life) between unskilled manual workers' families and the UK average rose from 13% to 19%. By 2003 infant mortality in unskilled manual workers' families was 69% higher than in managerial or professional families, a bigger

difference than at any time in the entire 20th century (Department of Health, 2005).

[18] Morris and Titmuss, 1944.

[19] Few now remember that when Aneurin Bevan was Minister of Health, he was also Minister for Housing. With 20% of British housing stock destroyed or seriously damaged by bombing, in 1948 this was a more pressing need than a new health service, and had corresponding priority. Bevan insisted on building only to the highest (full Parker-Morris) standard, so that council houses constructed before 1952 are for the most part still useful and in good condition. Later council housing reverted to the jerry-built standards considered adequate for the working class by politicians with less anger or conscience. The present government is attempting to eliminate council housing completely, but the need for social housing – particularly in London – is now so great that it is unlikely to succeed. Meanwhile, the Treasury, led by Blair's heir-apparent, Gordon Brown, is floating proposals for a 40% reduction in taxes on second homes.

[20] Morris, 1972.

[21] Welin et al, 1992.

[22] Yamey, 2002.

[23] Price et al, 1999.

[24] Jayasinghe, 2004; Nair, 2004.

[25] This was an important sub-plot in the run-up to referenda on the proposed new constitution for the European Union. This was better understood in France, which fortunately voted first, than in Britain. Even more than the original Treaty of Rome, part 3 of the proposed new constitution would have forced hitherto public service institutions into market competition, including multinational commercial providers. Though every EU country has at least one major political party claiming a future socialist society as its aim, this section of the new constitution would have made anything other than a neoliberal economy illegal. Large majorities against it

in referenda in France and the Netherlands have stalled this process for the time being, but the attack will certainly be renewed.

[26] Apparently exemption depends on whether health services are classified as economic or non-economic activity, evidently determined not by whether they have a useful product, but whether they operate for profit. Production of pornography, legal prostitution, gambling or advice on legal tax evasion are thus all classed as economic activities, while we have to pretend that the NHS is not.

[27] *Lancet* Editorial, 2000.

[28] When Margaret Thatcher became Prime Minister in 1979, the overall burden of taxation on GDP was already lower in Britain than the European Union average. Its relative position has hardly changed since, but there has been a substantial fall in taxation on the very rich (through reductions in top rates of income tax) and a relative rise in the tax burden on the poor (mainly through sales taxes). In 1995, under the last Conservative administration, the poorest 20% of UK households paid 39.3% of their income in taxes, whereas the richest 20% paid only 35.2% of their incomes in taxes (Hutton, 1995). By 1998-99, under the New Labour government, the poorest 20% paid 41.9% of their income in taxes, whereas the richest 20% paid 36.4% of their income in taxes (Table, 'Taxes as a percentage of gross income for non-retired households', *Economic Trends*, April 2000). In his *Enquiry into the Nature and Causes of the Wealth of Nations*, Adam Smith, patron saint of conservative economists, had this to say about taxes: 'Civil government, so far as it is instituted for the security of property, is in reality instituted for the defence of the rich against the poor, or of those who have some property against those who have none at all ...' ([1762] 1993, p 413). From this he concluded: 'The subjects of every state ought to contribute towards the support of the government, as nearly as possible in proportion to their respective abilities; that is, in proportion to the revenue which they respectively enjoy under the protection of the state' ([1762] 1993, p 451). North Americans might prefer the following quotation from Oliver Wendell Homes, still to be found above the entrance to the Inland Revenue Service in Washington: 'Taxes are the price we pay for a civilised society.'

[29] Leys, 2001b.

[30] Schweitzer, 1997. According to the same source, the US pharmaceutical industry workforce in the late 1980s was about 160,000 of whom 36% were in manufacturing, 28% in marketing and 23% in research and development.

[31] diMasi et al, 1991.

[32] Licensing decisions are based on trials involving an average of 1,500 patients. A serious reaction affecting one patient in 500 may therefore not only be undetected, but undetectable until used on a mass scale, and not even then unless clinicians remain always alert to this possibility, and use still inadequate notification machinery. Whistleblowers within the industry suffer the same fate as similar heroes anywhere else who threaten profits or management's peace of mind. The attitude of marketing departments to prescribing is revealed by the following passage from M.C. Smith's standard work *Principles of Pharmaceutical Marketing* (1968, quoted in Schweitzer, 1997):

> medical men are subject to they same kinds of stress, the same emotional influences that affect the layman. Physicians have, as part of their self-image, a determined feeling that they are rational and logical, particularly in their choice of pharmaceuticals. The advertiser must appeal to this rational self-image, and at the same time make a deeper appeal to the emotional factors which really influence sales.

Though the British record for sceptical prescribing compares favourably with colleagues elsewhere (Griffin and Griffin, 1992; Garratini and Garratini, 1993) and our proportion of generic prescribing rose from 16% in 1977 to 54% by 1994, and is still rising, most British doctors in practice still seem to believe they can let pharmaceutical companies sponsor most of their postgraduate education, without any effect on their clinical decisions.

[33] Hancher, 1990.

[34] Maynard, 1991.

[35] Liebenau, 1990.

[36] This seems an obvious opportunity for Wales, Scotland and both parts of Ireland, all in desperate need of new manufactures.

[37] Crick and Watson elucidated the molecular chemistry of DNA in 1953, the same year as I entered NHS practice. More than half a century later, though the entire human genome is now known, we are still waiting for the first practically useful products of that research. Informed people have no doubt whatever that it will eventually make medical practice immensely more effective in areas hitherto beyond the scope of science, and the scramble for patents has already been with us for more than a decade, but few investors will wait that long for their profits.

[38] Bekelman et al, 2003.

[39] House of Commons Health Committee, 2005. This committee has worked effectively despite a New Labour government apparently willing to do anything to ingratiate itself with big business, including the pharmaceutical industry. Its work, and that of the National Audit Office before it, seems to be leading toward a major shake-up at the Medicines and Healthcare Products Regulatory Agency, to be replaced by a Commission on Human Medicines, all of whose members will be prohibited from having any financial interest in health care-related companies, and with substantial lay representation (Collier, 2005).

[40] Sjöström and Nilsson, 1972.

[41] Though they did consider this option, it was discussed only to review evidence against this conclusion. However, the Labour Party did then, also for the first and last time, include in its shadow policy a nationalised component of the pharmaceutical industry to compete with the private sector. This vanished after the next election and has never been allowed by the party leaders to reappear. It remains a popular idea among the party membership, which could and should be revived.

[42] Berwick, 2002.

[43] 'Tony Blair speaks to Institute for Public Policy and Research', *Financial Times*, 15 January 1999.

44 Obviously, in this context, property means wealth as capital, not as objects for personal use, though a wheelbarrow or a car can come into either of these categories. For a large majority of people in developed economies, ownership of capital is almost or completely limited to ownership of their own home, which has both a personal use-value, and a market value. This has obvious implications for politicians eager to recruit as many people as possible to the sound views of property owners, from 'Two hectares and a cow' in the days of Thiers, to Margaret Thatcher's populist capitalism in the 1980s. By introducing her 'right to buy' policy for tenants of local government socially provided housing, she hoped to extend the ideology of people who live from what they own, to a large proportion of people who live from what they do. Houses were sold to tenants at prices far below their market value, followed by shares in previously nationalised industries available at similar knock-down prices. A generation of workers, formerly dependable Labour voters, became more receptive to the Conservative message. New Labour has followed the same course, accepting an end to all socially provided housing, as well as to nationalised industries and public utilities. The number of officially recognised homeless families in Britain consequently rose from 53,000 in 1978 to 287,000 by 1993. Large fortunes were made by estate agents, money lenders and speculative builders. People who profited from this looting of hitherto public property were left to wonder how they could help their children to pay the now astronomical price of getting a roof over their heads (OPCS, 1995; Victor, 1997). The Thatcher legacy includes transformation of houses from consumer commodities, places to live, into speculative investments, places to develop and sell profitably. As she intended, this has been socially divisive and politically confusing, and promoted growth of a third social category, people who live both from what they own and from what they do, with minds divided accordingly. Nevertheless, they must ultimately choose between these bases for their own lives and ideas.

This important story is not yet concluded. Speculative inflation of house values has continued since the 1970s, providing a basis for borrowing that supports rising consumer spending even where real wages are falling, as in the US. US national house prices today are still rising by 15% annually. Total value of house property in OECD countries has more than doubled over the past five years, from $30 billion to $70 billion, more than equal to their entire annual output of services and manufactures; in the words of 'The global housing boom: in come the waves', *The Economist*, 18 June 2005: 'Never before have real house prices risen so fast for so long in so many countries.' As rising house prices are almost entirely speculative and represent little material production, this is a bubble comparable to speculation preceding the US market collapse of 1929-33, which led to a world crisis of capitalism, fascism and the Second World War. There is today a growing divergence between real economies producing use-value, and notional economies apparently creating wealth, much of which could prove illusory,. The brunt of this will be felt by workers who accepted the illusion that they had become successful little capitalists.

[45] This seems to be a long-term trend in all imperial economies. Already by 1985, the gross profit share of all US manufacturing value added was only 24.8% of GDP (Glyn, 2005).

[46] Study of voting by social class, using detailed categories for turnout, shows no clear decline in cohesion of voting by the industrial working class since the 1930s in either Britain or France. The process of *embourgeoisement*, through which material affluence is supposed to make workers reallocate themselves to a middle class, seems confined to the US (Weakliem and Heath, 1995). Even there, the process is far less complete than most media comment implies. Commenting on the British general election in 2001, Professor Greg Philo (2001) of the Glasgow University Media Group thought the result reflected changes in class structure since Thatcher's deregulation measures in the 1980s. The top 10% of the population now earned as much as the bottom 50% put together, and 20 million adults had only a state pension. This meant that at least two-thirds of the population had to rely on the public sector, including many of the traditional middle class, who were now faced with the industrialisation of their work, as 'safe' occupations in banking and insurance turned into low-paid call-centre jobs. This was why health and education became the main concerns of the electorate, and why New Labour regained a 'natural' majority. He believed this could be sustained only by a wealth tax, with currency controls to prevent flight of capital. As a new party of big business, New Labour cannot provide such a tax or controls, so if it wants to sustain its natural majority, the Labour Party will have to revert to its former compromises.

SIX

The NHS as seed of future society

Throughout this book I have emphasised that the NHS, and public health services in all countries with economies ruled by the World Bank, World Trade Organisation (WTO) and International Monetary Fund (IMF), are being pushed off their previous slow, hesitant and always contested course toward socialised gift economies, back to the trade-cum-charity pattern from which they painfully emerged to work for all of the people, but with this trade transferred to multinational corporations, away from individual medical entrepreneurs. The neoliberal policy of marketisation is promoted by colossal concentrations of power and money, cutting across national frontiers, intimidating and seducing the leaders of nations. There is little convincing evidence that these policies of quasi-privatisation will improve either effectiveness or efficiency in producing health gain, and plenty of experience of their demoralising effects on staff, marginalisation of public health and diminished attention to people at highest risk. However, if governments continue to accept most of the market risks, and their laws are reformed or bent accordingly, this commercialising and industrialising process will continue to create offers few ambitious politicians can afford to refuse.

Faced with this pressure to industrialise and commercialise, how can any other path remain open? What real social and economic forces exist to renationalise the NHS, when all our traditional agents of progress seem either to have joined the enemy, or be heading for extinction?

Human history so far has been a sequence of economies, with cultures built upon them: from hunting and gathering through nomadic husbandry, tribal agriculture and slavery, feudal agriculture and serfdom, then first mercantile capitalism, followed by industrial capitalism, and finally our present rapidly changing economy, where the dominant commodity will be knowledge and ideas. If these ideas, formerly the proudest products of a gift economy centred on publicly funded universities, can be redefined as intellectual property and shrunk to commodity status, we shall fall into a morally impoverished society scarcely imaginable to Adam Smith, Tom Paine or Benjamin Franklin and other pioneers of the enlightenment.

History has not reached its end

As an ABC of human social history the last paragraph's grossly simplified sequence provides an outline, but its actual course has been enormously more complex, with huge overlaps between each of these stages of dominant economy. In every case, new economies and social classes have grown within the old. Obsolete economies and classes, though dethroned, have persisted wherever their continued fitness for function in particular niches could survive, without unduly impeding movement of capital or labour. Capitalism had a gestation lasting several hundred years, growing within feudal states long before it replaced them. Feudal habits of deference survive even today, wherever they serve the interests of capital accumulation more than they impede it.

Free trade in labour was both the foundation of industrial capitalism, and a corrosive force steadily eroding its predecessor, feudal economy and power derived from land ownership. Despite many violent and transiently successful attempts to suppress mobility and trade in labour, feudal landlords, slave owners and kings ultimately found this impossible. They needed the goods that wool merchants, manufacturers and traders could produce at a lower price with free labour, because factory labour was more productive than either slaves, or labourers tied to their land. They needed capital borrowed through usury, which their churches still condemned, to reinforce god-given supremacy of inherited property in land. Thus landed aristocrats ensured eventual supremacy of money over birth, and their own eclipse as a dominant class. Through these means of expansion and survival, they promoted their own downfall, though it has been a long time coming and is even today still incomplete.[1] We have to find the ways in which this latest form of exploitation contains within itself, indispensable to its own further growth, an entirely new and different future that could, with our intelligent action, eventually supersede it.

Revolutionary change neither falls from heaven nor rises from hell, but develops within the society that precedes it. Marx concentrated on evidence that it would develop within the process of commodity production. The brutalised, still unorganised workforce described by Friedrich Engels in Manchester would eventually provide an organised, literate revolutionary class, as after several more generations, and up to a point, it eventually did. The contradiction inherent in any system in which production itself is socialised, but the means of production remains in private hands, must eventually be resolved either through a more socialised and democratised society, or through 'the mutual destruction of the contending parties', as the first paragraph of the *Communist Manifesto* grimly and aptly reminds us. However, this takes a long time. If production of material commodities employs ever-diminishing labour, as in fully industrialised economies it increasingly appears to do, then labour alone cannot provide the army to win economic democracy.

I have found no indication that Marx took much interest in an alternative: that, added to these contradictions within the processes of commodity production, other forms of value production might grow outside, alongside and beyond the market economy, both serving some of its essential needs, and developing an alternative model for production of value, of non-commodity wealth. Marx seemed surprisingly uninterested in the strategies already adopted by Gladstone and Disraeli to secure popular assent to continued rule by the rich, shifting more or less painlessly from aristocrats owning land to plutocrats owning industry, merging the wealth and cultural power of both to redefine British nationality and common sense in ways that identified a sufficient proportion of industrial workers with the interests of their employers, to ensure continued rule by the few over the many, despite an eventually complete adult franchise. This redefinition increasingly depended on social stability achieved through consent rather than coercion. Public health care and education became important means for achieving this consent and stability, though they only became prominent in the early 20th century, 20 years after Marx's death.

There exists no value that cannot somehow be produced and marketed as a profitable commodity, though many then become almost unrecognisable in the process. Hollywood, Disney theme parks and the *Readers' Digest* relate to the world's accumulated knowledge and culture in much the same way as chicken factories, supermarkets and fast food relate to good farm produce and home cooking, but both these sets of relationships exist and continue to grow despite growing public suspicion that consumers are being deceived. Marketable commodities can include health care, education, sport and every other sort of cultural and creative activity. All of these can be passively consumed, and if consumers do not look too closely, can still appear much as they always were. If commodity production can produce and distribute these values more effectively and efficiently than socialised forms of production already developing in embryonic form from traditional pre-capitalist origins, and if people do not notice or care about the difference between creativity and passive consumption, or between difficult truths and plausible lies, then all these non-commodity modes of production can be drawn into commodity production by large corporations. Combination of these corporations with the state can then subordinate their social functions to the generation of profit, like everything else in commercial society. If, on the other hand, commodity production is seen not to increase productivity, if it subverts staff morale and generates distorted and untrustworthy products, then we have alternative economic models contending with capitalist commodity production. These non-commodity modes of production could then become an important new dimension for social struggle and change, with the outstanding and historically exceptional advantage that they are popular social institutions we already have, which we are learning to defend by adapting them to more participative and democratic forms.

Previous chapters suggest that commercialised production of health care as a commodity is in most ways much less efficient than socialised production of health care as a gift. This is therefore a potentially independent economy, using entirely different measures of input and output, setting entirely different tasks for health economists and policy formers, competing ideologically with the commodity economy but also providing the means to stabilise it in an otherwise disintegrating society – in Bevan's words, 'a new path entirely'. The commodity economy will still try to subordinate this socialised gift economy to itself, but its own continued growth may depend on accepting its rival as a necessary support, an inevitable competitor and even an eventually dominant successor.

Transition from physical to mental labour

All mature economies are now in transition from predominant manufacture of material commodities to predominant production of services, information and new knowledge and ideas. This entails social changes at least as great as their earlier transition from predominant agriculture to predominant manufacture. Transition to economies dominated by intellectual products also entails subtler social changes that are in some ways even more profound than the subordination of agriculture to industry.

Development of intelligent machines through chip technology has changed the character of labour from essentially mechanical tasks, which divided and subordinated human intelligence, to tasks requiring more imagination than these extremely fast and obedient, but still servile, machines are as yet able to undertake. These new tasks require relatively sophisticated, critical and imaginative human intelligence from an increasingly educated workforce, able to make complex judgements that still lie beyond the power even of intelligent machines. Employers now need workers possessing far more information than in the past, and able to make independent judgements once reserved for management.

The old boss's reply to '... but I thought' was that he did not pay his workers to think, he paid them to work. There was a general view among manual workers in heavy industry that work of any other kind was not really work at all. An entire working-class culture was built around physical skills, strength and endurance, necessary for work, but expressed in people's own lives through participation in sport, either on the field, or more often as appreciative and informed spectators. Successive generations struggled more or less successfully to rent their bodies to employers for the best price they could negotiate, which in turn depended on solidarity and keeping their minds for themselves. To employers, the sign of healthy minds in workers was that they accepted their weakness as free individual negotiators in a free market for labour. They could safely be encouraged to celebrate the strength of their bodies in their own terms through sport, but the only conventionally approved ways to celebrate the strength of their minds were in terms developed by owners of property, and rejected by most manual workers.

To workers, the signs of healthy minds were unity, solidarity and collective negotiation by organisations of their own. Protected by a mental barrier between their bodies rented to employers and their minds kept for themselves, industrial workers created the motive force for progress toward a more inclusive, less unequal, more stable society for everyone; not only for industrial workers but for all who lived from what they did rather than what they owned.

Starting in the 1970s, employers have changed the demands they make on education. Previously, for most of their workforce they needed only the three Rs, bare literacy and numeracy. Beyond these lay danger: workers who read books, asked their own questions and began searching for their own answers. Higher culture seemed accessible to workers only if they gave up their cultural independence and solidarity, creating barriers to education that still exist today and that governments see no way to overcome. The price commanded by skilled manual workers in the globalised labour market is sliding away from European toward Asian levels of subsistence, maybe not immediately, but in a future close enough to destroy the respect in which manual workers were formerly held, and their own confidence in themselves. This profound change in the way most people, particularly most men, earn their living, and consequent loss of confidence in independent working-class cultures, has initially divided generations, detaching young people from their own history and making old people doubt the value of their own past struggles.

To get employment at the leading edge of knowledge-based industry, workers must now acquire complex knowledge and ways of thinking previously reserved for the 5% or so of the population who in my youth reached a university. To do this on their own cultural terms, rather than the humiliating terms accepted by most of that old 5%, will be possible only when they have devised new ways to rent those parts of their minds that employers want and will pay for, while once again establishing a space for their own independent understanding and culture for themselves and their own future. Our planet is already dangerously close to midnight, so this task has greater urgency than ever before.

Two cultures

The core of this new economy is production, distribution and integration of information to produce profitable new knowledge, intellectual property as a marketable commodity. As technical applications come closer to their origins in new scientific knowledge, each successive innovation entails higher investment costs with ever-briefer periods of consequent profit. Each innovation creates more pressure to take new knowledge out of its traditional status as a shared gain for all humankind, and wrap it in commercial secrecy as intellectual property, profitable only so long as it is not shared. Contradictions inherent in all social production for private profit create a dilemma for employers in the new economy. The basic sciences from which new ideas must come can function effectively only when motivated by our common search for personal usefulness and significance in our society, now within global definitions. Discovery cannot be limited to what seems most immediately likely to yield a profit. It must have free access to discoveries by other people in other countries, unobstructed by copyright and commercial secrecy, a co-operative venture in which competition has become civilised into emulation, pursuing true honour (the real respect of our peers) rather than superfluous riches. In new knowledge-based industries, even the most stupid capitalists know that in the worlds of education and scientific discovery, motivation does not depend on anticipated profit.

Jean-Pierre Garnier, chief executive of GlaxoSmithKline pharmaceuticals, earned about £7m in 2001/02, making him the third highest-paid of all UK executives in that year. His company's profits had fallen from £18m when he took over in 2000 to £12.5m in 2002, and its share value had fallen from £18 to £12.50, but despite this failure, in November 2002 he asked for a 'massive increase' in pay for 2003. This was necessary, his boardroom supporters said, 'to keep him motivated', through earnings similar to those enjoyed by the same company's executives in the US.[2] Even Garnier must know that none of his company's best research pharmacologists, nor the university departments that create and develop the generation-long projects that must precede their work, nor the clinical researchers who must learn how to apply it in the field, can be so primitively motivated. Though we have entered an era that threatens to draw all higher education and research into a corrupting vortex of commercial secrecy, business ethics and ideological conformity, we still have two cultures; not the obvious but superficial division between arts and sciences described by C.P. Snow,[3] but the fundamental division, pushed to its limit by industrial capitalism, between pursuit of human needs and pursuit of profit.

Preconditions for growth in knowledge-based economies

Free development of socially inclusive education unconstrained by the culture of a dominant class, and free development of knowledge from independent universities unimpeded by commercial secrecy or commercial pressures for quick profit, are preconditions for optimal growth in knowledge-based economies. Commercial secrecy, preferential investment for quick profit, and neglect of long-term projects with high risks of short-term failure, are all inherent features of production for profit. These necessarily inhibit and distort growth, but successful competition demands optimal growth. From this contradiction it follows that though the dominant interests of large employers will certainly continue to fragment and distort education to produce the people they want, technically proficient and imaginative but socially and culturally blind, they cannot ultimately succeed. Any nation, or group of nations, that manages to defend its schools and universities from commercial pressures, will paradoxically gain a commercial advantage in the more rapid development of its knowledge-based economy, though it may also thereby hasten transition of that economy from ownership and control by private investors to ownership and control by the whole of society.

What has all this to do with the NHS? The NHS provides an organised, documented, personalised interface between the entire British population on the one hand, and new scientific knowledge on the other. Every NHS hospital is becoming a potential unit for teaching and research, and so is every NHS primary care unit. They have registered populations, continuing links allowing follow-up not only through lifetimes but also across several generations. They are staffed by university graduates with a basic understanding of scientific thought and evidence. A growing proportion of patients are engaged in mass education in the rudimentary elements of scientific learning and thinking. The NHS serves a population with experience of, and confidence in, a gift economy that was beginning to work – not perfectly, but more cost-effectively than any commercial economy. Memories of the former success of that economy will probably be long enough for many of them to recognise that retreat to the market has failed to achieve anything except to fill a new set of pockets. People will have to recognise a political mistake so profound that it amounts to a national betrayal, but that will not be difficult. It will be a treachery attributable to their preceding generation, which, as we saw in 1968, they will readily recognise.

Present British government policies are expressly designed to undo every one of these precious advantages, precious not only for development of more effective and efficient care, but also for advances in service that could become an increasingly important part of the wider British economy. They divide at every level those who plan and manage work from those who perform it. They divide once co-operative hospitals into jealous and secretive competitors, they divide continuing care into commodity-sized fragments that divide professionals from the consequences of their work, they divide the NHS by imposing unwanted choices to favour renewed growth of a once-moribund private sector, and they divide a nation of generous citizens into a gaggle of envious and recriminating consumers. However, all this takes time, creates its own new barriers to the cost-effectiveness and efficiency it claims to pursue, and becomes ever more vulnerable to an increasingly obvious alternative: simply to return to the path on which our feet were set in 1948, toward a widening gift economy wherever this offered solutions to problems the market had been unable to solve profitably, and had therefore ignored.

To have any future other than subordination of all human activity to profit, the whole class with a common interest in public services as a separate, not-for-profit economy needs to submerge its other differences, often profound and deeply felt, to create a common culture of social solidarity. This must have a very much wider base than the old and now shrinking industrial working class. It must include everyone who sees health care, education, performing and sporting arts as public services which, if they are not shared and used by everyone as participants rather than consumers, become distorted, degraded and unfit for their purpose.

Role of political parties in fundamental social change

Questions like these used to provide the core of politics. They moved generations of pioneering heroes and heroines to risk death and devote their lives to progressive change. The collapse of 20th-century socialism, correctly anticipated by Thatcher and Reagan in 1979, and confirmed by the transition of the USSR to bandit capitalism in 1990 and China to capitalist dictatorship, apparently signalled the end of political parties as vehicles for fundamentally different views of society and its future. By the end of the 20th century, all European political parties within reach of power had reached a single consensus view on the economic foundations of society, as major political parties in the US had already done since 1945. Major parties differ not on fundamental policies but on how this single consensus should be presented to the varying expectations of their still somewhat different social audiences – different ways to deceive the people. This is unstable and cannot last. What will succeed it?

Fundamental changes in the organisation of society depend on seismic shifts in the behaviour of dominant economies, which result from their own evolution and interactions between one another, including war. These shifts may be accelerated or delayed by political parties, but they cannot create them. It has long been obvious that such seismic shifts are now imminent. Either some major reorganisation of society must eventually follow, or society itself may collapse into banditry. The ruling classes in mature economies, particularly in the dominant economy in the US, do not rely on spontaneous support from the people, they organise it, but in so doing, they must show some material evidence that their rule provides at least some things that are necessary, even though they are not profitable. The mass of the people who live not from what they own, but from what they do, must organise themselves to ensure that this economy of needs expands at the expense of a shrinking economy of commodities.

The first-past-the-post electoral system shared by Britain and the US assures the alternating dominance of two large parties. In Britain, free speech has so far assured the existence of other small parties barking at their heels, but never credible contenders for power. They can say and think whatever they want, without endangering the property relations on which society now rests. The two big parties, on the other hand, can enjoy a so-called landslide victory with less than 50% of those who actually vote, and supported by less than 30% of people entitled to vote (New Labour retained power in the 2005 election supported by only about 20% of the electorate). Throughout the 19th century, as those qualified to vote came to include an increasing proportion of common people, they could choose which of two rich men they preferred to represent them, from either of two rich men's parties. This system persisted in the US, where the threat of a working-class party never fully materialised. In Britain it was threatened by advent of the Labour Party in 1903, and up to 1979, this threat never completely disappeared.

The few British working men who owned their homes got the right to vote in 1867, as Disraeli's alternative to the revolution either feared or anticipated by most people throughout the first half of the 19th century. By 1884 adult male suffrage was complete. The interests of industrial workers, so far as they reached Parliament at all, still did so through the Liberal Party, by then a party of industrialists contending with a Conservative Party representing aristocracy and landed gentry. During the last quarter of the 19th century, trade unions became a powerful social force, and a few trade unionists (mostly coal miners) got elected to Parliament as Liberal-Labour MPs (known as Lib-Labs), preaching a shared interest between workers and their employers in industrial prosperity. This has remained the central plank of Liberalism ever since. By the turn of the century the limits of this extremely unequal alliance seemed to have been reached. Socialism, the idea that production need not depend on private owners or private investors at all, but might work better through social investment for social purposes, became a popular idea in Britain from the mid-1880s. Thereafter it slowly penetrated the unions, creating demands for political action to influence law, as well as economic action to influence the price of labour. The Lib-Labs could still see no need for a party pursuing the interests of workers independently from the interests of employers, so in 1903 the Labour Party was born.

From its beginning, the British Labour Party was an alliance between a conservative majority aiming at a better deal for workers within the terms of a competitive market economy through trade union organisation and representation in parliament (reformists), and a radical minority aiming at a fundamental transformation of society and the social relations of work (revolutionaries). Though these aims were not necessarily or always incompatible in the here and now, they often appeared so. The Labour Party always contained division between these two trends, restrained mainly by a deeply rooted belief among industrial working-class communities, reinforced by experience, that unity was strength and division was fatal weakness. The reformist wing included equally powerful traditions of servility, the belief that at least in the short run, you may get the best deal from employers by agreeing with them, and that the long run can be left to posterity. The revolutionary wing included many who were in fact only rebels, discontented with society as it was but without any realistic plans for an alternative. Apart from keeping the idea of an alternative future alive, the main achievement of revolutionaries was to compel reformists actually to carry out their reforms, rather than just talk about them.

The British Labour Party differed from all other European socialist parties in containing affiliated trade unions as its major players, initially without any provision for individual membership, and without any agreed long-term political programme. Within its loose federal structure, the party included political groups with their own membership,[4] ranging from the Fabian Society of socialoid courtiers seeking friends in the corridors of power, to the sectarian Marxist Social Democratic Federation throwing pebbles at their windows. The party's de facto executive committee was the parliamentary Labour Party, MPs accepting the Labour whip in Parliament. Though delegates' votes at annual conferences of the party were supposed to determine its policy, they actually did so only once, when in 1944, led by Nye Bevan, they compelled Clement Attlee and his fellow ministers to break with Churchill's wartime coalition and contest the 1945 general election.[5] Otherwise, even massive majority votes at conference against policies pursued by Labour governments have always been ignored.

So far as a mass base for socialist ideas was ever created in Britain, this was achieved largely outside the Labour Party and against opposition from most of its leaders.[6] The only serious attempt to get the whole Labour Party nominally committed to transformation of society was in 1918, when Sidney Webb hastily composed the famous Clause 4 of the party's constitution, declaring that socialism was its objective, and defining this as 'the common ownership of the means of production, distribution and exchange'.[7] Even in 1945, this declared aim did not and could not lead Labour government policy. The nationalisations of that period largely confirmed de jure what had already begun de facto under Churchill's wartime coalition government (though they would certainly not have been made by a Conservative government). Although profit is supposed to be a reward for taking risks, once they became world bankers, British investors found safer and easier ways to make money than investment in manufacture, research or development. Britain therefore entered the war with a crumbling industrial infrastructure, with investment, research and development all grossly neglected. Market competition proved incapable of developing or maintaining the manufacturing base needed to prosecute the war, and had to be corrected by cooperation and collective investment for needs rather than profits, organised through the state.[8]

The common ownership referred to in Clause 4 assumed ownership by the state. Though there were examples of successful retail and agricultural producer cooperatives before 1914 in many parts of the world, and many more since, what really mattered was ownership of heavy industry and manufacturing, the model for which was created not by socialists but by Henry Ford, and the war industries coordinated by the German state during the First World War. These provided the prototype first for Lenin and Stalin after 1917,[9] then for Churchill and Franklin Roosevelt after 1941. Ironically, Hitler was too intoxicated by easy victories, and Mussolini was too corrupt, to take the firm hand with private investors that created the three more regulated economies victorious in the Second World War.[10]

Two forces have always been needed to create and maintain the Labour Party as a successful movement, in or close to power: first, demands for a better life here and now, in the economic and social system we already have, which experience has shown to require active and continuous struggle – never a gift, always an achievement. Second, hopes of a better life in the future, when the energies now required for political struggle could be devoted to a national and international cooperative economy in which everyone shares, without winners or losers. Both these forces, immediate demands and ultimate hopes, contemporary reform and revolutionary innovation, were and still are necessary, and should reinforce one another. The authors of the New Labour project distort the first by excluding struggle, and eliminate the second by erasing all prospects of alternative economy or society. A Labour Party thus shorn cannot long survive as a mass party. A party of big business cannot for long pass itself off as a party of labour. Its ageing generation of people who gave their lives to make the world happier for all of the people cannot, unnoticed by its members or voters, be replaced by a younger and far smaller generation of careerists aiming only to secure patronage for themselves. Even according to inflated official figures, membership of the Labour Party today is now half what it was in 1997. Even in the Labour heartlands in South Wales, in a constituency with an MP and an Assembly Member who both consistently resist New Labour policies, branches that had regular meetings of 30 members in 1997 have collapsed, merging with others to form ever-fewer branches, each of which now considers itself lucky if more than half a dozen members attend meetings, most of them pensioners. When the present generation of branch officers goes, there are few visible successors. Deleting socialism from the Labour Party's agenda has been fatal both to its own morale, and to the health of British politics.

Could the Labour Party ever become the organised force that the NHS needs to detach itself from business, and return to its developing gift economy? To anyone with inside experience of how the Labour Party machine actually works,[11] this is hard to believe, but we already know that any path other than capitulation to continued privatisation will be hard. I hope the answer is that it could and must somehow become such a force, given the continuing failure to invest in British manufacture and consequent decline in the real economy (now far inferior to France and Germany), and the increasingly visible failure of privatisation, commercialisation, fragmentation of responsibility and internal competition to deliver any of the economic or social advantages claimed for them.

These 'reforms' were applied first to our national railway system. Once the initial looting spree was over, we saw the consequences of privatisation: fragmented responsibility, reduction in experienced staff, experienced managers with industrial knowledge replaced by speculative accountants, out-sourcing to inexperienced contractors, a multitude of bureaucracies instead of a single agency, fatal accidents for which nobody would take responsibility, and higher state subsidies than ever before.[12] All this has led to a majority demand, both inside the Labour Party and among voters for all parties, for renationalisation (though not one of the major political parties has been willing to accept this aim).[13] Failure of privatisations, 'reform' and 'modernisation' to do anything other than line the pockets of shareholders and top management is now obvious to everyone except professional politicians loyal not to their voters, but to the World Bank, WTO, other agencies of multinational big business and their own leaders who hire and fire them. Once again, people are learning from their own experience that political democracy becomes meaningless without economic democracy, and that you cannot control what you do not own.

Every government elected since ordinary people got the vote has had a central problem hardly changed since Bagehot: how to maintain consent to continued rule in the interests of the few, while consent to legitimate government is measured by votes from the multitude. Whichever party best succeeded in this became the natural party of government. It is just possible that with its much wider social base, New Labour really could for a while become the chosen vehicle for big business, equally repellent but with a broader social base than the Conservative Party and with a younger and more able gang of careerists.[14] Yet even if that moment arrives, that broad base will shrink in consequence. The old Labour heartlands, industrial working-class communities that weighed rather than counted their votes, where a donkey could get elected if it was Labour, depended not on stupidity but on shared experience, rooted deeply enough to accept a few donkeys, but with a profound and lasting mistrust of the boss's party, whoever represented it. These heartlands are now changing, just as they changed after the First World War, when it was Liberal votes that had been weighed rather than counted, for as long as anyone could remember. In just two general elections, that Liberal ascendancy blew away.

Writing in 1944, on the eve of the 1945 Labour landslide that he, almost alone among British politicians, had confidently predicted, Nye Bevan wrote about the consequences of trying to preserve political democracy without economic democracy:

At each election power passes to the people, and each time they hand it back again to the same people who held it before.... A static democracy must die, if only because the people are blamed for the resultant nervelessness of government.... The people must be brought to see that social affairs are in a bad state, because the people themselves have not clothed the bones of political democracy with the flesh of economic power.... Parliament washes in public the linen which property dirties in private. It is a division of labour ultimately fatal to democratic representative government. It makes the public representative the scapegoat for the bandits of industry and finance, over whose actions he is denied effective control. Parliament is the professional mourner for private economic crimes.... If the deed lags too long behind the word, then the word itself turns sour. This is the psychological basis of Fascism.... the inevitable fate of a Parliament which denies itself the instruments of action, which are the industries and services of society.[15]

That remains as true today as it was in 1944. A few months ago Britain's last volume car production unit at Longbridge collapsed, together with about 20,000 jobs that depended on it. This was the inevitable conclusion of a story started more than a century before, when British investors discovered that in an imperial centre with its fingers into global finance, being clever with paper could be more profitable and less risky than investment in research, development or manufacture. For the entire 20th century British labour had to compete with less investment per employee in horsepower, in new machinery, or in engineering research and development, than any other industrialised nation, because the market offered easier ways to make big money fast and with less risk. Economies of comparable size in France, Germany, Italy, Japan and Korea have not yet lost their industrial base, because these governments promoted manufacture, even if this entailed lower rates of profit. British governments left investors to suit themselves, maximising profit, regardless of how it was made. The Thatcher era did not rebuild the British economy, but simply allowed the investment casino to operate as it pleased, which was to give up on manufacture and concentrate on a more immediately profitable paper economy, subordinating engineers to accountants. Because of that decision, apprenticeships in industry virtually vanished for a whole generation, and Britain lost its machine-tool industry, the foundation of industrial independence. The collapse of MG Rover, and shameless profiteering by its last set of directors, is a visible failure of a capitalist system led by market greed rather than planned by human intelligence. This could shift public understanding in ways that establishment commentators can no longer conceive.

Bevan famously declared that Labour's chief objective should be to secure public ownership and control of 'the commanding heights of industry'. From that victory, all else could follow. He underestimated the capacity of the owning class to co-opt state ownership of such infrastructural services and commodity-producing industries as coal, steel, docks and rail, road and air transport, without losing their control over the economy. Not one of these was profitable without huge state subsidies; all had suffered from gross under-investment when privately owned. The situation in 1945, when nationalisation was the only way to restore industrial infrastructure, could recur. But even if it did, experience has shown that it would provide few opportunities to develop the new social relations of production that socialists have always expected from a new society. The simplest and least vulnerable site from which to start building a road forward within capitalist society toward something better may be not the commanding heights of industry (through state capitalism), but the commanding depths of popular culture, including those that provided foundations for the NHS. This popular culture can initially be developed on a mass scale and to some extent spontaneously through democratised processes helping patients and their communities to develop shared adult roles. Of course, to bring about real change, this must also be organised by what must functionally be a political party. Whether this will be the Labour Party will depend on whether its membership reaches sufficient maturity to judge its leaders by what they actually do rather than what they say, and to recognise it will never get far so long as it takes all its ideas from its enemies.

On my Labour Party membership card these words appear: 'The Labour Party is a democratic socialist party'.[16] How can such a party in practice deny and denigrate the principal idea on which it claims to be based? The New Labour project has no secure foundation among members. It was imposed by a palace revolution in a party too long accustomed to its own monarchy and courtiers, but still popularly identified with the bottom rather than the top of a divided society. To reclaim the Labour Party for its members and core voters, and get it back on its old road with one wheel for hard bargaining and another for hope, we need the confidence in our own case that the mass of the people achieved in 1945. This would be immensely strengthened if we took more seriously what most Labour Party members have always believed: that the NHS and our comprehensive schools represent our own bits of socialism, the places where we can show what our future could be. Without these, we see only endless repetition of the same miserable sequence: Labour in power applies Conservative policies, so voters eventually settle for the organ grinder and discard his monkey.

Progress or cop-out?

Defending and extending the NHS as a gift economy, where we all can learn the new social skills we would need in a more generous future, meets the two essential requirements of the Labour Party as it was founded in 1903, and more or less remained until the New Labour project took control in 1994; it provides scope for reforms here and now, with revolutionary implications for the future.

If this Old Labour formula were restored, what would have changed? Would this not be just as deceptive as the present stance of New Labour, or the feeble capitulation of Callaghan's government on the eve of the neoliberal *Blitzkrieg* in 1979? Two things would have changed. First, global capitalism is now clearly heading for the buffers unless it can somehow achieve global regulation. Designs for a new society have therefore become an urgent matter for the immediate present, recognisable to a younger generation that has so far rejected the frameworks of any of the old major parties, and failed to agree on a new one. Global climate change and impending wars for resources are a visible abyss, compared with which the 1929 crash was a pothole. As Hugo Chávez has shown, the entire continent of Central and South America is now on the move, with a force Condoleezza Rice can find no way to resist. In most of the world, claims that the interests of big multinational investors are identical to the interests of the people are simply laughable, and young people are not deceived. A huge untapped reserve of support is already there for a Labour Party brave and honest enough to return to its own natural policies.

Second, we have the unstoppable process, already well under way, of intelligent participation by patients in the daily work of their NHS care, which will certainly continue because this is the central thrust of applied medical science. Effective prevention and treatment at their present level of sophistication depend on intelligent and informed participation by patients as co-producers, and on doctors and nurses who can welcome and encourage this as an essential new workforce. Of course, many patients, doctors and nurses have not yet learned to welcome or encourage such participation. Many patients just want to consume, many doctors are content with boutique medicine wherever customers can be found. Many doctors even in the NHS still just want to give orders, and many nurses are willing just to obey them – but none of these attitudes has much of a future or commands peer respect. Despite their long tradition of greed and servility, doctors as a group have moved steadily to the Left ever since Bevan set their feet on his new path. Medical science can no longer be applied in the crude ways possible when scientific knowledge itself was crude. The new ways have been both more effective and more attractive to their practitioners; they have been able to enjoy their work more, with more creativity and less drudgery, and greater confidence that they really make a difference to health.

If we win back the NHS as a gift economy, and drive the money changers from its temple, it will be a new, democratising NHS, impatient of its own hierarchies, willingly accountable not to managers too far above ordinary life to understand what they manage, but to the communities they serve. Working together, health workers have a huge political power, hitherto virtually unused. NHS staff serve the people: not anonymously, but knowing their names, their addresses, their telephone numbers and their infinite variety of qualities and limitations. When NHS staff are told to do absurd things just to conform to management protocols designed to make one health centre or hospital compete successfully with another, collectively they can refuse and confuse upwards, while still preserving their links with their patients: new, more imaginative and better-targeted forms of industrial action. If they have constructive ideas of their own about how their work could be done more effectively, collectively they can implement them, with or without higher authority: they are not yet mere machine minders, nor need they become machine smashers. Their work is of irresistible public interest. They can therefore be sure of media publicity, and through this of support from their local public, who still have votes in elections. Such actions have to be carefully considered, collectively organised, and cunningly applied (having been implemented even once, their threat becomes permanent) but their potential power will terrify not only politicians, but even World Bankers and the

WTO, once they understand that it will actually be used. Everything depends on solidarity, felt and seen.

This requires more than union organisation. It needs political campaigning and political education, organised at the workplace, understood by at least a large thoughtful minority of staff as essential to the development of their own work, and accepted by the workforce as a whole as essential to their common interest. Such groups must make themselves essential to improved functioning and morale of their whole unit by providing a big picture within which each can understand his or her own part.

Resistance at the point of production

Whether or not the British Labour movement regains the control over its own programme that it briefly enjoyed from 1944 to 1948, the contradictions inherent in any marketed public service will persist, and almost certainly intensify. An alliance between the BMA, RCN, UNISON and other NHS unions and the public they all serve is no longer unthinkable. 'Keep Our NHS Public' a larger, broader and above all more united alliance of health experts, professionals, staff and trade unionists than ever before is likely to become as big a force in British politics as its Spanish counterpart became a few years ago, eventually helping to unhorse a government.[17] A return to the path originally leading to democratised public services outside the market is now unthinkable only for people utterly sold to the marketeers. When the ideas underlying marketisation of health care were first advanced in the UK by Sir Keith Joseph in the 1970s, his Conservative Party leader Edward Heath described him as 'completely mad'.[18] Times change, and both ways.

How such an alliance should use its strength is a centrally important question. Strikes in the public sector, above all in health care, are a dangerously double-edged weapon, and have in the past been used at least as much by doctors trying to retain their grip on care as their own private property, as by health workers employed for humiliatingly low wages. New methods of struggle will have to be found, to unite a broad alliance around demands for return to the path on which the NHS embarked in 1948, away from the market and toward a higher form of economy and culture.

There seem to be two main ways in which such a new strategy might find practical expression: by finding components of information technology that serve management functions only remotely related to patient care, and taking concerted industrial action to impede or withdraw them; and by traditional NHS units competing so successfully against their newly imposed commercial components, that commercial providers are revealed for what they are, servants of their executives and shareholders, in search of profit wherever they can find it, rather than effective neighbourhood service. Some cooperative GP consortia are now forming or re-forming, compelled to compete with commercial providers for services, which might just do this.

A society founded on both solidarity and doubt

We have no map of the future, only a compass. The only road we can have to a more generous and sustainable future will be one we discover and make for ourselves, starting from where we actually are, with people we actually have, learning as we go. We can count on vigorous support from an overwhelming majority of people who live not from what they own, but what they do, and this will set limits to what our enemies can do to oppose us.

Clinical medicine is full of doubt. Nothing is ever completely certain, every judgement has possibilities of error. Yet our knowledge of this arises from another paradox: as never before, we can now face up to our weaknesses, because we can at last be confident of our real strength to control disease, our real ability to make life happier and less painful. When clinical medicine could do little to change the course of illness, health professionals spoke and behaved as if they were sure of everything. In public, and in front of their patients, they knew the answers to so much that there seemed to be little room for anything more that they did not know. They needed this dogmatism to conceal their ignorance, a professional duty because faith still seemed their best weapon, and both faith and fees depended on patients' continued collusion.

Honesty, doubt and respect for evidence regardless of personal consequences are the foundations of science. A scientific view of the world must recognise that everything in it is ultimately connected with everything else, in space and in time, so that our present can be understood only as a transient connection between our past and our future, providing our only opportunity to change the world to something better for our children, and thus contribute to the only eternal life worthy of an educated imagination. This implies that everyone who accepts such a view takes on an unlimited personal task; yet this task has in the past been successfully undertaken, with undeniably huge material results. Who performed this impossible task? It was, is, and always will be a collective undertaking, which will be done better as it engages a growing proportion of the whole of society. Obviously within this task there must be divisions of labour, but we have created these divisions only to help us to conceptualise our work and set ourselves achievable goals. These divisions do not exist in nature. Most major advances occur at their boundaries, at their interface with other specialised fields. They all require imagination within an overall big picture of the world as a whole, as it was, is, and is becoming. Each such advance leads to the definition of new fields, which for a while need consolidation by continued hard slogging at the centre, but then the breakthroughs come at the boundaries.

Is it not possible to develop a better big picture, a more useful common sense, within which fewer scientific ideas would seem counter-intuitive, and therefore appear irrelevant to everyday life? Daily life now poses many extremely serious scientific problems – human problems that are soluble only through scientific ways of thinking, through doubt, experiment, open and honest appraisal of consequent evidence. This attitude does not require acquisition of huge volumes of fact. It is said that the reason fewer school-leavers now choose to study sciences is that they see sciences as subjects requiring great feats of memory, large volumes of knowledge poured by didactic teachers into minds wrongly assumed to be empty, whereas traditional arts and humanities encourage creativity and judgement. Every mind already contains a set of working assumptions that we call common sense, arising from common experience. The products of science now engulf that experience. Our first and most urgent task should be to help first ourselves and then our children to make sense of it, rather than accept it as a kind of magic, allowing us to pretend we can have whatever world we wish, without regard to reality.

Development of this more mature common sense will entail doubt, participation in experiment and honesty about the results, on a mass scale and applied to the real world as it is, not within conventional compartments.[19] Conservatism, in its true sense of building on and conserving what we already have, can sometimes be a useful set of beliefs. Most revisions of established tradition fail, so people are rightly cautious in shifting from old devils they know to new devils they do not. They want convincing evidence before accepting any new practice. It was Margaret Thatcher who scrapped this – the only sound plank in the Conservative platform – to make way for her radical retreat to primitive classical economics. It is her New Labour disciples, the ever more radical 'reformers' and 'modernisers' of the NHS who insist on imposing options for private care on patients, competition on hospitals, division and discontinuity on staff, and tick-box medicine on clinical judgement. Safe doctoring depends on healthy scepticism when prescribing either medication or surgery, and respect for the extreme complexity of human biology and sociology rather than cocksure zeal, but none of these qualities can prosper within the consumerist paradigm.

Just as NHS experience has more to teach than to learn from the world of business, it may have the same relation to politics. The political illiteracy of most doctors (scarcely perceptible now that most other people have fallen into the same state) may make this hard to recognise, but for real politics, concerning social change rather than personal careers, politicians and parties could learn a lot from the developing culture of health care. Like politicians and their parties, health professionals inevitably make mistakes, and because in both cases they deal with human lives, the consequences may be serious. Unlike politicians and their parties, health professionals are at least beginning to develop a culture that learns from mistakes, by shifting routine practice toward the rules of organised experiment.

This provides a model that could begin to tackle the greatest problem so far encountered in real attempts to build sharing societies: the centralisation of peripheral decisions that has always followed central management of resources, ending with centralised beliefs and fossilised ideas. In the immediate aftermath of revolutions this has not been a serious problem, because first experience of a government ruling for the mass of the people rather than against them releases huge spontaneous social energy, often even greater at the periphery than at the centre. Ten years later it has been a different story. Chains of command conveying central policies to peripheral communities and places of work have become chains around imagination.

The nature of societies ultimately depends on the nature of social and property relationships at the point of production; how we think depends on how we work, who we work for and how we see ownership of the creative process. In humane public health services, the nature of work is fundamentally different from the nature of work in commodity production. It entails an exchange of information, and of interpretations of information and judgements, between two sets of players linked by trust, leading to creation of an added value, health gain — a social as well as personal asset, which cannot be exchanged or sold on as a commodity. For optimal productivity, this must depend on peripheral decisions. These can be oriented and encouraged by central policies, but can be centrally regulated only within limits wide enough to allow peripheral work to be done with imagination.[20] It is inherently democratic, in the true sense that everybody participates, and nobody can escape the consequences of their own decisions.

Errors are inevitable, so all decisions entail doubt. We can never eliminate it, not least because it is our chief source of new ideas and progress. Writing between 1938, when contemporary odds suggested that fascist ideas would soon dominate the world, and 1945, when his personal friends were producing the first nuclear weapons at Los Alamos and questioning their use, Bertolt Brecht wrote his play *The Life of Galileo*. This was a dramatic analysis of actual and potential social functions of science and their relation to state power. The play hinges on a central scene, where the chief inquisitor advises the new pope on how to handle Galileo's heresy, which has leaked out of the safe confines of discussion between academics, and become a subject of intense popular debate in the streets of Italy. While Cardinal Barberini, an intellectual previously known for his tolerance and enlightenment, is being robed for his coronation as Pope Urban VIII, layer by layer he acquires his new role as God's voice on earth, responsible for orderly conduct of society. The inquisitor speaks:

> They say it is their mathematical tables and not the spirit of denial and doubt. But it is not their tables. A horrid unrest has come into the world. It is this unrest in their own brains which these men impose upon the motionless earth. They cry, 'The figures compel us!' – but whence come these figures? They come from doubt, as everyone knows. These men doubt everything. Are we to found human society on doubt, and no longer on belief? (Brecht (1958), Scene 12, p 110 (my own translation))

It is time to say that we can, providing that doubt is always linked indissolubly with solidarity. We cannot do this at one stroke, but only by learning in a new field of social practice, its nascent culture protected from a surrounding economy still driven to maximise credulity for anything that is profitable, and to hold in contempt everything that is not profitable, with cocksure confidence in its own infallibility.[21] Science already builds on measured doubt, and our society now builds upon science as its material foundation. If we want to understand science rationally rather than fear it as magic, we must learn to take measured doubt into both our popular culture and our political culture, always remembering to link it with solidarity: everyone, everywhere, must be on board.

As a progressive force, doubt begins from not knowing, from understanding that we don't know, from designing increasingly precise hypotheses that can be tested in the real world, then revising our ideas, and thus progressively reducing our ignorance.[22] The doubt underlying science is not the infinite, nihilist doubt of mysticism or post-modern philosophy, abdicating responsibility for human progress yet open to any fashionable quackery that uses current key words.[23] Our doubt lies within confidence limits set by the accumulated experience of past generations, resulting in material advances whose growing power to change the real world surrounds us and cannot be deceived. No scientific hypothesis has eternal validity, no area of our knowledge is finite, but in every field our ignorance is diminishing and our understanding of nature is growing.

This is where Nye Bevan's new path has led. As every schoolchild knows, a crystal dropped into a super-saturated fluid solution quickly replicates itself, creating more and larger crystals, until suddenly fluid becomes solid. Our morally exhausted post-industrial society is already thick with generous and imaginative ideas about how everyone could live better, if the work and wealth now poured into stuffing people with things they do not need or even want, or into wars and threats of wars, were put to constructive use to meet human needs. While power commanded by those who own our economy is so overgrown that we can now hardly comprehend it, our own power to influence events seems to be vanishing. Stripped by disillusion, people everywhere are searching for something solid on which to set their feet, on which to stand up and regain control of their lives. The NHS could be our crystal, around which a material society of solidarity could form.

Summary and conclusions

History has seen a succession of societies, each organised around particular dominant techniques and social relations of production and ideas derived from them. If our society has no successor, this will not be because it has arrived at perfection, but because it is materially and socially unsustainable, and has destroyed even the beginnings of any alternative. The transition from predominantly physical to predominantly mental labour now impacting on old, advanced economies, and already beginning even in the least-developed economies, requires a profound political and cultural reorientation for that large majority of people who live from what they do rather than what they own, on whom all progress depends.

Public services for health care and education provide the most obvious growing points for a new mode of production of value, not producing commodity values for the market, but use-values for the whole of society according to need. The struggle to separate these from the primitive commodity economy and culture surrounding and now engulfing them provides the central ground for real political contention for the foreseeable future in mature economies. The struggle to develop them on socialist lines, bringing together the core traditions of self-critical science and participative democracy, provides the central ground for political action.

No major political parties in any of the world's advanced economies now provide a convincing vehicle for this necessary reorientation, but to the extent that they oppose the present drive to subordinate state health, welfare and educational services to competition for consumer markets, many might become so. In Britain and the US, the political parties originally responsible for distancing some or all of health care from the market – the Labour Party and the Democratic Party – now lead the drive toward fusion of business interests and the state, imposing commercial culture on science and public service. Either the memberships and electorates of these parties must find the understanding, confidence and courage to reclaim them, or broader coalitions must find new ways to organise.

Either way, health professionals of the 21st century will find that they have entered what must become politicised professions. There is nowhere else to go.

Notes

[1] The present continuing and possibly irreversible decline of the Conservative Party arises from its persisting association with aristocracy and inherited wealth, against which New Labour can successfully present itself as a party of all winners in a mature market society if (and only if) most people can still be persuaded that they will win in an increasingly fluid society. There is little evidence of any such shift toward increasing social mobility. Of eight developed economies (the UK, the US, West Germany, Canada, Norway,

Denmark, Sweden and Finland) compared in a recent study, the UK and the US had least intergenerational mobility. Comparing cohorts born in 1958 and 1970, social mobility showed little change in the US, but fell markedly in Britain despite rising average real incomes (Blanden et al, 2005). Between 1977 and 1997, the difference in long-term employee earnings between the top and bottom 10% of the income distribution rose by 275%. The lowest paid remained lowest paid, with longer periods of low pay or no pay (Department of Trade and Industry, 2000). Even in the US, the myth of rags to riches through hard work is probably losing credibility.

[2] This led to the first significant shareholders' revolt in modern UK business history, so that three years later Mr Garnier was still having to exist on only £7,815,360 a year. He still ranked third among the top ten company chief executives, but lagged well behind Sir Martin Sorrell of WPP (the world's largest communications, public relations and market research company) at £52m and Tony Ball of BSkyB at £13.9m (Finch and Treanor, 2005; Inman, 2005).

[3] Snow, 1959.

[4] Unlike the Labour Party, a loose federation of affiliated trade unions and substantially different political groups, the Independent Labour Party (ILP), formed in a decade earlier in 1893, was organised on European lines, with agreed objectives and individual membership. It later provided the Labour Party's first socialist MPs, notably Keir Hardie, James Ramsay Macdonald and virtually all Labour leaders until 1931. Following Macdonald's defection to Baldwin's Conservative coalition government, the ILP then lurched violently to the Left, even applying for affiliation to the Communist Third International (though it soon changed its mind). The ILP tradition remained powerful in Scotland, where it competed with the Communist Party for the militant traditions of the Clyde, and provided Nye Bevan with his wife and lifelong comrade-in-arms, Jenny Lee.

[5] The leaders of New Labour, Tony Blair, Gordon Brown and Peter Mandelson, were swept to power by two promises: to regain former Labour votes lost to the Conservatives during the Thatcher counter-revolution by adopting elements of Conservative policy – which they did; and to rescue the party from its own traditions of internal

corruption by introducing a system of one member one vote for all major internal elections – which, unremarked by news media, they have done only selectively since the first vote that gave them power.

[6] This occurred in four waves of rediscovered need for organisation. The first began in the 1890s, mainly through local branches of the ILP, Socialist League and other smaller groups gathered around Robert Blatchford, his weekly paper the *Clarion* and the cycling clubs that sold it, and his book *Merrie England* (see above, Chapter Four, n 10). Then came the Marxist and syndicalist mass movements in the South Wales coalfield and the Clyde from 1916 onwards, culminating in the huge international impact of the Russian Revolution in October 1917; then the mass anti-fascist movement from 1935 onwards, particularly in army units from 1942 to 1945, all led by the Communist Party. These movements underlay the landslide Labour victory of 1945 and mass refusal to return to the pre-war order of laissez-faire economics. Finally there were the romantic, often anarchic movements born in Europe and the US in 1968, gathered around opposition to America's war in Vietnam, but also reflecting the moral emptiness of newly emergent consumer culture. Serious, large-scale commitment to organisation on the Left disintegrated in Britain after the defeat of the miners' strike of 1984-85. For participants in this history, Helena Sheehan provides conclusions I share:

> I think that we should relate to the past of the socialist movement as we do personally to our own youth; as a time of naivete, excessive zeal, utopian flight, rash experiment, brash miscalculation, false friends; a time of healthy growth of instincts, which time would temper and further experience refine; a time of glory and terror and tragedy; a time of vulnerability and pain, spared those who dared not venture along such a dangerous road. (Sheehan, 1992)

[7] Sidney Webb, and the leaders who commissioned this work, were driven by events. The October Revolution of 1917 had suddenly put socialism back on the agenda of every party hoping to win or retain a mass base in the industrial working class. Whatever second thoughts they may have had later, in the third year of futile industrialised slaughter, 'peace, bread and socialism' was a slogan

no popular politician could afford to reject. There was no other way to satisfy the party's annual conference at that time.

[8] In Europe at least, the situation is similar today. As a percentage of GDP, growth in EU research and development investment has been slowing since 2000, and between 2002 and 2003, the latest year available, grew by only 0.2%, compared with about 10% a year in China. In 2003, EU spending on research and development was only 1.93% of GDP, compared with 2.6% in the US and 3.2% in Japan. Despite all the rhetoric, Europe is not now on course to become a leading knowledge-based world economy (EU Commission, 2005). However, this will certainly remain its aim, and will be the path pursued by the US economy when it escapes from its current celebration of ignorance.

[9] Lenin made it clear in 1918 that in his view, socialist industry had to start from centralised, quasi-monopolised, tightly managed industry with a disciplined and tightly managed workforce. Socialism was not a prior alternative, but a potential consequence. Such industry was most evolved in Germany and in Russia existed only in a few highly concentrated areas around Petrograd, Moscow and the Don basin, which became focal points for revolution within a much wider peasants' revolt, only seeking land ownership. His vision of socialism was a union between the economic achievement of wartime Germany and the political achievement of Russia in October 1917 (Carr, 1952, pp 97-102). Such a union depended on a revolution in Germany similar to that in Russia. By 1919 the mutinies in Germany's defeated armies were suppressed, the revolutionary threat to established power was in decline, and where it gained even a transient foothold, was descending to murderous farce. Hitler's accession to power received powerful assistance from the world's bankers to make sure such chaos would never return.

[10] This was confirmed by J.K. Galbraith from his experience as a successful leading economist in Roosevelt's wartime government, and through his postwar research into German war industry, both its tardy and incomplete transfer from consumer to war production after 1941, and its resilience against allied bombing after 1943. Nazi Germany developed no useful national accounting system comparable to the Soviet *Gosplan* or British and US central planning departments, nor even the concept of GNP, either during the war or in preparation for it. Civilian consumption and deployment of

manpower remained uncontrollably high for almost the whole war (Galbraith, 1987, pp 247-8). However, though British wartime industry became highly regulated, Churchill made sure that its ownership remained in private hands. There it would probably have remained if the membership revolt at the Labour Party conference in December 1944 had not forced Attlee, Morrison and Bevin to act – a situation not very different from the one faced by Sidney Webb in 1918.

[11] The great weakness of the Labour Party has been its consistent refusal to be anything other than a parliamentary or local government party, or to do anything outside Parliament or council chambers other than run elections. Throughout the bitter struggles of employed and unemployed workers against oppressive employers and their Conservative governments between the two World Wars – now generally recalled nostalgically as the vigorous youth of a party now senescent – virtually all campaigning between elections was in fact initiated by Britain's minuscule Communist Party, and was at least initially condemned by leaders both of the Labour Party and all the larger trade unions, until these began to acquire a democratic structure with some accountability to members in the 1960s. The Labour Party took no national action either in the general strike of 1926, or in the miners' strike of 1984-85, though many local branches ignored their leaders and did what they could to save the party's honour. The hunger marches of the unemployed in the 1930s were officially banned by the Labour Party (though usually locally supported by its branches) except for the last, the Jarrow march organised by Ellen Wilkinson and her local Labour Party, This became the party's sole historical claim to militancy. Bevan was expelled from the Labour Party in 1938 for sharing united front platforms with Communists, came close to expulsion in 1944 for daring to criticise Ernest Bevin's authoritarian management of coal miners, and again in 1953 for opposition to Attlee and Gaitskell's submission to the US. He was saved only by mass support in Ebbw Vale, his constituency. The Labour Party's occasional forays into political theory and education were provoked only by the need to develop some social democratic ideology to counter the influence of Communists and Trotskyists. Since the Soviet collapse, political education has ceased, other than training days to impart election and office skills. Political theory and policy development now lie almost entirely with 'independent' think tanks close to the New Labour project, hardly at all with either the party's annual conference,

or its National Executive Committee, and none of its leaders have any serious pretensions as theorists. In fact, their position rests on denial that any theory independent of capitalism is possible or necessary.

[12] Strangleman, 2005. Effects of replacing the established and stable work and safety-centred culture of railways by an unstable money-centred culture provide a close experimental parallel to the same process now being promoted in the NHS.

[13] Catalyst, ASLEF, RMT and TSSA, 2004. An ICM poll of 1,001 adults aged 18+ in March 2001 showed 76% of all voters, and 71% of Conservative voters, wanted railways to be renationalised (Travis, 2001).

[14] According to Colin Leys (interview with David Walton at Goldman Sachs and in issues of *Goldman Sachs' UK Economics Analyst*, quoted in Walton, 2001) financial analysts scanning the global market assign a 'political risk premium' to governments according to their friendliness to international capital. Wrongly anticipating a Labour victory led by Neil Kinnock in 1992, this was set at 2%. By 1997, anticipating a Blair victory, the risk premium fell to 0.5%. Since then company donations and gifts from the very rich have fallen steeply for the Conservative Party, and risen rather less for the Labour Party. At £41.1m in 2001-04, Labour's funds for the first time exceeded those of the Conservative Party at £28.7m, with the Liberal Democrats far behind at £6.3m. Though Blair has secured a few very wealthy personal donors (led by Lord Sainsbury with £4.5m in 2001-04 and another £2m for the recent election) 64% of Labour's funding still comes from trade unions, 32% from individual donations and only 3% from companies. The Conservative Party still gets 18% of its funding from companies, 33% from individual donations and 48% from public money supporting opposition parties, without which it would now be bankrupt. Proportionately, Liberal Democrats now get more of their funds from companies than the Conservatives, at 22%, with 12% from individual donations and a whacking 64% from public money ('Party cash', *Labour Research*, May 2005, pp 27-9). Trade unions have far more potential influence over Labour policy than they have so far chosen to use.

[15] 'Celticus', 1944, pp 82-4.

[16] Ironically, this line first appeared after a majority of the Labour Party membership voted to revise Clause 4 of the party's constitution, and to eliminate Sidney Webb's definition of socialism as common ownership of the means of production, distribution and exchange. It was a sprat offered to catch a mackerel. The Labour Party had never previously described itself as a socialist party. After 11 years' experience of leadership by an instinctive conservative, members could begin to take it more seriously.

[17] Sanchez Bayle and Beiras Cal, 2001.

[18] Heath's indiscretion was made, presumably off the record, to members of a royal commission on the NHS taking evidence from him some time between 1975, when it was set up, and 1979, when it reported. Members of the commission, having heard evidence from Sir Keith that the NHS should operate as a market, with its processes recast as commodities, asked Heath what he thought of this idea. Heath dismissed the question as absurd, saying 'Of course, he's completely mad'. I was told this by a member of the commission, my friend the late Dr Cyril Taylor. It could perhaps be confirmed by Ann Clwyd MP, also a member of that commission.

[19] Participation in trials has huge educational potential for communities, particularly if they participate repeatedly in different studies, because this becomes mass education in the nature of scientific reasoning and evidence. This potential is realised only in studies that stick to the same population through several generations, and so far as I know, nobody has ever measured the cumulative and collective effects of repeated community participation. Participants must be fully informed, and this should include discussion of trial design and its underlying logic. Randomisation of trial participants is particularly challenging and rewarding. In general, participants gain from scientific trials organised by bona fide independent agencies, like the Medical Research Council (MRC) or university departments, in that caring professionals who undertake them are highly motivated and work to obsessively high standards. However, there is no evidence that participants in trials either gain or lose compared with non-participants receiving the same care outside trials (Vist et al, 2005).

[20] Ironically, the pattern now being followed by NHS contracts both in primary and specialist care is one of central regulation through cybernetic control, pioneered by the late Stafford Beer in Chile, before the CIA-supported coup and murder of President Allende by Pinochet (Hanlon, 1973). This could never have worked, because it would have frozen all initiatives at points of production not centrally foreseen, and included in the central plan.

[21]   And each of them said, 'How wise we are!
    Though the sky be dark, and the voyage be long,
    Yet we never can think we were rash or wrong,
    While round and round in our sieve we spin!'
    Far and few, far and few,
    Are the lands where the Jumblies live.
    Their heads are green, and their hands are blue,
    And they went to sea in a sieve.

(Lear, 1947).

[22] Rosenhead, 1989.

[23] Fondness for mysticism and hostility to science has remained a weakness of the new Left ever since 1968. From 1936 to 1945 a social alliance between leading scientists and the Marxist Left appeared to have won the war against fascism but lost its way to socialism, so the new Left slid into a new alliance with mysticism and hedonism. We are still paying the price for that infantile response to bitter but necessary experience. Science eventually emerges from its first reductionist attempts to understand, but mysticism leads to no effective action, providing just those escapes from reality that our rulers need (Gillott and Kumar, 1993). Operational research, developed largely by these Left scientists in the Second World War, and significantly never conceived by the fascist powers, could have provided a basis for economic research in a planned economy after the war, if Britain had not quickly returned to business as usual (Rosenhead, 1991). In a new political context approaching that reached in 1944-45, it could also provide a basis for epidemiology as a more effective weapon for health care (Proctor, 1997).

Further reading

The works below are listed more or less in the same order as their ideas are discussed in the book.

For general background to any scientific approach to social development, see Jacob Bronowski's superb BBC series *The Ascent of Man*, now readily available on DVD (BBC). There is also a book of the series still in print, but viewing is better.

The best introduction to epidemiology and medicine as a social science is probably still Jerry Morris' classic *Uses of Epidemiology* (London: Gollancz, 1967; new edn, Bristol: The Policy Press, 2005). It contains virtually nothing about statistical techniques, and is none the worse for that. Students who become full-time epidemiologists will learn these techniques elsewhere, but the essentials required for study of populations are all here, with more conviction than you'll find in a couple of shelves of more recent textbooks.

For a conclusive assessment of what health care can or does contribute to health gain, see Ellen Nolte and Martin McKee's *Does Health Care Save Lives? Avoidable Mortality Revisited* (London: Nuffield Trust, 2004).

For economic development from a Keynesian liberal viewpoint read John Kenneth Galbraith's lucid and entertaining *A History of Economics: The Past as the Present* (London: Penguin Books, 1987). If an equally accessible book from a socialist viewpoint useful in the present era exists, I don't know of it, but would be glad to hear of any suggestions.

For a lively account of development of the pre-'reform' NHS from a non-socialist viewpoint by a central actor at the top of the civil service, read Geoffrey Rivett's *From Cradle to Grave: Fifty Years of the NHS* (London: King's Fund, 1998). He is particularly good at integrating development of clinical medicine with development of the NHS as a system. Charles Webster has written the official, definitive, detailed and excellent history of the pre-'reform' NHS in *The Health Services since the War. Vol 1. Problems of Health Care: The National Health Service before 1957* (London: HMSO, 1988). and *Vol 2. The National Health Service 1958-79* (London: HMSO, 1996). These also are easily readable.

For detailed analysis of commercialisation of the NHS since 1979 read Allyson Pollock's excellent *NHS plc: The Privatisation of our Health Care* (London: Verso, 2004). Jeremy Lee-Potter provides a very readable personal view of the early stages of this process from the point of view of an outraged gentleman in *A Damn Bad Business: The NHS Deformed* (London:Victor Gollancz, 1997). The only good account I know of what it is like to work in the NHS in the lower ranks of its hierarchy is Jonathan Neale's *Memoirs of a Callous Picket: Working for the NHS* (London: Pluto Press, 1983). Though now ancient, little has changed for the better, and his thoughtful account of primitive attempts to resist the forward march of managerialism and industrialisation are of great current relevance.

To understand how commercialisers of health care plan the strategies now being applied by government, read Nick Bosanquet and Steven Pollard's exceptionally frank and lucid explanation from a viewpoint exactly contrary to my own in their *Ready for Treatment: Popular Expectations and the Future of Health Care* (London: Social Market Foundation, 1997), pp 98-103).

The best analysis I know of similar developments in the US is David Himmelstein, Steffie Woolhandler and Ida Hellander's *Bleeding the Patient: The Consequences of Corporate Health Care* (Monroe, ME: Common Courage Press, 2001).

The best introduction to analysis of clinical medicine as a production system (though he does not call it that) is Alvan Feinstein's classic *Clinical Judgment* (New York: Robert E. Krieger, 1967). For origins of our dominant clinical philosophy, and indications of alternatives, read Foucault's classic *The Birth of the Clinic: An Archaeology of Medical Perception* (London: Tavistock Publications, 1973); first published as *Naissance de la Clinique* (Paris: Presses Universitaires de France, 1963). Though Foucault's prose is so dense as to be almost impenetrable to anyone with practical work to do, it's worth the effort. For a review of different Marxist approaches to science generally (with little reference to health sciences, but still very useful) see Helena Sheehan's *Marxism and the Philosophy of Science: A Critical History – the first hundred years* (New Jersey: Humanities Press, 1985, 1993). For an alternative view of clinical medicine in relation to public health, more sceptical than my own, read Geoff Rose's *Strategy of Preventive Medicine* (Oxford: Oxford University Press, 1992).

There are many good books designed to promote more effective cooperation between patients and professionals through improved consultation skills, but few pay much regard to constraints of time and other resources in everyday reality. Exceptions are Leonie Ridsdale's *Evidence-based General Practice: A Critical Reader* (London: WB Saunders, 1995) and Trisha Greenhalgh and Brian Hurwitz's

Narrative Based Medicine (London: BMA Books, 2002). A new generation of such books is now appearing, accepting – however reluctantly – the piecework-based contract now applied to all clinical work. None, so far as I know, explore the possibilities for resistance within this contract, above all at a community or political rather than personal level, but that must come.

Analysis of the role of information technology should still start from Lawrence Weed's classic *Medical Records, Medical Education and Patient Care: The Problem-oriented Record as a Basic Tool* (Cleveland, OH: Press of Case Western Reserve University, 1971).

Many authors have from time to time taken the lid off the multinational pharmaceutical industry, though few of them pose any alternative to getting our new treatments as a byproduct of profit for shareholders. The best introduction to the most dangerous trends in reification of disease is Charles Medawar's *Power and Dependence: Social Audit on the Safety of Medicines* (London: Social Audit, 1992). The more specific case of reification of dysfunctional behaviour in children is bravely and excellently presented by Sami Timimi in *Pathological Child Psychiatry and the Medicalisation of Childhood* (Hove: Brunner-Routledge, 2002). Recent experience of development and marketing of second-generation antidepressant drugs is excellently and very readably presented by David Healy in his *Let Them Eat Prozac: The Unhealthy Relationship between the Pharmaceutical Industry and Depression* (New York: New York University Press, 2004).

There is a good website critical of the industry at www.nofreelunch-uk.org, and an apologetic but responsible and reliable site for the Office of Health Economics at www.ohe.org.

Sebastian Mellanby gives an account of globalised capitalism in his *The World's Banker: A Story of Failed States, Financial Crises, and the Wealth and Poverty of Nations* (New Haven, CT: Yale University Press, 2005). Alternatively, you can read an even more authoritative account by the World Bank's most eminent defector, Joseph Stiglitz, in his *Globalization and its Discontents* (London: Penguin Books, 2002). Global responses to the neoliberal offensive on public health care systems are covered by the International Association for Health Policy, at www.healthp.org.

An excellent general guide to the neoliberal offensive and its impact on the British state is Colin Leys' *Market-driven Politics: Neoliberal Democracy and the Public Interest* (London: Verso, 2003).

For a general account of the British Labour movement from the industrial revolution to the end of the First World War, read Alan

Morton's and George Tate's *The British Labour Movement 1770-1920* (London: Lawrence & Wishart, 1956). For development of English (but not Scottish, Welsh or Irish) working-class culture read E.P. Thompson's classic *The Making of the English Working Class* (London: Penguin Books, 1963). The best general sources for history of the Welsh Labour movement are Gwyn Alf Williams' *When was Wales? A History of the Welsh* (London: Pelican Books, 1985) and Hywel Francis' and Dai Smith's *The Fed: A History of the South Wales Miners in the 20th Century* (London: Lawrence & Wishart, 1980). The most useful and readable analysis of the Labour Party's repeated paralysis whenever it gets close to power is still Ralph Miliband's *Parliamentary Socialism: A Study in the Politics of Labour* (London: George Allen & Unwin, 1961).

References

Abbasi, K. (1999) 'The World Bank and world health: changing sides', *British Medical Journal*, vol 318, pp 865-9.

Abramson, J.H., Gofin, J., Peritz, E. et al (1982) 'Clustering of chronic disorders – a community study of coprevalence in Jerusalem', *Journal of Chronic Diseases*, vol 35, pp 221-30.

Acheson, E.D. (1982) 'The impending crisis of old age: a challenge to ingenuity', *Lancet*, vol 2, pp 592-4.

Agdestein, K. and Roemer, M.I. (1994) 'Good health at a modest price: the fruit of primary care', *Journal of Public Health Policy*, vol 15, pp 485-90.

Albutt, T.C. (1912) 'The Act and the future of medicine', letter to *The Times*, 3 January.

American Psychiatric Association (1994) *Diagnostic and statistical manual of mental disorders* (4th edn), Washington, DC: American Psychiatric Association.

Anderson, G.F., Reinhardt, U.E., Hussey, P.S. and Petrosyan, V. (2003) 'It's the prices, stupid: why the United States is so different from other countries', *Health Affairs*, vol 22, pp 89-105.

Andersson, S.-O. and Mattsson, B. (1989) 'Length of consultations in general practice in Sweden: views of doctors and patients', *Family Practice*, vol 6, pp 130-4.

Anikin, A.V. (1975) *A Science in its Youth: Pre-Marxian Political Economy*, Moscow: Progress Publishers.

Appleby, J. (1996) 'Promoting efficiency in the NHS: problems with the labour productivity index', *British Medical Journal*, vol 313, pp 1319-21.

Appleby, J. (2005) 'Economic growth and NHS spending', *Health Service Journal*, 6 January, p 22.

Armstrong, C. (1997) 'Thousands of women sterilised in Sweden without consent', *British Medical Journal*, vol 15, p 563.

Arrow, K.J. (1963) 'Uncertainty and the welfare economics of medical care', *American Economic Review*, vol 53, pp 941-73.

Association of the British Pharmaceutical Industry (1999) *The Expert Patient Survey*, London: ABPI.

Aylin, P., Williams, S., Jarman, B. and Bottle, A. (2005) 'Dr Foster's case notes: variation in operation rates by Primary Care Trust, 1998-2004', *British Medical Journal*, vol 331, p 539.

Bagehot, W. ([1867] 1963) *The English Constitution*, London: Fontana.

Bagge, E., Bjelle, A., Eden, S. and Svanborg, A. (1991) 'Osteoarthritis in the elderly: clinical and radiological findings in 79 and 85 year olds', *Annals of the Rheumatic Diseases*, vol 50, pp 535-9.

Bagley, C. (2001) 'There is nothing postmodern in what people with schizophrenia want', *British Medical Journal*, vol 323, pp 449-50.

Barker, D.J.P, Gardner, M.J., Power, C. and Hutt, M.S.R. (1979) 'Prevalence of gallstones at necropsy in nine British towns', *British Medical Journal*, vol 2, pp 1389-92.

Barlow, J.H., Turner, A.P. and Wright, C.A. (2000) 'A randomised controlled study of the arthritis self-management programme in the UK', *Health Education Research*, vol 15, pp 665-80.

Barr, J. (1911) 'Some reasons why the public should oppose the National Insurance Act', *British Medical Journal*, vol 2, pp 1713-15.

Barr, J. (1912) 'What are we? What are we doing here? From whence do we come and whither do we go?', *British Medical Journal*, vol 2, pp 157-62.

Barsky, A.J. (1992) 'Amplification, somatization, and the somatiform disorders', *Psychosomatics*, vol 33, pp 28-34.

Battistella, R.M. and Southby, R.M.F. (1968) 'Crisis in American medicine', *Lancet*, vol 1, p 581.

Baumol, W.J. (1993) 'Social wants and dismal science: the curious case of the climbing costs of health and teaching', *Proceedings of the American Philosophical Society*, vol 137, pp 612-37.

Beckman, H.B. and Frankel, R.M. (1984) 'The effect of physician behavior on the collection of data', *Annals of Internal Medicine*, vol 101, pp 692-6.

Beecham, L. (1991) 'Yes, prime minister, it *is* underfunding', *British Medical Journal*, vol 302, pp 1108-9.

Beecher, H.K. (1961) 'Surgery as placebo: a quantitative study of bias', *Journal of the American Medical Association*, vol 176, pp 1102-7.

Bekelman, J.E., Li, Y. and Gross, C.P. (2003) 'Scope and impact of financial conflicts of interest in biomedical research: a systematic review', *Journal of the American Medical Association*, vol 289, pp 454-65.

Belsen, K. (2002) 'Executive pay: a special report: learning how to talk about salary in Japan', *New York Times*, 7 April, p 12.

Benson, H. and McCallie, D.P. (1979) 'Angina pectoris and the placebo effect', *New England Journal of Medicine*, vol 300, pp 1424-9.

Benson, P. (1979) 'And what is your fee, doctor?', *Modern Medicine*, vol 1, pp 77-9.

Benson, T. (2002a) 'Why general practitioners use computers and hospital doctors do not – Part 1: incentives', *British Medical Journal*, vol 325, pp 1086-9.

Benson, T. (2002b) 'Why general practitioners use computers and hospital doctors do not – Part 2: scalability', *British Medical Journal*, vol 325, pp 1090-3.

Berger, A. (1998) 'Human genome project to complete ahead of schedule', *British Medical Journal*, vol 317, p 85.

Berger, M.Y., Hartman, T.C.O., van der Velden, J.J.I.M. and Bohnen, A.M. (2004) 'Is biliary pain exclusively related to gallbladder stones? A controlled prospective study', *British Journal of General Practice*, vol 54, pp 574-9.

Bernal, P., Escroff, D.B., Aboudaram, J.F. et al (2000) 'Psychosocial morbidity: the economic burden in a pediatric health maintenance organisation sample', *Archives of Paediatric & Adolescent Medicine*, vol 154, pp 261-6.

Berwick, D. (2002) '"We all have AIDS": case for reducing the cost of HIV drugs to zero', *British Medical Journal*, vol 324, pp 214-18.

Berwick, D.M. (2005) 'Measuring NHS productivity: how much health for the pound, not how many events for the pound', *British Medical Journal*, vol 330, pp 975-6.

Blanden, J., Gregg, P. and Machin, S. (2005) *Intergenerational Mobility in Europe and North America: A Report Supported by the Sutton Trust*, London: Centre for Economic Performance.

Blass, T. (2004/05) *The Man who Shocked the World: The Life and Legacy of Stanley Milgram*, New York: Perseus Books and Basic Books.

Blatchford, R. ([1893] 1976) *Merrie England*, (facsimile edn with new foreword), London: Journeyman Press.

Bloor, D.U. (1980) 'The union doctor', *Journal of the Royal College of General Practitioners*, vol 30, pp 358-64.

Bosanquet, N. and Leese, B. (1986) 'Family doctors: their choice of practice strategy', *British Medical Journal*, vol 293, pp 667-70.

Bosanquet, N. and Pollard, S. (1997) *Ready for Treatment: Popular Expectations and the Future of Health Care*, London: Social Market Foundation.

Boseley, S. (2000) 'Cubans tell NHS the secret of £7 a head health care', *Guardian*, 2 October.

Branigan, T. and Glover, J. (2005) 'Stage to be set for public sector reform', *Guardian*, 24 August.

Brecht, B. (1958) *Leben des Galilei*, London: Heinemann German Texts.

Bridges, K.W. and Goldberg, D.P. (1985) 'Somatic presentation of DSM III psychiatric disorders in primary care', *Journal of Psychosomatic Research*, vol 29, pp 563-9.

Briggs, N. (1993) 'Illiteracy and maternal health: educate or die', *Lancet*, vol 341, pp 1063-4.

Brindle, D. (1994) 'Care ruling "could cost NHS dear"', *Guardian*, 3 February.

Brinkley, I. (2005) *China, Europe and UK Manufacturing*, London: Trades Union Congress.

Bristol, N. (2005) 'The muddle of US electronic medical records', *Lancet*, vol 365, pp 1610-11.

Brouwer, W.B.F., Niessen, L.W., Postma, M.J. and Rutten, F.F.H. (2005) 'Need for differential discounting of costs and health effects in cost effectiveness analyses', *British Medical Journal*, vol 551, pp 446-8.

Brownbridge, G., Evans, A. and Wall, T. (1985) 'Effect of computer use in the consultation on the delivery of care', *British Medical Journal*, vol 291, pp 639-41.

Brunner, E.J., Marmot, M.G., White, I.R., O'Brien, J.R., Etherington, M.D., Slavin, B.M. et al (1993) 'Gender and employment grade differences in blood cholesterol, apolipoproteins and haemostatic factors in the Whitehall II study', *Atherosclerosis*, vol 102, pp 195-207.

Bunker, J. (2001) *Medicine Matters After All: Measuring the Benefits of Medical Care, a Healthy Lifestyle, and a Just Social Environment*, Nuffield Trust series 15, London: Stationery Office.

Bunker, J.P., Barnes, B.A. and Mosteller, F. (1977) *Costs, Risks and Benefits of Surgery*, New York: Oxford University Press.

Bunting, M. (1995) *The Model Occupation: The Channel Islands under German rule, 1940-1945*, London: HarperCollins.

Burack, R.C. and Carpenter, R.R. (1983) 'The predictive value of the presenting complaint', *Journal of Family Practice*, vol 16, pp 749-54.

Burleigh, M. (2002) *Death and Deliverance: 'Euthanasia' in Germany 1900-1945*, Cambridge and London: Cambridge University Press and Pan Paperback.

Caines, E. (1993) 'Amputation is crucial to the patient's health: political cowardice is denying the NHS the medicine it needs: fewer professionals and greater productivity', *Guardian*, 11 May.

Campbell, E.J.M., Scadding, J.G. and Roberts, R.S. (1979) 'The concept of disease', *British Medical Journal*, vol 2, pp 757-62.

Cantlie, N. (1974) *A History of the Army Medical Department. Vol 1*, Edinburgh: Churchill Livingstone.

Carboni, D.K. (1982) *Geriatric medicine in the United States and Great Britain*, Contributions to the study of ageing 1, Westport, CT, and London: Greenwood, pp 1-97.

Carlisle, R. and Johnstone, S. (1996) 'Factors influencing the response to advertisements for general practice vacancies', *British Medical Journal*, vol 313, pp 468-71.

Carr, E.H. (1952) *A History of Soviet Russia: The Bolshevik Revolution 1917-1923. Vol 2*, London: Macmillan.

Carvel, J. (2003) 'Patients to choose their NHS hospital', *Guardian*, 17 July.

Catalyst, ASLEF, RMT and TSSA (2004) *Renaissance Delayed? New Labour and the Railways*, Catalyst working paper, free download from www.catalystforum.org.uk.

Caulfield, C. (1996) *Masters of Illusion: The World Bank and the Poverty of Nations*, London: Macmillan.

'Celticus' [Aneurin Bevan] (1944) *Why not Trust the Tories?*, London: Gollancz.

Chandna, S.M., Schultz, J., Lawrence, C., Greenwood, R.N. and Farrington, K. (1999) 'Is there a rationale for rationing dialysis? A hospital based cohort study of factors affecting survival and morbidity', *British Medical Journal*, vol 318, pp 217-23.

Charatan, F. (2001a) 'US settles biggest ever fraud case', *British Medical Journal*, vol 322, p 10.

Charatan, F. (2001b) 'Health maintenance organisations drop Medicare beneficiaries', *British Medical Journal*, vol 323, p 772.

Cherry, M.J. (2005) *Kidney for Sale by Owner: Human Organs, Transplantation and the Market*, Georgetown: Georgetown University Press.

Choudhry, N.K., Stelfox, H.T. and Detsky, A.S. (2002) 'Relationships between authors of clinical practice guidelines and the pharmaceutical industry', *Journal of the American Medical Association*, vol 287, pp 612-17.

Ciatto, S. (2003) 'Reliability of PSA testing remains unclear', *British Medical Journal*, vol 327, p 750.

Clarke, K. (1989) 'Working for patients: medical education, research and health', speech to medical profession, 10 July, official press release.

Cochrane, A.L. (1971) *Effectiveness and Efficiency: Random Reflections on Medical Care*, London: Nuffield Provincial Hospitals Trust.

Cochrane, A.L., St Leger, A.S. and Moore, F. (1978) 'Health service "input" and mortality "output" in developed countries', *Journal of Epidemiology & Community Health*, vol 32, pp 200-5.

Codman, E.A. (1914/1992) 'The product of a hospital', *Surgery, Gynaecology & Obstetrics*, vol 18, pp 491-6; reprinted in K.L. White, J. Frenk, C. Ordoñez et al, *Health Services Research: An Anthology*, Washington, DC: PAHO.

Coghill, D. (2004) 'Use of stimulants for attention deficit hyperactivity disorder: for'. *British Medical Journal*, vol 329, pp 907-8.

Cole, A. (2005) 'Interview with Iain Chalmers', *British Medical Journal*, vol 331, p 368.

Collier, J. (2005) 'New arrangements for the Medicines and Healthcare Products Regulatory Agency', *British Medical Journal*, vol 330, p 917.

Collings, J.S. (1950) 'General practice in England today', *Lancet*, vol 1, pp 555-85.

Committee of Inquiry (1956) *Report of the Committee of Inquiry into the Cost of the National Health Service*. Cmnd 9663, London: HMSO.

Cook, R.I., Render, M. and Woods, D.D. (2000) 'Gaps in the continuity of care and progress on patient safety', *British Medical Journal*, vol 320, pp 791-4.

Cooper, C. and Melton, L.J. (1992) 'Vertebral fractures: how large is the silent epidemic?', *British Medical Journal*, vol 304, pp 793-4.

Corney, R.H. (1990) 'A survey of professional help sought by patients for psychosocial problems', *British Journal of General Practice*, vol 40, pp 365-8.

Coulter, A., Klassen, A. and McPherson, K. (1995) 'How many hysterectomies should purchasers buy?', *European Journal of Public Health*, vol 5, pp 123-9.

Coulter, A., McPherson, K. and Vessey, M.P. (1988) 'Do British women undergo too many or too few hysterectomies?', *Social Science & Medicine*, vol 27, pp 987-94.

Coulter, A., Peto, V. and Jenkinson, C. (1994) 'Quality of life and patient satisfaction following treatment for menorrhagia', *Family Practice*, vol 11, pp 394-401.

Cox, A. (1966) *Among the Doctors*, London: Christopher Johnson.

Crawford, E.D. (2005) 'PSA testing: what is the use?', *Lancet*, vol 365, pp 1447-9.

Creese, A. (1997) 'User fees', *British Medical Journal*. vol 315, pp 202-3.

Crimlisk, H.L., Bhatia, K., Cope, H., David, A., Marsden, C.D. and Ron, M.A. (1998) 'Slater revisited: six year follow up study of patients with medically unexplained motor symptoms', *British Medical Journal*, vol 316, pp 582-6.

Cromarty. I. (1996) 'What do patients think about during their consultations? A qualitative study', *British Journal of General Practice*, vol 46, pp 525-8.

Crow, T.J., MacMillan, J.F., Johnson, A.L. and Johnstone, E.C. (1986) 'The Northwick Park study of first episodes of schizophrenia. II. A randomised controlled trial of prophylactic neuroleptic treatment', *British Journal of Psychiatry*, vol 148, pp 120-7.

Cunningham-Burley, S., Allbutt, H., Garraway, W.M., Lee, A. and Russell, E.B.A.W. (1996) 'Perceptions of urinary symptoms and health care seeking behaviour amongst men aged 40-79 years', *British Journal of General Practice*, vol 46, pp 349-52.

Darnborough, J. (1974) 'What price blood?', *Lancet*, vol 1, p 861.

Dash, P. (2004) 'New providers in UK health care: what effect will more competition have on the NHS?', *British Medical Journal*, vol 328, pp 340-2.

Davies, M. (ed) (1992) *The Valleys Autobiography: A People's History of the Garw, Llynfi and Ogmore Valleys*, Blaengarw: Valley and Vale.

Davies, N. (1998) 'The most secret crime', *Guardian*, 2 June.

Davies, R. (1995) 'Workers and medical services', in J. Edwards (ed) *Tinopolis: Aspects of Llanelli's Tinplate Trade*, Llanelli: Llanelli Borough Council, pp 162-9.

Davis, J. (2005) 'As doctors, we see the cancer that eats away at the NHS', *Guardian*, 27 June.

de Goulet, P., Ménard, J., Vu, H.-A. et al (1983) 'Factors predictive of attendance at clinic and blood pressure control in hypertensive patients', *British Medical Journal*, vol 287, pp 88-93.

De Gruy, F., Columbia, L. and Dickinson, P. (1987) 'Somatisation disorder in a family practice', *Journal of Family Practice*, vol 25, pp 45-51.

de Sardan, J.P.O. (2004) 'Africa: no money, no treatment', *Le Monde Diplomatique*, June, p 15.

de Vos, P., Dewitte, H. and van der Stuyft, P. (2004) 'Unhealthy European health policy', *International Journal of Health Services*, vol 34, pp 255-69.

Deber, R.B. (2003) *Delivering Health Care Services: Public, Not for Profit, or Private?*, Ottawa: Commission on the Future of Health Care in Canada.

deKare-Silver, N. (2005) 'Choose and book – whose choice is it anyway?', *British Medical Journal*, vol 330, p 1093.

Department of Health (1998) *The National Survey of NHS Patients: General Practice 1998*, at www.doh.gov.uk/public/nhssurvey.htm.

Department of Health (2001) *The Expert Patient*, London: Department of Health, August.

Department of Health (2005) , *Tackling Health Inequalities: Status Report on the Programme for Action*, at www.dh.gov.uk/.

Department of Trade and Industry (2000) *Trends in Earnings Inequality and Earnings Mobility, 1977-1997: The Impact of Mobility on Long-term Inequality*, London: Department of Trade and Industry.

Devereux, P.J., Choi, P.T.I., Lacchetti, C., Weaver, B., Schünemann, H.J., Haines, T., Lavis, N.J., Grant, B.J.B., Haslam, D.R., Bhandari, M., Sullivan, T., Cook, D.J., Walter, S.D., Meade, M., Khan, H., Bhatnagar, N. and Guyatt, G.H. (2002) 'A systematic review and meta-analysis of studies comparing mortality rates of private for-profit and private not-for-profit hospitals', *Canadian Medical Association Journal*, vol 166, pp 1399-1406.

Di Blasi, Z., Harkness, E., Ernst, E., Georgiou, A. and Kleijnen, J. (2001) 'Influence of context effects on health outcomes: a systematic review', *Lancet*, vol 357, pp 757-62.

diMasi, J.A., Hansen, R.W., Grabowski, H.G. and Lasagna, L. (1991) 'Cost of innovation in the pharmaceutical industry', *Journal of Health Economics*, vol 10, pp 107-42.

Doll, W.R.S. (1973) 'Monitoring the National Health Service', *Journal of the Royal Society of Medicine*, vol 66, pp 729-40.

Dove, G.A.W., Wigg, P., Clarke, J.H.C. et al (1977) 'The therapeutic effect of taking a patient's history by computer', *Journal of the Royal College of General Practitioners*, vol 27, pp 477-81.

Dowrick, C., May, C., Richardson, M. and Bundred, P. (1996) 'The biopsychosocial model of general practice: rhetoric or reality?', *British Journal of General Practice*, vol 46, pp 105-7.

Doyal, L. and Pennell, I. (1979) *The Political Economy of Health* London: Pluto Press.

Dunea, G. (1991) 'Nonsenserine', *British Medical Journal*, vol 303, p 253.

Dyer, O. (2005) 'Doctors protest over Bush's nomination for top legal post', *British Medical Journal*, vol 330, p 60.

Eagle, K.A., Goodman, S.G., Avezum, A., Budaj, A., Sullivan, C.M. and Lopez-Sendón, J. (2002) 'Practice variation and missed opportunities for reperfusion in ST-segment-elevation myocardial infarction: findings from the Global Registry of Acute Coronary Events (GRACE)', *Lancet*, vol 359, pp 373-7.

Earwicker, R. (1981) 'Miners' medical services before the First World War: the South Wales coalfield', *Llafur*, vol 3, no 2, pp 39-52.

Eckel, R.H., Grundy, S.M. and Zimmer, P.Z. (2005) 'The metabolic syndrome', *Lancet*, vol 365, pp 1415-28.

Egan, D. (1987) *Coal Society: A History of the South Wales Mining Valleys 1840-1980*, Llandyssul: Gomer Press.

Eisenberg, L. (1988) 'Science in medicine: too much, or too little and too limited in scope?', *American Journal of Medicine*, vol 84, pp 483-91.

Enterline, P.E., Salter, V. and McDonald, J.C. (1973) 'The distribution of medical services before and after "free" medical care – the Quebec experience', *New England Journal of Medicine*, vol 289, pp 1224-9.

Enthoven, A. (1990) 'International comparisons of health care systems: what can Europeans learn from Americans?', in OECD, *Health Care Systems in Transition*, Social Policy Studies 7, Paris: OECD, pp 57-71.

Enthoven, A.C. (1993) 'Why managed care has failed to contain health costs', *Health Affairs*, vol 12, pp 27-43.

Escobar, J.L., Golding, J.M. and Hough, R.L. et al (1987) 'Somatisation in the community: relationship to disability and use of services', *American Journal of Public Health*, vol 77, pp 837-40.

EU Commission (2005), report at europa.eu.int/comm./research/press/2005/pr 1907en.cfm.

Evans, R.G. and Barer, M.L. (1990) 'The American predicament', in OECD, *Health care systems in transition*, Policy Studies 7, Paris: OECD, pp 80-5.

Fairfield, G., Hunter, D.J., Mechanic, D. and Rosleff, F. (1997) 'Managed care: origins, principles and evolution', *British Medical Journal*, vol 314, pp 1823-6.

Falk, L.J. (1966) 'Coal miners' prepaid medical care in the United States, and some British relationships 1792-1964', *Medical Care*, vol 4, pp 37-42.

Feachem, G.A., Sekhri, N.K. and White, K.L. (2002) 'Getting more for their dollar: a comparison of the NHS with California's Kaiser Permanente', *British Medical Journal*, vol 324, pp 135-43.

Feder, G., Griffiths, C., Highton, C., Eldridge, S., Spence, M. and Southgate, L. (1995) 'Do clinical guidelines introduced with practice based education improve care of asthmatic and diabetic patients? A randomised controlled trial in general practice in East London', *British Medical Journal*, vol 311, pp 1473-8.

Ferguson, T. and McPhail, A.N. (1954) *Hospital and Community*, London: Oxford University Press.

Fijten, G.H., Muris, J.W.M., Starmans, R., Knottnerus, J.A., Blijham, G.H. and Krebber, T.F.W.A. (1993) 'The incidence and outcome of rectal bleeding in general practice', *Family Practice*, vol 10, pp 283-7.

Finch, J. and Treanor, J. (2005) 'Profits down, shares sinking, but boss on £7m says it's not enough', *Guardian*, 18 November.

Fink, P. (1992) 'Surgery and medical treatment in persistent somatising patients', *Journal of Psychosomatic Research*, vol 36, pp 439-47.

Foot, M. (1973) *Aneurin Bevan: A Biography. Vol 2, 1945-1960*, London: Davis-Poynter.

Ford, P. and Walsh, M. (1994) *New Rituals for Old: Nursing through the Looking Glass*, Oxford: Butterworth-Heinemann.

Forrest, C.B., Majeed, A., Weiner, J.P., Carroll, K. and Bindman, A.B. (2002) 'Comparison of specialty referral rates in the United Kingdom and the United States: retrospective cohort analysis', *British Medical Journal*, vol 325, pp 370-1.

Forrest, C.B., Majeed, A., Weiner, J.P., Carroll, K. and Bindman, A.B. (2003) 'Referral of children to specialists in the United States and the United Kingdom', *Archives of Paediatric & Adolescent Medicine*, vol 157, pp 279-85.

Forssas, E., Keskimäki, I., Reunanen, A. and Kosskinen, S. (2003) 'Widening socioeconomic mortality disparity among diabetic people in Finland', *European Journal of Public Health*, vol 13, pp 38-43.

Foucault, M. (1973) *The birth of the clinic: An archaeology of medical perception* (originally published as *Naissance de la clinique*, Paris: Presses Universitaires de France, 1963), London: Tavistock Publications.

Francis, H. and Smith, D. (1980) *The Fed: A History of the South Wales Miners in the 20th Century*, London: Lawrence & Wishart.

Frank, J.D. (1983) 'The placebo is psychotherapy', *The Behavioral & Brain Sciences*, vol 6, pp 291-2.

Frankel, S., Eachus, J., Pearson, N., Greenwood, R., Chan, P., Peters, T.J., Donovan, J., Smith G.D. and Dieppe, P. (1999) 'Population requirement for primary hip-replacement surgery: a cross-sectional study', *Lancet*, vol 353, pp 1304-9.

Frankel, S., Ebrahim, S. and Smith, G.D. (2000) 'The limits to demand for health care', *British Medical Journal*, vol 321, pp 40-5.

Fraser, S., Bunce, C., Wormald, R. and Brunner, E. (2001) 'Deprivation and late presentation of glaucoma: case-control study', *British Medical Journal*, vol 322, pp 639-43.

Freeman, G.K., Horder, J.P., Howie, J.G.R., Hungin, A.P., Hill, A.P., Shah, N.C. and Wilson, A. (2002) 'Evolving general practice consultation in Britain: issues of length and context', *British Medical Journal*, vol 324, pp 880-2.

Friedman, M. and Friedman, R.D. (1962) *Capitalism and Freedom*, Chicago: University of Chicago Press.

Frow, J. (1996) 'Information as gift and commodity', *New Left Review*, vol 219, pp 89-108.

Fulton, W.W. (1961) 'General practice in the USA', *British Medical Journal*, vol 1, pp 275-82.

Gaffney, D., Pollock, A.M., Price, D. and Shaoul, J. (1999a) 'The politics of the private finance initiative and the new NHS', *British Medical Journal*, vol 319, pp 249-53.

Gaffney, D., Pollock, A.M., Price, D. and Shaoul J. (1999b) 'PFI in the NHS – is there an economic case?', *British Medical Journal*, vol 319, pp 116-19.

Gaffney, D., Pollock, A.M. and Shaoul, J. (1999) 'NHS capital expenditure and the Private Finance Initiative – expansion or contraction?', *British Medical Journal*, vol 319, pp 48-51.

Galbraith, J.K. (1987) *A History of Economics: The Past as the Present*, London: Penguin/Hamish Hamilton.

Gannon, C. (2005) 'Will the lead clinician please stand up?', *British Medical Journal*, vol 330, p 737.

Garratini, S. and Garratini, L. (1993) 'Pharmaceutical prescriptions in four European countries', *Lancet*, vol 342, pp 1191-2.

Garratt, A.M., Ruta, D.A., Abdalla, M.I. et al (1993) 'The SF36 health survey questionnaire: an outcome measure suitable for routine use within the NHS?', *British Medical Journal*, vol 306, pp 1440-4.

Geiringer, E. (1959) 'Murder at the crossroads: or the decapitation of general practice', *Lancet*, vol 1, pp 1039-45.

Gene-Macdaniel, C. (1996) 'US could ban patents on medical procedures', *British Medical Journal*, vol 312, p 997.

General Municipal and Boilermakers' Union (2001) *PFI in the NHS: A Dossier*, London: GMB.

Gillott, J. and Kumar, M. (1993) *Science and the Retreat from Reason*, London: Merlin Press.

Gilson, L. (1993) 'Health care reform in developing countries', *Lancet*, vol 342, p 800.

Glasser, R.J. (1998) 'The doctor is not in: on the managed failure of managed medical care', *Harper's Magazine*, March, pp 35-41.

Glyn, A. (2005) 'Imbalances of the global economy', *New Left Review*, vol 34, July/Aug, pp 5–37.

Godber, G. (1980) 'An endangered thesis. Review of McKeown T. *The role of medicine: dream, mirage or nemesis?* Oxford: Blackwell, 1979', *British Medical Journal*, vol 280, p 102.

Godfrey, K. (2005) 'Delays in implementing e-booking threaten patient choice agenda', *British Medical Journal*, vol 330, p 166

Goldberg, D. and Williams, P. (1988) *A User's Guide to the General Health Questionnaire (GHQ)*, Windsor: NFER-Nelson Publishing.

Gottlieb, B. (1969) 'Non-organic disease in medical outpatients', *Update*, vol 5, pp 917-22.

Gracie, W.A. and Ranschoff, D.F. (1982) 'The natural history of silent gallstones: the innocent gallstone is not a myth', *New England Journal of Medicine*, vol 307, pp 794-800.

Greenfield, S., Kaplan, S.H., Ware, J.E., Yano, E.M. and Frank, J.H. (1988) 'Patients' participation in medical care', *Journal of General Internal Medicine*, vol 3, pp 448-57.

Greenhalgh, T. (1998) 'Research methods 2: Whose evidence is it anyway?', *British Journal of General Practice*, vol 48, pp 1448-9.

Greenhalgh, T. (2005) 'Early life risk factors for obesity in childhood: the hand that rocks the cradle rules the world', *British Medical Journal*, vol 331, p 453.

Grey, M.R. (1999) *New Deal Medicine: The Rural Health Programs of the Farm Security Administration*, Baltimore: Johns Hopkins University Press.

Griffin, J.P. and Griffin, T.D. (1992) 'The economic implications of therapeutic conservatism', in G.T. Smith (ed) *Innovative Competition in Medicine: A Schumpeterian Analysis of the Pharmaceutical Industry and the NHS*, London: Office of Health Economics, pp 85-96.

Grigg, J. (1978) *Lloyd George: The People's Champion, 1902-1911*, London: Eyre Methuen.

Grol, R., Wensing, M., Mainz, J., Ferreira, P., Hearnshaw, H., Hjortdahl, P., Oleson, F., Ribacke, M., Spenser, T. and Szécsényi, J. (1999) 'Patients' priorities with respect to general practice care: an international comparison', *Family Practice*, vol 16, pp 4-11.

Guevara, J.P. and Stein, M.T. (2001) 'Evidence based management of attention deficit hyperactivity disorder', *British Medical Journal*, vol 323, pp 1232-5.

Gunstone, C. (2005) 'Cancer in the elderly – a case for informed pessimism?', *British Journal of General Practice*, vol 55, p 648.

Habel, J. (2004) 'Cuba: what will happen after Castro?', *Le Monde Diplomatique*, June, pp 8-9.

Hampton, J.R., Harrison, M.J.G., Mitchell, J.R.A., Prichard, J.S. and Seymour, C. (1975) 'Relative contributions of history-taking, physical examination, and laboratory investigation to diagnosis and management of medical outpatients', *British Medical Journal*, vol 2, pp 486-9.

Hancher, L. (1990) *Regulating for Competition: Government, Law, and the Pharmaceutical Industry in the United Kingdom and France*, Oxford: Oxford University Press.

Hanlon, J. (1973) 'Chile leaps into cybernetic future', *New Scientist*, 15 February, pp 363-4.

Hannay, D.R. (1997) 'Deprivation payments and workload', *British Journal of General Practice*, vol 47, pp 663-4.

Harding, M.-L. (2005) 'Patients could get their own budgets, Number 10 says', *Health Services Journal*, 19 May, p 5.

Hart, J.T. (1970) 'Semicontinuous screening of a whole community for hypertension', *Lancet*, vol 2, pp 223-7.

Hart, J.T. (1971) 'The inverse care law', *Lancet*, vol 1, pp 405-12.

Hart, J.T. (1973) 'An assault on all custom: Cochrane's "Effectiveness and efficiency"', *International Journal of Health Services*, vol 3, pp 101-4.

Hart, J.T. (1974) 'The marriage of primary care and epidemiology: continuous anticipatory care of whole populations in a state medical service. (Milroy lecture)', *Journal of the Royal College of Physicians of London*, vol 8, pp 299-314.

Hart, J.T. (1984) 'Hidden agendas of earlier diagnosis', in L. Zander (ed) *Change: The Challenge for the Future*, Royal College of General Practitioners Annual Symposium 1983, London: RCGP, pp 54-63.

Hart, J.T. (1988) *A New Kind of Doctor: The General Practitioner's Part in the Health of the Community*, London: Merlin Press.

Hart, J.T. (1992a) 'Rule of halves: implications of underdiagnosis and dropout for future workload and prescribing costs in primary care', *British Journal of General Practice*, vol 42, pp 116-19.

Hart J.T. (1992b) 'Two paths for medical practice', *Lancet*, vol 340, pp 772-5.

Hart, J.T. (1993) *Hypertension: Community Control of High Blood Pressure* (3rd edn), Oxford: Radcliffe Medical Press.

Hart, J.T. (1995a) 'Clinical and economic consequences of patients as producers', *Journal of Public Health Medicine*, vol 17, pp 383-6.

Hart, J.T. (1995b) 'Innovative consultation time as a common European currency', *European Journal of General Practice*, vol 1, pp 34-7.

Hart, J.T. (1997) 'What evidence do we need for evidence based medicine? (Cochrane lecture)', *Journal of Epidemiology & Community Health*, vol 51, pp 623-9.

Hart, J.T. and Dieppe, P. (1996) 'Caring effects', *Lancet*, vol 347, pp 1606-8.

Hart, J.T. and Humphreys, C. (1987) 'Be your own coroner: an audit of 500 consecutive deaths in a general practice', *British Medical Journal*, vol 294, pp 871-4.

Hart, J.T. and Smith, G.D. (1997) 'Response rates in south Wales 1950-1996: changing requirements for mass participation in human research', in I. Chalmers and A. Maynard (eds) *Non Random Reflections on Health Services Research: On the 25th Anniversary of Archie Cochrane's Effectiveness and Efficiency*, London: BMJ Publishing Group, pp 31-57.

Hart, J.T., Thomas, C., Gibbons, B., Edwards, C., Hart, M., Jones, J., Jones, M. and Walton, P. (1991) 'Twenty five years of audited screening in a socially deprived community', *British Medical Journal*, vol 302, pp 1509-13.

Heath, I. (1995) 'The perils of checklist medicine', *British Medical Journal*, vol 311, p 373.

Hensher, M. and Edwards, N. (1999) 'Hospital provision, activity, and productivity in England since the 1980s', *British Medical Journal*, vol 319, pp 911-14.

Herxheimer, A. (2003) 'Gathering and assessing narrative evidence', paper read at the Conference on Integration of Narrative with Science in Medicine, London, 3 December.

Hill, A.B. (1951) 'The doctor's day and pay', *Journal of the Royal Statistical Society*, series A, vol 114, pp 1-37.

Hin, H., Bird, G., Fisher, P. et al (1999) 'Coeliac disease in primary care: case finding study', *British Medical Journal*, vol 318, pp 164-7.

Hobsbawm, E. (1987) *The age of empire 1875-1914*, London: Weidenfeld & Nicolson.

Hoffman, C., Rice, D. and Sung, H.Y. (1997) 'Persons with chronic conditions: their prevalence and costs', *Journal of the American Medical Association*, vol 277, pp 1473-9.

Hooper, P.D. (1990) 'Psychological sequelae of sexual abuse in childhood', *British Journal of General Practice*, vol 40, pp 29-31.

Horder, J.P. (1977) 'Physicians and family doctors: a new relationship', *Journal of the Royal College of General Practitioners*, vol 27, pp 391-7.

House of Commons Health Committee (1995) *First Report. Long-term Care: NHS Responsibilities for Meeting Continuing Health Care Needs*, London: HMSO.

House of Commons Health Committee (2005), *The Influence of the Pharmaceutical Industry*, at www.parliament.the-stationery-office.co.uk/pa/cm200405/cmselect/cmhealth/42/42/pdf.

Howden-Chapman, P., Carter, J. and Woods, N. (1996) 'Blood money: blood donors' attitudes to changes in the New Zealand blood transfusion service', *British Medical Journal*, vol 312, pp 1131-2.

Howe, A. (1996) '"I know what to do, but it's not possible to do it"– general practitioners' perceptions of their ability to detect psychological distress', *Family Practice*, vol 13, pp 127-32.

Hrobjartsson, A. and Gotzsche, P.C. (2001) 'Is the placebo powerless? An analysis of clinical trials comparing placebo with no treatment', *New England Journal of Medicine*, vol 344, pp 1594-602.

Hull, C.H. (ed) (1963) *The Economic Writings of Sir William Petty, together with the Observations upon the Bills of Mortality, more probably by Capt. John Graunt*, New York: A.M. Kelley.

Hunter, D.J. and Harrison, S. (1997) 'Democracy, accountability and consumerism', in S. Iliffe and J. Munro (eds) *Healthy Choices: Future Options for the NHS*, London: Lawrence & Wishart, pp 120-54.

Hutton, W. (1995) 'Poorest pay more tax than rich', *Guardian*, 20 November.

Idler, E.L. (1992) 'Subjective assessments of health and mortality: a review of studies', *International Review of Health Psychology*, vol 1, pp 33-54.

Idler, E.L. and Angel, R.J. (1990) 'Self-rated health and mortality in the NHANES-I epidemiologic follow-up study', *American Journal of Public Health*, vol 80, pp 446-52.

Illich, I. (1976) *Medical nemesis: Limits to medicine: the expropriation of health*, London: Marion Boyars.

Inman, P. (2005) 'Executive bonuses influence pensions row', *Guardian*, 4 August.

Irvine, D. and Jeffreys, M. (1971) 'BMA planning unit survey of general practice 1969', *British Medical Journal*, vol 4, pp 535-43.

Isometså, E., Henriksson, M., Heikkinen, M., Aro, H., Lonnqvist, J., Owen, A., O'Hare,T., Goode, H., Matthews, K., Isacsson, G., Holungren, P., Wasserman, D. and Bergman, U. (1994) 'Suicide and the use of antidepressants: drug treatment of depression is inadequate', *British Medical Journal*, vol 308, pp 915-6.

James, J. (1979) 'Impacts of the medical malpractice slowdown in Los Angeles County: January', *American Journal of Public Health*, vol 69, pp 437-43.

Jayasinghe, S. (2004) 'Health in South Asia: Sri Lanka needs to build on its strengths and gains', *British Medical Journal*, vol 328, p 1497.

Jeffreys, M. (1983) 'The over-eighties in Britain: the social construction of a panic', *Journal of Public Health Policy*, vol 4, pp 367-72.

Jess, P., Jess, T., Beck, H. and Beck, P. (1998) 'Neuroticism in relation to recovery and persisting pain after laparoscopic cholecystectomy', *Scandinavian Journal of Gastroenterology*, vol 33, pp 550-3.

Jick, H., Kaye, J.A. and Black, C. (2004) 'Incidence and prevalence of drug-treated attention deficit disorder among boys in the UK', *British Journal of General Practice*, vol 54, pp 345-7.

Johansson, S.R. (1994) 'Food for thought: rhetoric and reality in modern mortality history', *Historical Methods*, vol 27, pp 101-25.

Johnstone, E.C., Crow, T.J., Johnson, A.L. and MacMillan, J.F. (1986) 'The Northwick Park study of first episodes of schizophrenia. I. Presentation of the illness and problems relating to admission', *British Journal of Psychiatry*, vol 148, pp 115-20.

Jolly, R. (ed) (1996) *United Nations Report on Human Development 1996*, Geneva: UNO.

Jones, A. (1994) 'Screening for asthma in children', *British Journal of General Practice*, vol 44, pp 179-83.

Jones, K., Lane, D., Holgate, S.T. and Price, J. (1991) 'Asthma: a diagnostic and therapeutic challenge', *Family Practice*, vol 8, pp 97-9.

Kassem, A. (2004) 'Rise in spending on NHS has not been matched by rise in activity', *British Medical Journal*, vol 329, p 700.

Katon, W., Kleinman, A. and Rosen, G. (1982) 'Depression and somatization: a review. Part 1', *American Journal of Medicine*, vol 72, pp 127-35.

Katon, W.J. and Walker, E.A. (1998) 'Medically unexplained symptoms in primary care', *Journal of Clinical Psychiatry*, vol 59 (suppl 20), pp 15-21.

Kaul, S. (1991) 'Twenty five years of case finding and audit', *British Medical Journal*, vol 303, pp 524-5.

Kerrison, S.H. and Pollock, A. (2001) 'Caring for older people in the private sector in England', *British Medical Journal*, vol 323, pp 566-9.

Kewley, G.D. (1998) 'Personal paper: attention deficit hyperactivity disorder is underdiagnosed and undertreated in Britain', *British Medical Journal*, vol 316, pp 1594-6.

King, M. and Nazareth, I. (1996) 'Community care of patients with schizophrenia: the role of the primary care team', *British Journal of General Practice*, vol 46, pp 231-7.

Kinmonth, A.L., Murphy, E. and Marteau, T. (1989) 'Diabetes and its care – what do patients expect?', *Journal of the Royal College of General Practitioners*, vol 39, pp 324-7.

Kosskinen, S.V.P., Martelin, T.P. and Valkonen, T. (1996) 'Socioeconomic differences in mortality among diabetic people in Finland: five year follow up', *British Medical Journal*, vol 313, pp 975-8

Kotz, D. and Weir, F. (1997) *Revolution from Above: The Demise of the Soviet System*, London: Routledge.

Kovac, C. (2001) 'Drug company breaks 30-year agreement on patient advertising'. *British Medical Journal*, vol 323, p 470.

Kroenke, K. and Mangelsdorff, D. (1989) 'Common symptoms in ambulatory care: incidence, evaluation, therapy and outcome', *American Journal of Medicine*, vol 86, pp 262-6.

Kunst, A.E., Geurts, J.J.M. and van den Berg, J. (1995) 'International variation in socioeconomic inequalities in self reported health', *International Journal of Epidemiology & Community Health*, vol 49, pp 117-23

Kunst, A.E. and Mackenbach, J.P. (1994a) 'The size of mortality differences associated with educational level. A comparison of 9 industrialized countries', *American Journal of Public Health*, vol 84, pp 932-7

Kunst, A.E. and Mackenbach, J.P. (1994b) 'International variation in the size of mortality differences associated with occupational status', *International Journal of Epidemiology*, vol 23, pp 742-50.

Kuvietowicz, Z. (2003), 'NICE is told to break its close links with pharmaceutical industry by WHO adviser Kees de Joncheere', *British Medical Journal*, vol 327, p 637.

Lakhani, A., Coles, J., Eayres, D., Spence, C. and Rachet, B. (2005a) 'Creative use of existing clinical and health outcomes data to assess NHS performance in England: Part 1 – performance indicators closely linked to clinical care', *British Medical Journal*, vol 330, pp 1426-31.

Lakhani, A., Coles, J., Eayres, D., Spence, C. and Rachet, B. (2005b) 'Creative use of existing clinical and health outcomes data to assess NHS performance in England: Part 2 – more challenging aspects of monitoring', *British Medical Journal*, vol 330, pp 1486-92.

Lam, C.-M., Cuschieri, A. and Murray, F.E. (1995) 'Rate of surgery for gallstones is increasing', *British Medical Journal*, vol 311, p 1092.

Lambert, R.J. (1963) *Sir John Simon 1816-1904, and English social administration*, London: McGibbon & Kee.

Lancet Editorial (1989) 'Dying with their rights on', *Lancet*, vol 2, p 1492.

Lancet Editorial (1992) 'Charging for health services in the third world', *Lancet*, vol 340, pp 458-9.

Lancet Editorial (2000) 'A manipulated dichotomy in global health policy', *Lancet*, vol 356, p 1923.

Langton, A. (2003) 'Sharing patient information electronically throughout the NHS: change of culture is needed', *British Medical Journal*, vol 327, pp 622-3.

Lear, E. (1947) *Collected Nonsense Songs of Edward Lear*, London: Crown Classics.

Lee-Potter, J. (1993) '"Honeymoon for medicine" is over, warns chairman of council', *British Medical Journal*, vol 306, p 1073.

Lenzer, J. (2004) 'FDA's counsel accused of being too close to drug industry', *British Medical Journal*, vol 329, p 189.

Levine, M.D. and Oberklaid, F. (1980) 'Hyperactivity: symptom complex or complex symptom?', *American Journal of Diseases in Childhood*, vol 134, pp 409-14.

Leys, C. (2001a) *Market-driven Politics: Neoliberal Democracy and the Public Interest*, London: Verso.

Leys, C. (2001b) 'Missed connections', *Red Pepper*, April.

Liebenau, J. (1990) 'The rise of the British pharmaceutical industry', *British Medical Journal*, vol 301, pp 724-8, 733.

Lilford, R.J. (1997) 'Hysterectomy: will it pay the bills in 2007?', *British Medical Journal*, vol 314, pp 160-1.

Lilienfeld, A.M. and Lilienfeld, D.E. (1982) 'Epidemiology and the public health movement: a historical perspective', *Journal of Public Health Policy*, vol 3, pp 140-9.

Lister, J. (2005) 'The reinvention of failure', *Guardian*, 20 July.

Lloyd, K.R., Jenkins, R. and Mann, A. (1996) 'Long term outcome of patients with neurotic illness in general practice', *British Medical Journal*, vol 313, pp 26-8.

Lorig, K.R., Sobel, D.S., Stewart, A.L., Brown, B.W., Bandura, A., Ritter, P., Gonzalex, V.M., Laurent, D.D. and Holman, H.R. (1999) 'Evidence suggesting that a chronic disease self-management programme can improve health status while reducing hospitalisation. A randomised trial', *Medical Care*, vol 37, pp 5-14.

Lynch, J.W., Kaplan, G.A., Cohen, R.D. et al (1994) 'Childhood and adult socioeconomic status as predictors of mortality in Finland', *Lancet*, vol 343, pp 524-7.

MacDonald, T. (1997) *Hippocrates in Havana: Cuba's Health Care System*, Knebworth: Bolivar Books.

MacGregor, D. (2000/01) 'Jobs in the Public and Private Sectors', *Economic Trends*, June.

McKee, M. (2004) 'Not everything that counts can be counted: not everything that can be counted counts', *British Medical Journal*, vol 328, p 153.

McKeown, T. (1979) *The Role of Medicine*, Oxford: Blackwell.

MacMahon, S., Neal, B. and Rodgers, A. (2005) 'Hypertension – time to move on', *Lancet*, vol 365, pp 1108-9.

MacMillan, J.F., Crow, T.J., Johnson, A.L. and Johnstone, E.C. (1986a) 'The Northwick Park study of first episodes of schizophrenia. III. Short-term outcome in trial entrants and trial eligible patients', *British Journal of Psychiatry*, vol 148, pp 128-33.

MacMillan, J.F., Crow, T.J., Johnson, A.L. and Johnstone, E.C. (1986b) 'The Northwick Park study of first episodes of schizophrenia. IV. Expressed emotion and relapse', *British Journal of Psychiatry*, vol 148, pp 133-43.

McNeill, W.H. (1979) *Plagues and Peoples* (first published New York: Doubleday/Anchor, 1976; Oxford: Blackwell, 1977), London: Penguin Books.

Mair, F.S., Crowley, T.S. and Bundred, P.E. (1996) 'Prevalence, aetiology and management of heart failure in general practice', *British Journal of General Practice*, vol 46, pp 77-9.

Marcovitch, H. (2004) 'Use of stimulants for attention deficit hyperactivity disorder: against'. *British Medical Journal*, vol 329, pp 908-9.

Maricle, R.A., Hoffman, W.F., Bloom, J.D., Faulkner, L.R. and Keepers, G.A. (1987) 'The prevalence and significance of medical illness among chronic mentally ill outpatients', *Community Mental Health Journal*, vol 23, pp 81-90.

Marinker, M. (1973) 'On the boundary', *Journal of the Royal College of General Practitioners*, vol 23, pp 83-94.

Market & Opinion Research International, for Developing Patient Partnerships, formerly the Doctor Patient Partnership (DPP) (2003) *Medicines and the British*, London: MORI.

Marvel, M.K., Epstein, R.M., Flowers, K. and Beckman, B. (1999) 'Soliciting the patient's agenda: have we improved?', *Journal of the American Medical Association*, vol 281, pp 283-7.

Marwick, C. (2003) 'Drug companies defend rewards to doctors for switching treatments'. *British Medical Journal*, vol 326, p 67.

Mathieson, S.A. (2005) 'NHS continues open service software trials', *Guardian*, 5 July.

Maylett Smith, F. (1981) *The Surgery at Aberffrwd*, Hythe: Volturna Press.

Maynard, A. (1991) 'Review of Hancher, *Regulating for competition*', *Lancet*, vol 337, pp 601-2.

Maynard, A. (1994) 'Taking on the health clinicians: the National Health market', *New Economy* (Institute for Public Policy Research), Autumn.

Mayor, S. (1996) 'Warning against overuse of drugs for inattentive children', *British Medical Journal*, vol 313, p 770.

Mechanic, D. (2001) 'How long should hamsters run? Some observations about sufficient patient time in primary care', *British Medical Journal*, vol 323, pp 266-8.

Medawar, C. (1992) *Power and dependence: Social Audit on the Safety of Medicines*, London: Social Audit.

Mellanby, S. (2005) *The World's Banker: A Story of Failed States, Financial Crises, and the Wealth and Poverty of Nations*, New Haven, CT: Yale University Press.

Menendez, R. (1999) Correspondence, *New England Journal of Medicine*, vol 341, p 1769.

Michell, E. and Smith, G. (2003) 'An oral history of general practice 9: record keepers', *British Journal of General Practice*, vol 53, pp 166-7.

Mold, J.W. and Stein, J.F. (1986) 'The cascade effect in the clinical care of patients', *New England Journal of Medicine*, vol 314, pp 512-14.

Moncrieff, J. and Kirsch, I. (2005) 'Efficacy of antidepressants in adults', *British Medical Journal*, vol 331, pp 155-9.

Moore, S. and Molyneux, D. (1997) 'Chronic disease in institutionalised patients', *British Medical Journal*, vol 315, p 1539.

Morabia, A. (1996) 'PCA Louis and the birth of clinical epidemiology', *Journal of Clinical Epidemiology*, vol 49, pp 1327-33.

Morris, J.N. (1972) 'Four cheers for prevention', *Proceedings of the Royal Society of Medicine*, vol 66, pp 225-32.

Morris, J.N. and Titmuss, R.M. (1944) 'Health and social change: I.–The recent history of rheumatic heart disease', *The Medical Officer*, 26 August, pp 69-71.

Moses, S., Manji, F. and Bradley, J.E. (1992) 'Impact of user fees on attendance at a referral centre for sexually transmitted diseases in Kenya', *Lancet*, vol 340, pp 463-6.

Murray, S.A., Boyd, K., Sheikh, A., Thomas, K. and Higginson, I.J. (2004) 'Developing primary palliative care: people with terminal conditions should be able to die at home with dignity', *British Medical Journal*, vol 329, p 1056.

Nair, V.M. (2004) 'Health in South Asia: future of Kerala depends on its willingness to learn from past', *British Medical Journal*, vol 328, p 1497.

Navarro, V. (1976) *Medicine under Capitalism*, New York, NY/London: Prodist/Croom Helm.

Naylor, C.D. and Williams, J.I. (1996) 'The Ontario panel on Hip and Knee Arthroplasty. Primary hip and knee replacement surgery: Ontario criteria for case selection and surgical priority', *Quality in Health Care*, vol 5, pp 20-30.

Neale, J. (1983) *Memoirs of a Callous Picket: Working for the NHS*, London: Pluto Press.

Needham, C. and Murray, A. (2005) 'The future of public services in Europe', prepared by Catalyst and the Centre for European Reform for UNISON and Ver.di, at www.catalystforum.org.uk/pubs/paper30.html, May.

Netherlands Central Bureau for Statistics, Erasmus University, Rotterdam (1992) *International Variation in Socioeconomic Inequalities in Self Reported Health*, The Hague: SDU Publishers/CBS Publications.

Nilsson, M. (1993) 'Sweden's health reform', *Lancet*, vol 342, p 979.

Nolte, E. and McKee, M. (2003) 'Measuring the health of nations: analysis of mortality amenable to health care', *British Medical Journal*, vol 327, pp 1129-32.

Nolte, E. and McKee, M. (2004) *Does Health Care Save Lives? Avoidable Mortality Revisited*, London: Nuffield Trust.

North, R.D. (2005) *Rich is Beautiful: A Very Personal Defence of Mass Affluence*, London: Social Affairs Unit.

Nuffield Trust (2005) *Governance of Foundation Trusts*, London: Nuffield Trust.

Oakley, A. (1996) 'Blood donation – altruism or profit?', *British Medical Journal*, vol 312, p 1114.

Ochoa, F.R. (2003) 'Situacion, sistema y recursos humanos en salud para el desarollo en Cuba', *Revista Cubana de Salud Pública*, vol 29, pp 157-69.

OECD (1994) 'Economic survey, United Kingdom 1994', *LRD Fact Service*, vol 56, pp 143-4.

OECD (2003) *Health at a Glance*, Paris: OECD.

Oeppen, J. and Vaupel, J.W. (2002) 'Broken limits to life expectancy', *Science*, vol 296, pp 1029-31.

OPCS (1995) *The Health of our Children*, London: HMSO.

Oye, R.K. and Bellamy, P.E. (1991) 'Patterns of resource consumption in medical intensive care', *Chest*, vol 99, pp 685-9.

Page, B. (2004a) 'The vision thing', *Health Service Journal*, vol 114 (5901), pp 14-15.

Page, B. (2004b) 'What they really really want', *Health Service Journal*, vol 114 (5900), pp 16-17.

Paterson, C. (1996) 'Measuring outcomes in primary care: a patient-generated measure, MYMOP, compared with the SF-36 health survey', *British Medical Journal*, vol 312, pp 1016-20 and 626-7.

Peterson, M.C., Holbrook, J.H., Hales, D.V. et al (1992) 'Contributions of the history, of physical examination, and of laboratory investigation in making medical diagnosis', *Western Journal of Medicine*, vol 156, pp 163-5.

Philo, G. (2001) Letters, *Guardian*, 13 June.

Pollard, S. (2005) 'Tories need a Clause 4', *Guardian*, 24 August.

Pollock, A. (2004) *NHS plc: The Privatisation of our Health Care*, London: Verso.

Pollock, A.M. and Whitty, P.M. (1990) 'Crisis in our hospital kitchens: ancillary staffing levels during an outbreak of food poisoning in a long stay hospital', *British Medical Journal*, vol 300, pp 383-5.

Pollock, K. and Grime, J. (2002) 'Patients' perceptions of entitlement to time in general practice consultations for depression: qualitative study', *British Medical Journal*, vol 325, pp 687-90.

Portegijs, P.J.M., Jeuken, F.M.H., van der Horst, F., Kraan, H.F. and Knottnerus, J.A. (1996) 'A troubled youth: relations with somatization, depression and anxiety in adulthood', *Family Practice*, vol 13, pp 1-11.

Powell, J.E. (1966) *A New Look at Medicine and Politics*, London: Pitman Medical.

Powell, M. (2000) 'Wales and the National Health Service', *Llafur*, vol 8, no 1, p 34.

Price, D., Pollock, A.M. and Shaoul, J. (1999) 'How the World Trade Organisation is shaping domestic policies in health care', *Lancet*, vol 354, pp 1889-92.

Pringle, J. (1974) *Living with Schizophrenia – by the Relatives*, Surbiton: National Schizophrenia Fellowship.

Proctor, S. (1997) 'Is this the end of research as we know it?', *British Medical Journal*, vol 315, p 388.

Prosser, S. and Dobbs, F. (1997) 'Case-finding incontinence in the over-75s', *British Journal of General Practice*, vol 47, pp 498-500.

Punglia, R.S., D'Amico, A.V., Catalona, W.J., Roehl, K.A. and Kuntz, K.M. (2003) 'Effect of verification bias on screening for prostate cancer by measurement of prostate-specific antigen', *New England Journal of Medicine*, vol 349, pp 335-42.

Pyper, C., Amery, J., Watson, M. and Crook, C. (2004) 'Patients' experiences when accessing their on-line electronic patient records in primary care', *British Journal of General Practice*, vol 54, pp 38-43.

Quintana. J.M., Catoriada, J., López de Tejada, I., Perdigo, L., Aróstegui, I., Bilbao, A. and Garay, I. (2004) 'Appropriateness variation in cholecystectomy', *European Journal of Public Health*, vol 14, pp 252-7.

Rayner, G. (1997) 'The "New Mandarins" and the monetarisation of the NHS', in S. Iliffe and J. Munro (eds) *Healthy Choices: Future Options for the NHS*, London: Lawrence & Wishart, pp 18-52.

Reaven, G.M. (1988) 'The role of insulin resistance in human disease. Banting lecture 1988', *Diabetes*, vol 37, pp 1595-607.

Rees, M.C.P. (1991) 'Role of menstrual blood loss in management of complaints of excessive menstrual bleeding', *British Journal of Obstetrics & Gynaecology*, vol 98, pp 327-8.

Reid, P.C. and Mukri, F. (2005) 'Trends in number of hysterectomies performed in England for menorrhagia: examination of health episode statistics, 1989 to 2002-3', *British Medical Journal*, vol 330, pp 938-9.

Richardson, J. and Feder, G. (1995) 'Domestic violence against women', *British Medical Journal*, vol 311, pp 964-5.

Richardson, J. and Feder, G. (1996) 'Domestic violence: a hidden problem for general practice', *British Journal of General Practice*, vol 46, pp 239-42.

Riddle, M.C. (1980) 'A strategy for chronic disease', *Lancet*, vol 2, pp 734-6.

Ridsdale, L., Carruthers, M., Morris, R. and Ridsdale, J. (1989) 'Study of the effect of time availability on the consultation', *Journal of the Royal College of General Practitioners*, vol 39, pp 488-91.

Ridsdale, L. and Hudd, S. (1994) 'Computers in the consultation: the patients' view', *British Journal of General Practice*, vol 44, pp 367-9.

Rivett, G. (1998) *From Cradle to Grave: Fifty Years of the NHS*, London: King's Fund.

Roberts, Ff. (1952) *The Cost of Health*, London: Turnstile Press.

Roberts, J. (1994) 'Oregon overwhelmed in its first three weeks', *British Medical Journal*, vol 308, p 618.

Roberts, J. (1996) 'Behavioural disorders are overdiagnosed in the US', *British Medical Journal*, vol 312, p 657.

Roberts, J. (1997) 'Washington: political allies and enemies take on junior doctor surplus', *British Medical Journal*, vol 314, p 774.

Rodgers, J.S. and Gray, J.A.M. (1982) 'Long stay care for elderly people: its continuing evolution', *British Medical Journal*, vol 285, pp 707-9.

Roemer, M.I. and Schwartz, J.L. (1979) 'Doctor slowdown: effects on the population of Los Angeles County', *Social Science & Medicine*, vol 130, pp 213-18.

Rollin, H. (1979) 'In my own time: schizophrenia', *British Medical Journal*, vol 1, pp 1773-5.

Rosen, G. (1958/1993)*History of Public Health*, New York: MD Publications; expanded edn, Baltimore: Johns Hopkins University Press.

Rosenhan, D.L. (1973) 'On being sane in insane places', *Science*, vol 179, pp 250-8.

Rosenhead, J. (1989) *Rational Analysis for a Problematic World: Problem Structuring Methods for Complexity, Uncertainty and Conflict*, New York: John Wiley.

Rosenhead, J. (1991) 'Swords into ploughshares: Cecil Gordon's role in the post-war transition of operational research to civilian use', *Public Administration*, vol 69, pp 481-501.

Roslyn, J.J., Binns, G.S., Hughes, E.F.X., Saunders-Kirkwood, K., Zinner, M.J. and Cates, J.A. (1993) 'Open cholecystectomy: a contemporary analysis of 42,474 patients', *Annals of Surgery*, vol 218, pp 129-37.

Sackett, D.L., Rosenberg, W.M.C., Gray, J.A.M., Haynes, R.B. and Richardson, W.S. (1996) 'Evidence based medicine: what it is and what it isn't', *British Medical Journal*, vol 312, pp 71-2.

Saltman, R.B. (1994) 'A conceptual overview of recent health care reforms', *European Journal of Public Health*, vol 4, pp 287-93.

Saltman, R.B. (2003) 'Melting public–private boundaries in European health systems', *European Journal of Public Health*, vol 13, pp 24-9.

Sanchez Bayle, M. and Beiras Cal, H. (2001) 'The people's campaign against health care counter-reforms in Spain', *Journal of Public Health Policy*, vol 22, pp 139-52.

Schieber, G.J. and Poullier, J.-P. (1990) 'Overview of international comparisons of health care expenditures', in OECD, *Health Care Systems in Transition*, Policy Studies 7, Paris: OECD, pp 9-15.

Schulz, R., Beach, S.R., Ives, D.G., Martire, L.M., Ariyo, A.A. and Kop, W.J. (2000) 'Association between depression and mortality in older adults: the Cardiovascular Health Study', *Archives of Internal Medicine*, vol 160, pp 1761-8.

Schweitzer, S. (1997) *Pharmaceutical Economics and Policy*, Oxford: Oxford University Press.

Scott, E.A. and Black, N. (1992) 'Appropriateness of cholecystectomy: the public and private sectors compared', *Annals of the Royal College of Surgeons of England*, vol 74, pp 97-101.

Scottish Executive (2005) *Delivering for Health*, November, p 25.

Select Committee on Medical Relief (1854) *Report of the Select Committee on Medical Relief*, Shannon: Irish University Press.

Shaw, G.B. (1907) *The Doctor's Dilemma*, London: John Constable.

Shaw, J. and Baker, M. (2004) '"Expert patient" – dream or nightmare?', *British Medical Journal*, vol 328, pp 723-4.

Shaw, M., Smith, G.D. and Dorling, D. (2005) 'Health inequalities and New Labour: how the promises compare with real progress', *British Medical Journal*, vol 330, pp 1016-21.

Sheehan, H. (1992) *European socialism: A blind alley, or a long and winding road?*, Dublin: Movement for a Socialist Future.

Sheehan, N. (1989/90) *A bright shining lie: John Paul Vann & America in Vietnam*, London: Jonathan Cape/Picador.

Shi, L., Macinko, J., Starfield, B., Politzer, R. and Xu, J. (2005) 'Primary care, race and mortality in US states', *Social Science & Medicine*, vol 61, pp 65-75.

Shock, M. (1994) 'Medicine at the centre of the nation's affairs: doctors and their institutions are failing to adapt to the modern world', *British Medical Journal*, vol 309, pp 1730-3.

Silverman, E.M., Skinner, J.S. and Fisher, E.S. (1999) 'The association between for-profit hospital ownership and increased Medicare spending', *New England Journal of Medicine*, vol 341, pp 420-6.

Sims, A. (1973) 'Mortality in neurosis', *Lancet*, vol 2, pp 1072-5

Sims, A. and Prior, P. (1978) 'The pattern of mortality in severe neuroses', *British Journal of Psychiatry*, vol 133, pp 299-305.

Sjöström, H. and Nilsson, R. (1972) *Thalidomide and the Power of the Drug Companies*, London: Penguin.

Slater, E. (1965) 'Diagnosis of "hysteria"', *British Medical Journal*, vol 1, pp 1395-9.

Slater, P.E. and Ever-Hadani, P. (1983) 'Mortality in Jerusalem during the 1983 doctors' strike', *Lancet*, vol 2, p 1306.

Smee, C.H. (2002) 'What have we really learned from the NHS v Kaiser comparison?', *British Medical Journal*, website letters, 31 January.

Smith, A. ([1762] 1993) *Enquiry into the nature and causes of the wealth of nations*, Oxford: Oxford University Press.

Smith, G.D., Hart, C., Blane, D. and Hole, D. (1998) 'Adverse socioeconomic conditions in childhood and cause specific adult mortality: prospective observational study', *British Medical Journal*, vol 316, pp 1631-5.

Smith, M.C. (1968) *Principles of pharmaceutical marketing*, Philadelphia: Lea Febiger.

Smith, R. (1994) 'The rise of Stalinism in the NHS: an unfree NHS and medical press in an unfree society', *British Medical Journal*, vol 309, pp 1644-5.

Smith, R. (1996) 'Global competition in health care', *British Medical Journal*, vol 313, pp 764-5.

Smith, R. (1999) 'PFI: perfidious financial idiocy. A "free lunch" that could destroy the NHS', *British Medical Journal*, vol 319, pp 2-3.

Smith, R. (2002) 'Review of new printing of Illich I. *Limits to medicine. Medical Nemesis: the expropriation of health*. London: Marion Boyars, 1974', *British Medical Journal*, vol 324, p 923.

Snow, C.P. (1959) *The Two Cultures and the Scientific Revolution*, Cambridge: Cambridge University Press.

Sorum, P.C. (2005) 'France tries to save its ailing national health insurance system', *Journal of Public Health Policy*, vol 26, pp 231-45.

Sparrow, M.K. (2000) *License to Steal: How Fraud Bleeds America's Health Care System*, Boulder, CO: Westview Press.

Speckens, A.E.M., van Hemert, A.M., Spinhoven, P., Hawton, K.E., Bolk, J.H. and Rooijmans, H.G.M. (1995) 'Cognitive behavioural therapy for medically unexplained physical symptoms: a randomised controlled trial', *British Medical Journal*, vol 311, pp 1328-32.

Spence, J. (1960) 'The need for understanding the individual as part of the training and function of doctors and nurses', in *The Purpose and Practice of Medicine*, London: Oxford University Press, pp 271-80.

Spenser, T. (1993) 'Guidelines as an integral stage in quality development', *Family Physician (Israel)*, vol 21, pp 37-9.

Spurgeon, D. (2005) 'Canadian Supreme Court upholds right to take out private health insurance', *British Medical Journal*, vol 330, p 1408.

Squires, B. and Learmonth, I. (2003) 'Empowerment of patients: fact or fiction', *British Medical Journal*, vol 326, p 710.

Starfield, B. (2001) 'New paradigms for quality in primary care', *British Journal of General Practice*, vol 51, pp 303-9.

Starfield, B., Wray, C., Hess, K., Gross, R., Birk, P.S. and D'Lugaff, B.C. (1981) 'The influence of patient-practitioner agreement on outcome of care', *American Journal of Public Health*, vol 71, pp 127-31.

Stephens, D. (1988) 'Hearing aids – making the system work', *Soundbarrier*, December, p 4.

Stevens, R. (1966) *Medical Practice in Modern England*, New Haven, CT: Yale University Press.

Stewart, A.L., Greenfield, S., Wells, K., Rogers, W.H., Berry, S.D., McGlynn, E.A. and Ware, J.E. (1989) 'Functional status and well-being of patients with chronic conditions: results from the medical outcomes study', *Journal of the American Medical Association*, vol 262, pp 907-13.

Stewart-Brown, S. and Layte, R. (1997) 'Emotional health problems are the most important cause of disability in adults of working age: a study in the four Counties of the old Oxford region', *Journal of Epidemiology & Community Health*, vol 51, pp 672-5.

Stirling, A.M., Wilson, P. and McConnachie, A. (2001) 'Deprivation, psychological distress, and consultation length in general practice', *British Journal of General Practice*, vol 51, pp 456-60.

Strangleman, T. (2005) *Work Identity at the End of the Line? Privatisation and Culture Change in the UK Rail Industry*, London: Palgrave Macmillan.

Sudlow, M., Thomson, R., Kenny, R.A. and Rodgers, R. (1998) 'A community survey of patients with atrial fibrillation: associated disabilities and treatment preferences', *British Journal of General Practice*, vol 48, pp 1775-8.

Sullivan, F. and Mitchell, E. (1995) 'Has general practice computing made a difference to patient care? A systematic review of published reports', *British Medical Journal*, vol 311, pp 848-52.

Švab, I. and Katic, M. (1991) 'Let the patients speak', *Family Practice*, vol 8, pp 182-3.

Taylor, E., Sandberg, S., Thorley, C. and Giles, S. (1991) *The Epidemiology of Childhood Hyperactivity*, Oxford: Oxford University Press.

Taylor, J.S. (2005) *Stakes and Kidneys: Why Markets in Human Body Parts are Morally Imperative*, Aldershot: Ashgate.

Terris, M. (2002) 'The changing relationships of epidemiology and society', *Journal of Public Health Policy*, vol 22, pp 441–63.

Thomas, S.M., Davies, A.R.W., Birtwhistle, N.J., Crowther, S.M. and Burke, J.F. (1996) 'Ownership of the human genome', *Nature*, vol 380, pp 387-8.

Thompson, S. (2006, forthcoming) 'A proletarian public sphere: working class provision of medical services and care in south Wales, c.1900-1948', in A. Borsay (ed) *Public/Private: Medicine, Power and Identity in Wales, c.1800-2000*, Cardiff: University of Wales Press, ch 5.

Timimi, S. (2002) *Pathological Child Psychiatry and the Medicalisation of Childhood*, Hove: Brunner-Routledge.

Timimi, S. (2005) 'Effect of globalisation on children's mental health', *British Medical Journal*, vol 331, pp 37-9.

Titmuss, R.M. (1997) *The Gift Relationship: From Human Blood to Social Policy*, edited by A. Oakley and J. Ashton (original edn 1970) with new chapters by Virginia Berridge, Vanessa Martlew, Gillian Weaver, Susan Williams and Julian Le Grand, London: London School of Economics and Political Science.

Torgerson, D.J. and Raftery, J. (1999) 'Discounting', *British Medical Journal*, vol 319, pp 914-15.

Townsend, P. (1962) *The Last Refuge*, London: Routledge & Kegan Paul.

Townsend, P. (1981) 'The structured dependency of the elderly: a creation of social policy in the 20th century', *Ageing & Society*, vol 1, pp 5-28.

Towse, R. (ed) (1997) *Baumol's Cost Disease: The Arts and Other Victims*, Cheltenham and Northampton, MA: Edward Elgar.

Trades Union Congress (TUC) (2004) *Work till you drop*, London: TUC.

Travis, A. (2001) 'Vote of confidence in public services', *Guardian*, 20 March.

Turner, T.H. (2004) 'Long term outcome of treating schizophrenia: antipsychotics probably help – but we badly need more long term studies', *British Medical Journal*, vol 329, pp 1058-9.

Tymms, P. and Wiggins, A. (2000) 'Schools' experience of league tables should make doctors think again', *British Medical Journal*. vol 321, p 1467.

Ulrich, R.S. (1984) 'View through a window may influence recovery from surgery', *Science*, vol 224, pp 420-1.

van den Acker, M., Buntinx, F. and Knottnerus, J.A. (1996) 'Morbidity and co-morbidity: what's in a name? A review of literature', *European Journal of General Practice*, vol 2, pp 65-70.

van den Bos, G.A.M. (1995) 'The burden of chronic diseases in terms of disability, use of health care and healthy life expectancies', *European Journal of Public Health*, vol 5, pp 29-34.

Verby, J.E., Holden, P. and Davis, R.H. (1979) 'Peer review of consultations in primary care: the use of audio-visual recordings', *British Medical Journal*, vol 1, pp 1686-8.

Verheijden, M.W., Bakx, J.C., Delemarre, I.C.G., Wanders, A.J., van Woudenbergh, N.M., Bottema, B.J.A.M., van Weel, C. and van Staveren, W.A. (2005) 'GPs' assessment of patients' readiness to change diet, activity and smoking', *British Journal of General Practice*, vol 55, pp 452-7.

Victor, C.R. (1997) 'The health of homeless people in Britain: a review', *European Journal of Public Health*, vol 7, pp 398-404.

Vist, G.E., Hagen, K.B., Devereaux, P.J., Bryant, D., Kristoffersen, D.T. and Oxman, A.D. (2005) 'Systematic review to determine whether participation in a trial influences outcome', *British Medical Journal*, vol 330, pp 1175-9.

Vogt, T.M. (1993) 'Paradigms and prevention', *American Journal of Public Health*, vol 83, pp 795-6.

Waitzkin, H. (1994) 'The strange career of managed competition: military failure to medical success?', *Journal of the American Public Health Association*, vol 84, pp 482-9.

Walker, A. (1991) 'Erosion of Swedish welfare state', *British Medical Journal*, vol 303, p 267.

Wall, A. (1993) 'Reforming the reforms', in S. Iliffe, J. Mostyn and R. Ross (eds) *From Market Chaos to Common Sense: Papers on Future Policies for Health*, London: Medical World/Socialist Health Association, pp 2-3.

Wallace, R. and Wallace, D. (1997) 'Socioeconomic determinants of health: community marginalisation and the diffusion of disease and disorder in the United States', *British Medical Journal*, vol 314, pp 1341-5.

Walton, D. (2001) 'What works: public services publicly provided', at www.catalyst-trust.co.uk.

Ward, L. and Innes, M. (2003) 'Electronic summaries in general practice: considering the patient's contribution', *British Journal of General Practice*, vol 53, pp 293-7.

Weakliem, D.L. and Heath, A. (1995) *The Secret Life of Class Voting: Britain, France and the United States since the 1930s*, Centre for Research Into Elections and Social Trends, Working Paper 31, Glasgow: University of Strathclyde, Glasgow.

Webster, C. (1976) 'The crisis of subsistence and health of the puritan revolution', *Bulletin of the Society for Social History of Medicine*, vol 17, pp 8-10.

Webster, C. (1988) *The Health Services since the War. Vol. 1. Problems of Health Care: The National Health Service before 1957*, London: HMSO.

Weich, S., Lewis, G., Donmall, R. and Mann, A. (1995) 'Somatic presentation of psychiatric morbidity in general practice', *British Journal of General Practice*, vol 45, pp 143-7.

Weindling, P. (1989) *Health, Race, and German Politics between National Unification and Nazism, 1870-1945*, New York: Cambridge University Press.

Welin, L., Larsson, B., Svardsudd, K., Tibblin, B. and Tibblin, G. (1992) 'Social network and activities in relation to mortality from cardiovascular diseases, cancer and other causes: a 12 year follow up of the study of men born in 1913 and 1923', *Journal of Epidemiology & Community Health*, vol 46, pp 127-32.

Welsh Assembly (2005) *Informing Healthcare: the National Case*, Cardiff: Welsh Assembly Government.

Westin, S. (1995) 'Challenges of changing political and socioeconomic structures', keynote speech at WONCA Conference, Hong Kong.

Whitehead, M. (1990) 'Health inequalities in Britain and Sweden', *Lancet*, vol 335, p 331.

Whitehead, M., Evandrou, M., Haglund, B. and Diderichsen, F. (1997) 'As the health divide widens in Sweden and Britain, what's happening to access to care?', *British Medical Journal*, vol 315, pp 1006-9.

Whitehead, M., Gustafsson, R.A. and Diderichsen, F. (1997) 'Why is Sweden rethinking its NHS style reforms?', *British Medical Journal*, vol 315, pp 935-9.

Wiersma, D. et al (1998) 'Natural course of schizophrenic disorders: a 15-year follow-up of a Dutch incidence cohort', *Schizophrenia Bulletin*, vol 24, pp 75-85.

Wilber, J.A. and Barrow, J.G. (1972) 'Hypertension – a community problem', *American Journal of Medicine*, vol 52, pp 653-63.

Wilheim, D. and Metcalfe, D.H.H. (1984) 'List size and patient contact in general medical practice', *British Medical Journal*, vol 189, pp 1501-5.

Williams, A. (1989) *Creating a Health Care Market: Ideology, Efficiency, Ethics and Clinical Freedom. NHS White Paper*, Occasional Paper 5, York: York Centre for Health Economics Consortium.

Williams, B. (1994) 'Insulin resistance: the shape of things to come', *Lancet*, vol 344, pp 521-4.

Williams, B., Poulter, N.R., Brown, M.J., Davis, M., McInnes, G.T., Potter, J.F., Seven, P.S. and Thom, S.M. (2004) 'British Hypertension Society guidelines for hypertension management 2004 (BHS-IV): summary', *British Medical Journal*, vol 328, pp 634-40.

Williams, C. (1996) *Democratic Rhondda: Politics and Society 1885-1951*, Cardiff: University of Wales Press.

Williams, J. (2005) 'National programme for IT: the £30 billion question' *British Journal of General Practice* , vol 55, pp 340-2.

Williams, P., Tarnspolsky, A., Hand, D. and Shepherd, M. (1986) 'Minor psychiatric morbidity and general practice consultation', *Psychological Medicine*, monograph supplement 9.

Williamson, C. (1995) 'Ensuring that guidelines are effective: give them to the patient', *British Medical Journal*, vol 311, p 1023.

Wing, J.K. (1987) 'Epidemiology of schizophrenia', *Journal of the Royal Society of Medicine*, vol 80, pp 134-5.

Wintour, P. (2004) 'Voters turn against choice in public services', *Guardian*, 27 March.

Wolinsky, H. (1995) 'Ethics in managed care', *Lancet*, vol 346, p 1499.

Woolhandler, S., Campbell, T. and Himmelstein, D.U. (2003) 'Costs of health care administration in the United States and Canada', *New England Medical Journal*, vol 349, pp 768-75.

Woolhandler, S. and Himmelstein, D.U. (1999) 'When money is the mission – the high costs of investor owned care', *New England Journal of Medicine*, vol 341, pp 444-6.

Wormald, W.P.L., Wright, L.A., Courtney, P., Beaumont, B. and Haines, A.P. (1992) 'Visual problems in the elderly population and implications for services', *British Medical Journal*, vol 304, pp 1226-9.

Yamey, G. (2002) 'Why does the world still need WHO?', *British Medical Journal*, vol 325, pp 1294-8.

Yates, J. (1995) *Private Eye, Heart and Hip: Surgical Consultants, the National Health Service and Private Medicine*, London: Churchill Livingstone.

Yelin, E. (1986) 'The myth of malingering: why individuals withdraw from work in the presence of illness', *Milbank Quarterly*, vol 64, pp 622-49.

Young, J.B. (2001) 'The primary care stroke gap', *British Journal of General Practice*, vol 51, pp 787-8.

Index of names

Index of subjects